KEY TOPICS IN

OTOLARYNGOLOGY

and Head and Neck Surgery

Second Edition

N.J. ROLAND
MD, FRCS
Consultant in Otolaryngology and Head and Neck Surgery,
Honorary Lecturer, Liverpool University, University Hospital Aintree, Liverpool, UK

R.D.R. McRAE
FRCS
Consultant in Otolaryngology and Head and Neck Surgery,
Colchester General Hospital, Colchester, Essex, UK

A.W. McCOMBE
MD, FRCS
Consultant in Otolaryngology and Head and Neck Surgery,
Frimley Park Hospital, Surrey, UK

BIOS

First published 1995
Second Edition 2001

A CIP catalogue record for this book is available from the British Library.

ISBN 1 85996 198 3

BIOS Scientific Publishers Ltd
9 Newtec Place, Magdalen Road, Oxford OX4 1RE, UK
Tel. +44 (0)1865 726286. Fax +44 (0)1865 246823
World Wide Web home page: http://www.bios.co.uk/

Important Note from the Publisher

The information contained within this book was obtained by BIOS Scientific Publishers Ltd from sources believed by us to be reliable. However, while every effort has been made to ensure its accuracy, no responsibility for loss or injury whatsoever occasioned to any person acting or refraining from action as a result of information contained herein can be accepted by the authors or publishers.

The reader should remember that medicine is a constantly evolving science and while the authors and publishers have ensured that all dosages, applications and practices are based on current indications, there may be specific practices which differ between communities. You should always follow the guidelines laid down by the manufacturers of specific products and the relevant authorities in the country in which you are practising.

Production Editor: Paul Barlass.
Typeset by Jayvee Computer Services, Trivandrum, India
Printed by Cambrian Printers, Aberystwyth, Wales, UK

CONTENTS

CONTRIBUTORS

P. Bradley
Consultant Otolaryngologist, Queens Medical Centre, Nottingham, UK

George Browning
Professor of Otolaryngology, Glasgow Royal Infirmary, Glasgow, UK

P. Charters
Consultant Anaesthetist, University Hospital Aintree, Liverpool, UK

Austin Leach
Consultant Anaesthetist, Royal Liverpool University Hospital, Liverpool, UK

T. H. J. Lesser
Consultant ENT Surgeon, University Hospital Aintree, Liverpool, UK

Huw Lewis-Jones
Consultant Radiologist, University Hospital Aintree, Liverpool, UK

N. S. Niranjan
Consultant Plastic and Reconstructive Surgeon, Colchester General Hospital, Colchester, Essex, UK

Michael Pringle
Consultant Otolaryngologist, Queen Alexandra Hospital, Portsmouth, UK

M. F. Ramadan
Consultant ENT Surgeon, University Hospital Aintree, Liverpool, UK

S. R. Saeed
Consultant Otolaryngologist, Manchester Royal Infirmary, Manchester, UK

A. Shenoy
Consultant Oncologist, Clatterbridge Centre for Oncology, Bebington, Wirral, UK

J. C. Watkinson
Consultant Head and Neck and Thyroid Surgeon, Queen Elizabeth Hospital, Queen Elizabeth Medical Centre, Birmingham, UK

Pam Young
Senior Speech and Language Therapist, Royal Liverpool University Hospital, Liverpool, UK

ABBREVIATIONS

AA	androgenic alopecia
AJC	American Joint Committee
ANCA	anti-neutrophil cytoplasmic antibody
ASA	American Society of Anesthesiologists
ASOM	Acute suppurative otitis media
BAHA	bone-anchored hearing aid
BDNF	brain-derived neurotrophic factor
BERA	brainstem evoked response audiometry
BEHA	behind the ear hearing aid
BIPP	bismuth iodoform paraffin paste
BW	body-worn hearing aid
c-ANCA	cytoplasmic anti-neutrophil cytoplasmic antibody
CHARGE	colobama, heart disease, atresia choanae, retarded growth and development, genital anomalies, ear abnormalities and deafness
CHI	Commission for Health Improvement
CHOP	cyclophosphamide, hydroxydaunorubicin, oncovine (vincristine) and prednisolone
CJD	Creutzfeldt Jakob disease
COWS	cold-opposite, warm-same
CPU	central processing unit
CROS	contralateral routing of signal
CSF	cerebro-spinal fluid
CSOM	chronic suppurative otitis media
CT	computerized tomography
DSF	delayed speech feedback
DSP	digital signal processing
EAM	external auditory meatus
EBV	Epstein–Barr virus
ECochG	electrocochleography
ECS	extra-capsular spread
EEMG	evoked electromyogram
EMLA	eutectic mixture of local anaesthetic
EPS	exophthalmos producing substance
Er:YAG	erbium: YAG (laser)
ESR	erythrocyte sedimentation rate
EUA	examination under anaesthetic
FBC	full blood count
FESS	functional endoscopic sinus surgery
FNA	fine needle aspiration
FNAC	fine needle aspiration cytology
FTA	fluorescent treponemal antibody test
GASH	gender, age, stage and histology
GDNF	glial cell line-derived neurotrophic factor

GPN	glossopharyngeal neuralgia
HIB	*Haemophilus influenzae* type B
HL	hearing level
Ho:YAG	holmium: YAG (laser)
HPL	half-peak level
HPLE	half-peak level elevation
HPV	human papillomavirus
HSV	herpes simplex virus
IAM	internal auditory meatus
IHC	inner hair cell
IR	intrinsic rhinitis
ITC	'in the canal'
ITE	'in the ear'
KTP	potassium titanyl phosphate (laser)
MEN	multiple endocrine neoplasia
MRI	magnetic resonance imaging
MSGC	minor salivary gland carcinoma
NARTI	nucleoside analogue
NCEPOD	National Confidential Enquiry into Perioperative Deaths
Nd-YAG	neodymium doped-yttrium aluminium garnet (laser)
NF2	neurofibromatosis type 2
NHL	non-Hodgkin's lymphoma
NICE	National Institute for Clinical Excellence
NIHL	noise-induced hearing loss
NNRTI	non-nucleoside
NOHL	non-organic hearing loss
NPC	nasopharyngeal carcinoma
OAE	otoacoustic emission
ODS	optimum discrimination score
OHC	outer hair cell
p-ANCA	perinuclear anti-neutrophil cytoplasmic antibody
PCT	percutaneous tracheostomy
PE	pharyngo-oesophageal
PI	protease inhibitors
PHN	postherpetic neuralgia
PLF	perilymph fistula
PORP	partial ossicular replacement prosthesis
PRIST	plasma radioimmunosorbent test
pTNM	pathological staging
PTS	permanent threshold shift
RAST	radioallergosorbent test
SCC	squamous cell carcinoma
SCPL	supracricoid partial laryngectomy
SMAS	superficial muscle and aponeurotic system
SMR	submucosal resection
SNHL	sensorineural hearing loss

SRT	speech reception threshold
STIR	short tau inversion recovery
SVR	surgical voice restoration
TENS	transcutaneous electrical nerve stimulation
TEOAE	transient evoked otoacoustic emission
TGN	trigeminal neuralgia
TMJ	temperomandibular joint
TORP	total ossicular replacement prosthesis
TPHA	treponema pallidum haemagglutination test
TSH	thyroid stimulating hormone
TTS	temporary threshold shift
UICC	International Union Against Cancer
URTI	upper respiratory tract infection
USS	ultrasound scan
VAPEL-B	vincristine, adreomycin, prednisolone, etoposide, cyclophosphamide and bleomycin
VMA	vanillylmandelic acid
WG	Wegener's granulomatosis
WHO	World Health Organization
WNG	White Noise Generators

NAMES OF MEDICAL SUBSTANCES

In accordance with directive 92/27/EEC, this book adheres to the following guidelines on naming of medicinal substances (rINN, Recommended International Non-proprietary Name; BAN, British Approved Name).

List 1 – Both names to appear

UK Name	rINN
[2]adrenaline	epinephrine
amethocaine	tetracaine
bendrofluazide	bendroflumethiazide
benzhexol	trihexyphenidyl
chlorpheniramine	chlorphenamine
dicyclomine	dicycloverine
dothiepin	dosulepin
eformoterole	formoterol
flurandrenolone	fludroxycortide
frusemide	furosemide
hydroxyurea	hydroxycarbamide
lignocaine	lidocaine
methotrimeprazine	levomepromazine
methylene blue	methylthoninium
mitozantrone	mitoxantrone
mustine	chlormethine
nicoumalone	acenocoumarol
[2]noradrenaline	norepinephrine
oxypentifylline	pentoxyifylline
procaine penicillin	procaine benzylpenicillin
salcatonin	calcitonin (salmon)
thymoxamine	moxisylyte
thyroxine sodium	levothyroxine sodium
trimeprazine	alimemazine

List 2 – rINN to appear exclusively

Former BAN	rINN/new BAN
amoxycillin	amoxicillin
amphetamine	amfetamine
amylobarbitone	amobarbital
amylobarbitone sodium	amobarbital sodium
beclomethasone	beclometasone
benorylate	benorilate
busulphan	busulfan
butobarbitone	butobarbital
carticaine	articane
cephalexin	cefalexin
cephamandole nafate	cefamandole nafate
cephazolin	cefazolin
cephradine	cefradine
chloral betaine	cloral betaine
chlorbutol	chlorobutanol
chlormethiazole	clomethiazole
chlorathalidone	chlortalidone
cholecalciferol	colecalciferol
cholestyramine	colestyramine
clomiphene	clomifene
colistin sulphomethate sodium	colistimethate sodium
corticotrophin	corticotropin
cysteamine	mercaptamine
danthron	dantron
desoxymethasone	desoximetasone
dexamphetamine	dexamfetamine
dibromopropamidine	dibrompropamidine
dienoestrol	dienestrol
dimethicone(s)	dimeticone
dimethyl sulphoxide	dimethyl sulfoxide
doxycycline hydrochloride (hemihydrate hemiethanolate)	doxycycline hyclate
ethancrynic acid	etacrynic acid
ethamsylate	etamsylate
ethinyloestradiol	ethinylestradiol
ethynodiol	etynodiol
flumethasone	flumetasone
flupenthixol	flupentixol
gestronol	gestonorone
guaiphenesin	guaifenesin
hexachlorophane	hexachlorophene
hexamine hippurate	methenamine hippurate
hydrosyprogesterone	hydroxyprogesterone

hexanoate	caproate	sodium calciumedetate	sodium calcium edetate
indomethacin	indometacin		
lysuride	lisuride	sodium cromoglycate	sodium cromoglicate
methyl cysteine	mecysteine	sodium ironedetate	sodium feredetate
methylphenobarbitone	methylphenobarbital	sodium picosulphate	sodium picosulfate
oestradiol	estradiol	sorbitan monostearate	sorbitan stearate
oestriol	estriol	stilboestrol	diethylstilbestrol
oestrone	estrone	sulphacetamide	sulfacetamide
oxethazaine	oxetacaine	sulphadiazine	sulfadiazine
pentaerythritol tetranitrate	pentaerithrityl tetranitrate	sulphadimidine	sulfadimidine
		sulphaguanadine	sulfaguanadine
phenobarbitone	phenobarbital	sulphamethoxazole	sulfamethoxazole
pipothiazine	pipotiazine	sulphasalazine	sulfasalazine
polyhexanide	polihexanide	sulphathiazole	sulfathiazole
potassium cloazepate	dipotassium clorazepate	sulphinpyrazone	sulfinpyrazone
		tetracosactrin	tetracosactide
pramoxine	pramocaine	thiabendazole	tiabendazole
prothionamide	protionamide	thioguanine	tioguanine
quinalbarbitone	secobarbital	thiopentone	thiopental
riboflavine	riboflavin	urofollitrophin	urofollitropin

ACOUSTIC NEUROMA

Acoustic neuroma represents 8% of all intracranial tumours and 80% of cerebellopontine angle tumours. They arise from Schwann (neurolemmal) cells. The commonest nerve of origin is the superior vestibular nerve, followed by the inferior vestibular and then, rarely, the cochlear nerve. Many surgeons prefer therefore the term vestibular schwannoma to acoustic neuroma.

Pathology

The medial portions of the cranial nerves are covered with glial stroma. Acoustic neuromas originate at the junction of the glial and Schwann cells, which for the vestibular nerve is usually within the internal auditory meatus. The sexes are equally affected and, whatever the time of onset and rate of progression, the presentation is most often between the ages of 40 and 60. The annual incidence is approximately 1 in 100 000. The majority of these tumours are unilateral, and the small proportion that are bilateral (5%) are seen in multiple neurofibromatosis type 2 (NF2). This is an autosomal dominant disease due to an aberration on the long arm of chromosome 22.

Macroscopically the tumour appears as a firm yellowish encapsulated mass with the nerve splayed out on its surface. Histologically the tumour consists of packed sheaves of connective tissue cells (fasciculated) or may be composed of a disorderly loose network of cells with intercellular vacuoles and cysts (reticular pattern). Haemorrhage can occur (particularly in the reticular type), leading to a sudden increase in size and therefore marked symptoms such as acute vertigo or sudden deafness.

Clinical features

Clinically, two phases can be recognized: an *otological phase* in which a small tumour compresses structures in the meatus; and a *neurological phase* as the tumour expands medially into the cerebellopontine angle.

1. Otological symptoms. Gradual and progressive unilateral deafness is the usual presenting symptom (90%). The deafness is often associated with tinnitus (70%). Sudden onset hearing loss can occur (10%). Some patients have normal hearing (5%). Vertigo is an unusual complaint as compensation for vestibular nerve damage usually keeps pace with the slow rate of neural destruction.

2. Trigeminal nerve symptoms. Facial pain, numbness and paraesthesiae may all occur.

3. Headache. Discomfort and dull aching around the ear and mastoid area are probably caused by posterior fossa dura irritation due to the enlarging tumour.

4. Late symptoms. Like most motor nerves, the facial nerve is resistant to pressure deformity and symptoms of (facial weakness or hemifacial spasm are uncommon). Ataxia and unsteadiness develop with progressive brain stem displacement and cerebellar involvement. Diplopia due to pressure on the VIth cranial nerve, and hoarseness with dysphagia due to involvement of the IXth and Xth nerves is (rare.)

5. Terminal symptoms. The raised CSF pressure causes failing vision due to papilloedema, headache, alteration in conscious level and eventually coma.

In the otological phase, general examination will usually reveal no abnormalities. The patient may have a unilateral neural hearing loss. Hypaesthesia of the posterior external ear canal on the side of the hearing loss should raise the index of suspicion (Hitselberger sign). Loss of the corneal reflex is an early sign of trigeminal nerve impairment. Nystagmus when present may be of the vestibular or cerebellar type. Facial nerve impairment is usually of the sensory element and can be elicited as a lack of taste on electrogustometry or loss of lacrimation on Schirmer's test. Slight facial weakness may show as a delay in the blink reflex. Later the patient may have evidence of ataxia. Neurological signs of the other cranial nerve palsies will eventually become apparent.

Investigations

1. Radiological investigations. The most accurate means of identifying small intracanalicular tumours is magnetic resonance imaging (MRI) with gadolinium enhancement. This is therefore the investigation of choice and is used for screening. Computerized tomography (CT) scanning with high definition and enhancement techniques will accurately diagnose and delineate most tumours, but should only be used when MRI is unavailable.

2. Audiometry. A unilateral or asymmetrical sensorineural hearing loss can usually be demonstrated by a pure tone audiogram. The hearing loss is classically a neural lesion with no loudness recruitment, abnormally rapid adaptation and disproportionately poor speech discrimination. Stapedial reflex decay can be measured using impedance audiometry, and this gives a low-false negative rate of around 5%. Brainstem electric response audiometry has only a 3% false-negative rate. It demonstrates a retrocochlear lesion by an increased latency between N1 and N5 waves. If the pure tone threshold hearing loss is greater than 70 dB, the accuracy of audiometric testing is poor.

3. Vestibular investigations. Caloric responses are usually reduced in or absent from the affected side, but there is no abnormality in some patients with small tumours. Special audiometric and vestibular testing are now rarely, if ever, used for the diagnosis of an acoustic neuroma.

Differential diagnosis of a tumour at the cerebellopontine angle

1. *Acoustic neuromas* (constitute 80% of cerebellopontine angle tumours).
2. *Meningioma.*
3. *Neuroma of the VIIth nerve.*
4. *Congenital cholesteatoma.*
5. *Aneurysm of the basilar or vertebral arteries.*
6. *Cholesterol granuloma of the petrous apex.*
7. *Cerebellar tumour.*

Management

The ideal management is a single stage total removal of the lesion, with preservation of all neural function and with minimal morbidity and mortality. However, this ideal is not always possible. Each case must be assessed on its own merits, with careful consideration of the age and general condition of the patient and the size, site and rate of growth of the lesion.

1. **Conservative management.** Small, slow-growing tumours in elderly patients can be watched by carrying out CT or MRI scanning at regular intervals to gauge the rate of expansion. Annual MRI scans show that around 60% of acoustic neuromas are not growing.

2. **Radiosurgery or radiotherapy.** These are popular treatments with patient self-help groups and are increasingly advocated in the USA. Hyperfractionated stereotactic radiotherapy is considered by some to be the primary treatment modality of choice. Stereotactic radiosurgery (gamma knife) has been applied to the tumour margin to control growth. Opponents to this view argue that future microsurgery may be more difficult and there is a theoretical risk of inducing malignant change.

3. **Microsurgery.** Removal of acoustic neuroma is associated most commonly with injury to the VIIth and VIIIth cranial nerves. Cerebrospinal fluid leak (often down the Eustachian tube) and meningitis are also relatively common. The morbidity and mortality from both tumour growth and its operative removal increase with large tumours. A small tumour can be extracted from the meatus with negligible hazard and preservation of the facial nerve. Early diagnosis and removal of these tumours should therefore be the rule.

There are three surgical approaches to the cerebellopontine angle and the choice depends on the position and size of the tumour and preoperative assessment by the otoneurologist and neurosurgeon.

1. **Translabyrinthine approach.** This is the most common approach. The facial nerve can be preserved but all hearing is lost. The approach tends to be used for patients with a severe sensorineural hearing loss (less than 70% speech discrimination).

2. **Middle fossa route.** This gives a limited access and is usually used for small intrameatal tumours, but an extended middle fossa approach can be used for larger ones. Hearing and the facial nerve can be preserved. The main disadvantage is that there is a 15% risk of the patient developing epilepsy. In the UK, driving is banned for 1 year following this procedure.

3. **Retrosigmoid approach.** This route is feasible when there is CSF between the lateral margin of the tumour and the lateral margin of the IAM (cochlea). The patient's hearing and facial nerve can be preserved, so this approach is also used for tumours when there is good hearing.

Further reading

Chandler CL, Ramsden RT. Acoustic schwannoma. *British Journal of Hospital Medicine*, 1993; **49**(5): 3–16; 335–343.

Kveton JF. Evaluation and management of acoustic neuroma. *Current Opinion in Otolaryngology and Head and Neck Surgery*, 1993; **1**: 53–63.

Brackmann D, Syms C. Tumours of the auditory-vestibular nerve. In: Ludman H, Wright T (eds) *Diseases of the Ear*, 6th edn. London: Arnold, 1998; 535–547.

Van Roijen L. Costs and effects of microsurgery versus radiosurgery in treating acoustic neuroma. *Acta Neurochir* 1997; **139**: 942–945.

Wilson J (ed). *Effective Head and Neck Cancer Management. Second Consensus.* British Association of Otolaryngologists, Head and Neck Surgeons, 2000.

Related topics of interest

ACUTE SUPPURATIVE OTITIS MEDIA

Definition

Otitis media is an inflammation of part or all of the mucosa of the middle-ear cleft, the collective term for the eustachian tube, tympanic cavity, attic, aditus, antrum and mastoid air cells.

Classification

It may be classified as acute or chronic with the suffix suppurative or non-suppurative. A third category, 'specific otitis media' has been used to describe tuberculous and syphilitic otitis media as it may present acutely or chronically, with or without suppuration and a fourth category namely 'adhesive otitis media' has been used to describe tympanosclerosis (hyaline degeneration and calcification) and adhesion formation within the tympanic cavity but should more accurately be regarded as a sequelae of otitis media.

Acute suppurative otitis media (ASOM)

Aetiology

This is a bacterial disease caused by pus forming organisms, *Streptococcus pneumoniae* (40%), *Haemophilus influenzae* (30%) and *Branhamella* (*Moraxella*) *catarrhalis* (10%) being the most commonly implicated. It may occur as a primary or a secondary infection after a viral acute non-suppurative otitis media. Bacteria enter the middle-ear cleft via the eustachian tube, a perforated tympanic membrane or more rarely be blood-borne. Infants have a short, wide more horizontally placed eustachian tube, allowing contamination from the regurgitation of feed and when actively vomiting. Teething increases the incidence of infection. Poor sanitation and hygiene, overcrowding and malnutrition are predisposing factors. Children aged 3–7 years have the highest incidence, direct extension from a bacterial or secondary to a viral upper respiratory tract infection being the most common aetiological factor. Risk factors in all age groups are recurrent or chronic rhinosinusitis, adenoiditis, chest disease and eustachian tube dysfunction. Causes of the latter are nasopharyngeal tumours including adenoidal hypertrophy, abnormal eustachian patency, cleft palate and submucous cleft palate. Pathogenic bacteria have been isolated from the nasopharynx in up to 97% of children with ASOM.

Clinical features

The two main symptoms are:

- *Pain*, which may increase rapidly in intensity to become deep and throbbing.
- *Deafness*, initially described as a blocked ear and secondary to Eustachian tube dysfunction.

Deafness progresses as suppuration occurs and both symptoms may rapidly improve if rupture of the tympanic membrane produces a mucopurulent otorrhoea.

The initial event after infection is mucosal oedema causing Eustachian tube occlusion and a dull tympanic membrane on examination. Hyperaemia rapidly follows and leashes of vessels may be seen running along or parallel to the malleus handle. Soon radial vessels are visible on the drumhead and a middle ear effusion occurs. The drumhead takes on a full (i.e. opposite to retraction), red, angry appearance and pus may be seen bulging postero-inferiorly. Pressure necrosis of this region may cause the drumhead to rupture allowing mucopus to drain into the external ear canal. Children are usually fretful with a high pyrexia ($> 39°C$) and there may be signs of complications of ASOM.

Treatment

1. *Rest* in a warm, well humidified room.
2. *Antibiotics* in an adequate dose administered until resolution. Amoxicillin will cover the most common pathogens provided the patient is not allergic to penicillin and the organisms are not resistant, the latter occurring in about 14% of cases but resistance is increasing. In these circumstances, gleaned from bacterial sensitivity studies or lack of clinical response, a β-lactamase resistant antibiotic should be chosen, for example coamoxiclav. Oral medication is adequate in the absence of complications.
3. *Systemic and topical decongestants* have a theoretical adjuvant role; they have not been proven to be of significant value.
4. Conditions predisposing to ASOM should be treated on their own merit after resolution.

Complications

- *Mucositis may progress to an osteomyelitis*, namely acute mastoiditis, if the mastoid air cells are affected and acute petrositis should the petrous apex become involved. Gradenigo's syndrome, comprising signs of ASOM, an ipsilateral abducent nerve palsy causing paralysis of the external rectus and pain in the distribution of the ipsilateral trigeminal nerve, is a classic feature of petrositis. The respective cranial nerves are only separated from the petrous apex by a layer of dura so that an extradural abscess or pachymeningitis (meningitis extending to the dural layer) of this region from a generalized meningitis may also cause the combined cranial nerve signs.
- *Meningitis*.
- *Citelli's abscess* (a subperiosteal abscess which has spread through the medial aspect of the mastoid, into the digastric fossa) or *Bezold's abscess* (an abscess which has tracked inferiorly within the sheath of sternomastoid to form a fluctuant mass along its anterior border).
- *Extradural and subdural abscess*.
- *Cerebellar, temporal lobe and perisinus abscess*.
- *Lateral sinus thrombosis*, rarely extending in an antegrade direction to thrombose the internal jugular vein and in a retrograde direction causing a cavernous sinus thrombosis.

6 ACUTE SUPPURATIVE OTITIS MEDIA

- *Otitic hydrocephalus.*
- *Lower motor neurone facial nerve paralysis.* The at-risk population (6%) are that group of patients with a congenital dehiscence of the horizontal portion of the facial nerve.
- *Serous and suppurative labyrinthitis.*

Sequelae of ASOM

- *Non-suppurative middle-ear effusion.* These persist for over 30 days in 40% of children and for over 3 months in 10%.
- *High-tone sensorineural hearing loss*, perhaps secondary to bacterial toxins migrating across the round window.
- *Tympanic membrane perforation.*
- *Adhesions* between the tympanic membrane, ossicles and the medial wall of the middle ear.
- *Tympanosclerosis* which may spread from the tympanic membrane to the ossicular chain, fixing the latter.
- *Erosion of the ossicular chain*, in particular the long process of the incus, especially following recurrent episodes of ASOM.
- Sequelae of ASOM complications.

Further reading

Haddad J Jr. Treatment of acute otitis media and its complications in pediatric otology. *Otolaryngologic Clinics of North America*, 1994; **6**: 431–441.

Pichichero ME. Assessing the treatment alternatives for acute otitis media. *Paediatric Infectious Diseases Journal*, 1994; **13**: 27–34.

Stutman HR, Arguedas AG. Comparison of cefprozil with other antibiotic regimes in the treatment of children with acute otitis media. *Clinical Infectious Diseases*, 1992; **14**(suppl 2): 204–208.

Related topics of interest

Tympanoplasty, p. 341; Cholesteatoma, p. 35; Chronic suppurative otitis media, p. 38; Chronic suppurative otitis media – complications, p. 42.

ADENOIDS

The adenoids are a mass of lymphoid tissue found at the junction of the roof and posterior wall of the nasopharynx. They are a normal structure with a function in the production of antibodies (IgA, IgG and IgM). The size of the adenoids varies, but in general they attain their maximum size between the ages of 3 and 8 years and then regress.

Pathology

Inflammation due to acute viral and bacterial infections results in hyperplasia with enlargement and multiplication of the lymphoid follicles. Most of the pathological effects related to the adenoids are due to this increase in size. The symptoms caused by hypertrophy result not from the actual size of the lymphoid mass, but from the relative disproportion in size between the adenoids and the cavity of the nasopharynx. The effect of the enlargement is to produce obstruction of the nasal airways and possibly obstruction of the Eustachian tubes.

Clinical features

1. Nasal obstruction leads to mouth breathing, snoring and hyponasal speech. Infants may have difficulty in feeding because they have to stop sucking intermittently to take a breath. Nasal discharge and postnasal drip or catarrh may develop as a result of secondary chronic rhinitis and sinusitis. Besides snoring, some children may suffer from episodes of sleep apnoea. The child with the 'classic' adenoid facies appearance (an open lip posture, prominent upper incisors, a short upper lip, a thin nose and a hypoplastic maxilla with a high arched palate) is rarely seen.

2. Eustachian tube obstruction may result in earache and deafness due to recurrent bouts of acute otitis media and otitis media with effusion (glue ear).

The clinical features of adenoid hypertrophy are not always clear cut, and unfortunately the parents' history is not always reliable. Symptoms are frequently wrongly attributed to enlarged adenoids. In some children examination of the nasopharynx with a postnasal mirror will identify large adenoids, but in many children it is impossible to assess the adenoids in this way. Fibreoptic endoscopy is useful if tolerated by the child.

Investigations

The only reliable means of assessing the size of the adenoid is examination under general anaesthetic, but some preoperative investigations may suggest enlargement. The most useful investigation is a lateral soft-tissue radiograph. This will give a measure of the absolute size of the adenoids and an assessment of their proportion in relation to the size of the airway. This is not always accurate and some children will still need an examination of the postnasal space under general anaesthetic. If enlarged adenoids are present they can then be curetted.

Indications for adenoidectomy

Generally speaking, an adenoidectomy is only indicated if troublesome symptoms can be attributed to abnormal adenoid hypertrophy. The indications for adenoidectomy are as follows:

- Nasal obstruction.
- Otitis media with effusion (glue ear).
- Recurrent acute otitis media.
- Chronic rhinosinusitis.
- Sleep apnoea.

Contraindications for adenoidectomy

- Recent upper respiratory tract infection.
- An uncontrolled bleeding disorder.
- Cleft palate. The adenoids assist in closure of the nasopharynx from the oropharynx during speech and deglutition. They should never be removed in a child who has had a cleft palate repair or a congenitally short palate. All children who have a bifid uvula should have a submucous cleft excluded.

Complications

1. *Immediate.*
- Anaesthetic complications.
- Soft palate damage.
- Dislocation of the cervical spine.
- Reactionary haemorrhage.

2. *Intermediate.*
- Secondary haemorrhage.
- Subluxation of the atlanto-occipital joint (secondary to infection).

3. *Late.*
- Eustachian tube stenosis.
- Hypernasal speech (rhinolalia aperta).
- Persistence of symptoms.

The most serious complication is reactionary haemorrhage. This is treated in the same manner as post-tonsillectomy haemorrhage. The child should be returned to theatre and an attempt made to localize and diathermy the bleeding point. A post-nasal pack should be inserted if necessary. Hypernasal speech can be a troublesome complication in some children. It often improves with time and speech therapy but may be sufficiently severe to require a pharyngoplasty to correct the problem. It is less likely to occur if children with palatal abnormalities are excluded from operation. Some surgeons advocate removal of the upper part of the adenoid mass leaving a lower ridge of adenoid tissue against which the defective palate may continue to make contact.

Follow-up and aftercare

In view of the problems with accurate diagnosis and the potential long-term complications it is worthwhile reviewing adenoidectomy children in the outpatient clinic 6 months postoperatively.

Further reading

Hotaling AJ, Silva AB. Advances in adenotonsillar disease. *Current Opinion in Otolaryngology and Head and Neck Surgery*, 1993; **1**: 177–184.

Potsic WP. Assessment and treatment of adenotonsillar hypertrophy in children. *American Journal of Otolaryngology*, 1992; **13**: 259–264.

Related topics of interest

ALLERGIC RHINITIS

Allergic rhinitis is an IgE-mediated, type 1 hypersensitivity reaction in the mucous membranes of the nasal airways. The disease is very common, affecting approximately 30% of the Western population. It can be either seasonal (summer hayfever) or perennial (sometimes with seasonal exacerbations).

Aetiology

Allergy is a hypersensitivity reaction of tissues to certain substances called allergens. The commonest allergens are highly soluble proteins or glycoproteins with a molecular weight in the range of 10000–40000. Typical allergens include pollens, moulds, house dust mite (*Dermatophagoides pteronyssinus* and *D. forinae*) and animal epithelia.

Pathogenesis

Immunoglobulin E is formed by plasma cells which are regulated by T-suppressor lymphocytes and T-helper cells. In normal individuals this system maintains a constant function. In allergic patients the IgE T-helper cells appear to promote overproduction at times of exposure to the allergen, or suppressor T cells may not be functioning correctly. The IgE antibody is composed of an Fc and an Fab portion. The Fc portion of IgE has an affinity for mast cells and basophils, which have receptors for the immunoglobulin on their cell membrane. The Fab portion of IgE is free to combine with an allergen. The allergen is thought to interact with two adjacent cell-bound IgE antibody molecules, so forming a cross-link composed of IgE–allergen–IgE. This triggers a chain of events with the synthesis and release of arachidonic acid metabolites (prostaglandin D, leukotrienes and other chemotactic factors) and initiates disruption of the mast cell with degranulation of lysosomes (releasing histamine, proteases and more chemotactic factors). The effect is that capillaries become more permeable, the ground substance viscosity is reduced by enzymes such as hyaluronidase, eosinophils infiltrate the tissues and oedema occurs. This produces the typical features of vascular congestion, oedema, rhinorrhoea and irritation.

Clinical features

Seasonal rhinitis usually occurs any time from early summer to early autumn depending on the specific allergen. The patient suffers from rhinorrhoea, nasal irritation and sneezing, associated with itchy and watering eyes. Some individuals (described as atopic) will have a strong family history of allergy or a previous history of eczema or asthma. Long-standing cases of perennial allergy may not display all these features, but they often have nasal obstruction due to hypertrophy of the turbinates sometimes associated with hyposmia. Patients with perennial rhinitis are almost invariably allergic to house-dust mite and typically have more than one allergy.

On examination, the nasal mucosa classically appears moist, pale and swollen, and the turbinates hypertrophied. Sometimes the mucosa is red and the turbinates may have a blue hue. Polyps may be present, but they are more often seen in intrinsic rhinitis.

Investigations

There are many investigations available, but clinically the most useful are the skin tests and plasma IgE measurements.

1. Skin tests. The epidermal prick test and the intradermal injection test use an allergen placed on the skin of the flexor aspect of the forearm. If the patient has an allergy to this then a wheal and flare will come up within 20 minutes. A negative control (carrier substance) and a histamine-containing solution (positive control) are used to ensure that the patient is not allergic to the carrier substance and does react in the normal fashion to histamine. A battery of common allergens (e.g. pollens, moulds, feathers, house dust mite, animal epithelia, etc.) are compared with the controls by the wheal they produce. Specific substances can be used depending on the history. If the patient is highly sensitive a widespread or even an anaphylactic reaction may result. Resuscitation equipment must always be available although the epidermal prick test is safe if properly performed. If an adverse reaction occurs, a tourniquet should be placed proximally to contain it and the patient given intravenous hydrocortisone, chlorpheniramine (chlorphenamine) and adrenaline (epinephrine).

2. Blood tests. Total plasma IgE levels may be measured in the plasma radio-immunosorbent test (PRIST) and IgE to specific allergens in the radioallergosorbent test (RAST). These tests are more convenient, do not expose the patient to the risks of the skin tests and do not rely on the use of a specific allergen. However, they are more expensive and have no diagnostic superiority over skin tests. An eosinophilia may occur in an acute allergic reaction but is unusual in allergic rhinitis.

3. Nasal smears. An increase in eosinophils in a nasal smear indicates an allergic rhinitis but is not diagnostic.

4. Provocation tests. A drop of the suspected allergen squeezed into the nose may cause symptoms (rhinorrhoea, sneezing, etc.). The effect can be measured objectively by rhinomanometry.

Management

1. Avoidance of the precipitating allergen is obviously helpful, but not always possible.

2. Oral antihistamines which selectively block histamine receptors, cause minimal or no drowsiness and can be given once daily are now available (e.g. astemizole, cetirizine, fexofenadine, loratidine). Some patients still prefer the older antihistamines which may cause drowsiness (e.g. chlorpheniramine and triprolidine) and they should be warned of this. Intranasal antihistamine sprays (e.g. azelastine hydrochloride) have the advantage of minimal systemic absorption.

3. Topical steroid sprays and drops are now considered to be the cornerstone in the treatment of rhinitis. They are safe and effective. Crusting and bleeding are the main side-effects. Systemic absorption is negligible, as is the chance of promoting fungal infections. Examples include fluticasone, mometasone, and triamcinolone sprays.

4. *Depot intramuscular injections of steroids* (e.g. triamcinolone acetonide) should be reserved for when symptoms interfere with special events (e.g. school examinations). Oral steroids are similarly indicated, but only in short courses.

5. *Topical anticholinergic drugs* (e.g. ipratropium bromide) are useful in the treatment of patients in whom rhinorrhoea is the predominant symptom.

6. *Sodium cromoglycate* stabilizes mast-cell membranes and therefore prevents the release of the allergic response mediators. It has few side-effects, but needs to be used five to six times per day for adequate prophylaxis, so compliance is poor. It works in relatively few people, but may be effective in children and can be used for allergic conjunctivitis.

7. *Desensitization* involves a series of injections of small amounts of the proven allergens in a purified form, in the hope that blocking IgG antibodies will be produced. It is really only of use in patients who are sensitive to only one or two allergens, in particular pollen allergy. The main complication of this treatment is anaphylaxis, and for this reason its use in the UK has been discouraged. Resuscitation equipment must always be available where this therapy is performed, and in case of anaphylaxis there must be a supply of intravenous hydrocortisone, chlorpheniramine and adrenaline.

8. *Leukotriene synthesis inhibitors and receptor antagonists* are not marketed for the treatment of allergic rhinitis, but they show promise for the future treatment of the disease.

9. *Surgical treatment* has a role to play other than in symptom control, especially turbinate surgery when there are symptoms of nasal obstruction.

Follow-up and aftercare

Most cases of allergic rhinitis can be managed by the patient's general practitioner. If the offending allergen is identified by any of the tests then the patient should be given general advice on avoidance. When there are any nasal abnormalities (e.g. deflected nasal septum or turbinate hypertrophy) or concomitant disease of the sinuses that complicate and exaggerate the symptoms of the rhinitis, they should be treated on their own merit.

Further reading

Norman PS. Allergic rhinitis. *Journal of Allergy and Clinical Immunology*, 1985; **75**: 531–545.
Baroody FM. Developments in the drug treatment of allergic rhinitis. *Current Opinion in Otolaryngology and Head and Neck Surgery*, 1998; **6**: 6–17.

Related topics of interest

Sinusitis, p. 285; Intrinsic rhinitis, p. 131.

ANAESTHESIA – GENERAL

P. Charters

Principles

In providing general anaesthesia for ENT surgery an anaesthetist will aim to render a patient:

- unresponsive to the stress of the surgical stimulus;
- amnesic for the event;
- free from pain post-operatively.

Safety during the procedure depends on the pre-morbid medical state of the patient, effect of the anaesthetic agents used and the particular requirements of the surgery. When surgery involves the airway itself, the anaesthetist must ensure continuous patency and adequate measures to deal with any contamination (e.g. blood or infected material). Liaison between the surgeon and anaesthetist is mandatory to anticipate and minimize critical operative events.

Pre-operative assessment

Most ENT surgery can be regarded as relatively superficial procedures performed on fit young patients. At the other extreme, there are also quite lengthy procedures performed on rather infirm elderly subjects. Upper airway tumours are associated with longstanding cigarette consumption and patients who have already suffered for many years from chronic pulmonary and cardiovascular disease. In these cases a thorough medical workup will assess risk and potential for improvement prior to surgery. Optimization of pulmonary function may be helped with pre-operative physiotherapy and medications review, especially bronchodilators. Cardiovascular workup may require referral for left ventricular function assessment by echocardiography and exercise tests in angina patients. Nutritional correction by naso-gastric or parentral feeding may substantially improve pre-operative status of patients with swallowing difficulty. Airway assessment by clinical, fibreoptic and radiological imaging should involve the anaesthetist in that the appropriate measures for operative management should be planned rather than haphazard as a result of insufficient information. Obstructive sleep symptoms and a history of nocturnal apnoeas are easily overlooked on routine clerking. It is important to determine pre-operatively which patients should be singled out for post-operative oximetry monitoring and the setting most appropriate for their nursing care.

Routine haematological and biochemical investigations are generally limited to the following:

- FBC (females of menstrual age; patients over 60 years; prior to major operations; after significant blood loss).
- U&E (patients over 60 years; prior to major operations; patients with diabetes, renal or hepatic impairment, hypertension, or on medications such as diuretics and anti-hypertensives).

- ECG (patients over 60 years; cardiac symptoms including palpitations and fainting).
- Chest radiography (patients with cardio-respiratory symptoms; cancer screening especially in patients with upper airway tumours).

These guidelines are modified for the less well patient. Urea and electrolytes are mandatory when deliberate hypotension is to be part of the anaesthetic technique. Medical treatments should be optimised preoperatively. Steroid cover is required when patients have received steroids in the past 12 months and antibiotic prophylaxis for patients with valvular heart disease. Hospitals normally have prescribed protocols for peri-operative care of diabetic subjects.

Premedication

Premedication may be used to reduce anxiety and decrease the incidence of nausea and vomiting. A benzodiazepine with an anti-emetic is a suitable combination, although patients with a compromised airway should not be sedated and appropriate reassurance may be an alternative. Oral sedative agents are often used in children and local anaesthetic cream (e.g. EMLA, a eutectic mixture of local anaesthetic: lignocaine 2.5% with prilocaine 2.5%) is applied to potential venepuncture sites under an occlusive dressing. Anticholinergics may be given as an anti-sialogogue, glycopyrolate being the best as it causes less tachycardia and does not cross the blood–brain barrier thus avoiding confusion. They are not given if hypotension is required as the resulting tachycardia antagonizes this effect.

Anaesthetic agents and technique

The usual intravenous agents to induce anaesthesia are thiopentone, etomidate and propofol. These drugs are all short-acting and it is usual to continue anaesthesia by a volatile anaesthetic agent, e.g. enflurane, isoflurane or desflurane in a mixture of nitrous oxide in oxygen. Induction of anaesthesia by breathing volatile anaesthetic agents remains common in paediatric practice where halothane and sevoflurane are usually preferred. Pharmacological muscle paralysis is not usually mandatory for ENT surgery but can be used to facilitate tracheal intubation and to lessen the requirement for 'deep anaesthesia' with volatile agents alone. Use of muscle relaxants in patients with difficult airways can lead to disaster when patients are rendered apnoeic and assisted ventilation is not possible. Patients at risk of aspiration or gastric contents on induction of anaesthesia usually have a rapid induction sequence with cricoid pressure applied. 'Total intravenous anaesthesia' refers to techniques where the use of inhalation agents are avoided and drugs combinations such as propofol and remifentanil (a very short acting opiate) are administered by infusion pump.

Nitrous oxide (N₂O)

This has been in use for 120 years as a general anaesthetic. It is 35 times more soluble in blood than nitrogen, and thus diffuses into air-containing spaces such as the middle ear, leading to an increase in pressure. This is maximal after 40 min of anaesthesia and is implicated in the adverse positioning of grafts, altered appearance of the tympanic membrane and postoperative nausea and vomiting. Nitrous oxide may be excluded by substituting air or by total intravenous anaesthesia. It has been suggested that packing the middle ear during surgery reduces the clinical significance of nitrous oxide-induced pressure changes.

Induced hypotension

This can reduce blood loss during head and neck operations. It may result in cerebral or myocardial ischaemia and renal or hepatic hypoperfusion. It is contraindicated in patients with coexisting hypertension, ischaemic heart disease, previous cerebrovascular accident, pregnancy, anaemia, hypovolaemia or impaired renal or hepatic function.

Techniques of inducing hypotension include:

- the prevention of anxiety-related tachycardia by good premedication;
- the avoidance of hypertension during laryngoscopy and intubation;
- volatile agent-induced vasodilatation;
- the use of head-up positioning to encourage venous drainage from the operative site.

Specific drugs used to induce hypotension include:

- sodium nitroprusside, which directly dilates arterioles and venules;
- glyceryl trinitrate, which dilates capacitance vessels;
- trimetaphan, which releases histamine, blocks ganglia and directly reduces peripheral vascular resistance;
- labetolol, which reduces arteriolar tone (by its alpha-blocking effect) and heart rate (by its beta-blocker effect, useful in preventing the reflex tachycardia seen in response to hypotension).

Large-bore intravenous access (to allow fluid correction of precipitous fall in blood pressure) and an arterial cannula for direct blood pressure monitoring are required if profound hypotension is to be induced. This is however, rarely, if ever, warranted in ENT surgery.

Per-operative monitoring

Apart from recommended minimum standards (HR, ECG, non-invasive BP and pulse oximetry), major operations will usually require invasive blood pressure monitoring, central venous cannulation and bladder catheterization. This should also apply when hypotensive anaesthesia is planned. Blood loss measurement per-operatively often simply involves weighing swabs and measurement of the suction container. Ideal post-operative haemoglobin is a compromise between a low haemoglobin (e.g. 8 mg per 100 ml) which favours blood flow through free flaps versus higher levels which may improve oxygen delivery.

Care of the airway

The airway can be a particular problem in ENT operations and difficulties may be due to:

- morphological derangement;
- soiling (by blood or infected material);
- surgery to alter the airway itself (e.g. laryngeal laser surgery and tumour debulking).

In all these situations the most important aspect is that the anaesthetist be as fully informed of the situation as possible pre-operatively. Where a patient presents acutely in a state of distress, relief of symptoms should be considered while determining what investigations are feasible. Helium and oxygen mixtures may relieve symptoms as may bronchodilators and nebulised adrenalin. Anxiety can potentiate as well as result from respiratory difficulty and reassurance may help but even small dose of anxiolytic can induce respiratory arrest.

Surgery for abscesses involving part of the upper airway must always be seen in context. Antibiotics alone may resolve some situations and good drainage will usually only be effective in well organised abscess cavities. External drainage under local anaesthesia may be appropriate and normally negates the risk of airway contamination. Where airway instrumentation does need to be considered, good radiological imaging may delineate precise morphological changes and also indicate where the abscess wall is thinnest and in danger of disruption.

Acute airway obstruction usually means that the patient presents with an airway that is not severely narrowed, i.e. even with mild stridor a 4-mm microlaryngoscopy tube can usually be advanced into the trachea. However, when airway obstruction has been longstanding (weeks or months), adaptation over time may mean that very small airways are encountered. In young children and adults less than 30 years of age, pinhole glottis narrowing is not infrequently encountered. The nature of the relevant pathology is important because chronic obstruction tends to be a relatively 'solid' processes (e.g. fibrosis following radiation treatment, sessile ulcerative tumour and granulation/deposition diseases). By comparison, acute obstruction is usually associated with a more 'fluidic' processes such as friable or cystic tumours, oedema, infection or haemorrhage into normal or abnormal tissue.

Management of these cases does depend on the experience of the doctors concerned. Tracheotomy under local anaesthesia is commonly regarded as a final fallback position but success may be difficult in an extremely restless patient who is fighting for breath. It should also be remembered that there is no guarantee that the trachea and in particular the subglottis will be free of pathology when there has been little time for formal investigations. Because the view with a fibreoptic laryngoscope can be quite restricted, the endoscopist needs to have a good general idea as to where to expect to find the relevant anatomical landmarks. Experience will guide in the choice as to whether or not awake fibreoptic laryngoscopy should be considered. Patient co-operation is important when sedation is inadvisable. When general anaesthesia is considered necessary the anaesthetist will usually consider techniques which allow sedation to be gradually increased. In the case of the airway worsening, the sedation can then be lightened and if necessary the patient is woken up. If the airway pathology is not a relative contraindication, the use of airway devices such as the laryngeal mask airway (LMA) and cuffed oro-pharyngeal airway (COPA) may help to control the immediate airway difficulty. Then either can be used as a means to tracheal intubation using an exchange catheter (e.g. the Aintree intubation catheter) over a fibreoptic laryngoscope.

Airway debulking is a particular problem for the anaesthetist. This is used in patients presenting with acute airway obstruction where the immediate surgical aim is to improve the airway and acquire histology before considering formal treatment. This usually proceeds shortly after the histology becomes available. Tumours that are papilliferous are easier to debulk than sessile ulcers. Bleeding after surgery is possible as is the risk of laryngeal oedema. The surgeon and anaesthetist need to agree on a suitable end point for this surgery, i.e. when the airway will be adequate in the post-operative period. Surgical debulking may be augmented by intravenous steroids and antibiotics. Post-operative care needs to be in an environment where the nursing and medical staff are aware of the risk of post-operative problems and their management.

Laser surgery carries a risk of an airway fire after ignition of the tracheal tube or the fresh gas mixture. The tracheal tube should be flexo-metallic, wrapped in aluminium foil or laser-proof. The tracheal tube cuff is filled with saline or preformed with foam. If airway fire occurs, the surgery must be discontinued and ventilation stopped until the fire is extinguished with a pre-filled syringe of saline. The tracheal tube should then be replaced, the patient ventilated with 100% oxygen, a bronchoscopy performed, steroids commenced and antibiotics and prolonged ventilatory support provided as necessary.

Related topics of interest

Anaesthesia – local, p. 19; Hypopharyngeal carcinoma, p. 124; Laryngeal carcinoma p. 138; Paediatric airway problems, p. 232; Stridor and stertor, p. 311; Tracheostomy, p. 336.

ANAESTHESIA – LOCAL

P. Charters

Mode of Action

Local anaesthetic (LA) agents produce a reversible block in the transmission of impulses along nerve fibres. They vary in terms of potency, toxicity, water solubility, ability to penetrate mucous membranes and duration of action. When applied to different sites their efficacy is influenced by these properties and the local blood supply can have implications for both duration of action and liability to toxic effects. Removal from the site of action tends to be by the circulation, diffusion, metabolism or dilution which reduce local tissue concentration of the LA to restore nerve function. Local anaesthetics are weak bases and the degree of ionization depends on the individual drug's pKa and the surrounding pH. At a low pH, more of the drug remains in the ionized form, preventing it from diffusing across the axonal membrane and therefore reducing efficacy.

Classification

There are two broad classes of LA:

- esters (e.g. benzocaine, cocaine and procaine);
- amides (e.g. lignocaine, prilocaine, bupivacaine, ropivacaine and levobupivacaine).

Complications

Complications associated with the use of local anaesthesia may not be common but can be life threatening and for this reason their use should be restricted to areas where resuscitation facilities are to hand.

1. Toxicity. This depends on the dose of the agent and speed of uptake into the circulation. Where the circulation is poor or when vasoconstrictors (e.g. adrenaline) are administered with the LA, larger doses can be tolerated. For ENT surgery, toxicity most commonly results from inadvertent direct intravascular injection or rapid absorption via mucous membranes and toxicity from any concomitant vasoconstrictor is likely. The blood supply may be increased in infected tissue where the choice of local anaesthesia must be questioned. Manifestations of toxicity usually start during drug administration or very shortly afterwards. They include:

- CNS: lightheadedness, perioral paraesthesia, slurred speech, tinnitus, facial twitching, convulsions and coma.
- CVS: bradycardia, hypotension and cardiac arrest.
- RS: an initial increase in respiratory rate followed by respiratory depression, hypoxia and respiratory arrest.

If any of these symptoms occur during the injection, drug administration should be stopped immediately and the situation assessed. Toxic effects are usually self-limiting but fitting and cardiovascular collapse should be treated with oxygen administration. CPR may be required. Longer acting drugs (e.g. bupivacaine) can have a prolonged effect on the heart, necessitating prolonged cardiac massage. Anyone who has had a severe reaction should be observed on a High Dependency or Intensive Care Unit to monitor cardiovascular and renal function even when immediate recovery appears complete.

2. Allergic reactions.   The onset of a reaction is more immediate and more severe with inadvertent intravenous administration. Reactions are more common with esters than amides. Clinical manifestations include cardiovascular collapse, bronchospasm, generalized (and laryngeal) oedema and there may be an urticarial rash. The airway should be secured and the subject positioned horizontally. Cardiopulmonary collapse requires ventilation with 100% oxygen, IV fluids and adrenaline 1 : 10000 in 1 ml aliquots. Bronchodilators may be required. Antihistamines should be considered and if hypotension and bronchospasm persist steroids should also be considered. Continuing care (or observation and monitoring in the case of apparent recovery) in ICU or HDU is mandatory.

Specific LA agents

1. Cocaine.   An ester hydrolysed by plasma cholinesterases. It has vasoconstrictive properties and is rapidly effective on mucous membranes. It potentiates catecholamine activity and sensitizes the myocardium to adrenaline. Concern about toxicity has recently restricted its availability to a 10% spray used topically to facilitate nasal surgery. Maximum dose 1.5 mg/kg or total 100 mg in a fit adult. Duration of action: 30–60 min.

2. Lignocaine.   An amide metabolized in the liver. It is available in injectable form as 0.5–2%, sprays as 4% or 10% and ointments of 2–5%. It is a mild vasodilator and is often given with a vasopressor, e.g. adrenaline 1 : 200000. Maximum dose: 3 mg/kg or 7 mg/kg with adrenaline. Duration of action (when infiltrated): 90 min without adrenaline.

3. Prilocaine.   An amide with no vasodilating effect and lower systemic toxicity. Metabolism to o-toluidine may cause methaemoglobinaemia. Maximum dose: 5 mg/kg or 7 mg/kg with adrenaline. Duration of action: 140 min.

4. Bupivacaine.   A vasodilating amide with a long duration, useful for postoperative analgesia. At toxic levels cardiac events, especially ventricular fibrillation, may precede neurological events. Max dose: 2 mg/kg or 3 mg/kg with adrenaline. Duration of action: 240 min without adrenaline.

5. Ropivacaine.   A single isomer and propyl homologue of bipivacaine (itself a racemic mixture). Levo isomers of amide local anaesthetics in general tend to have lower potential for systemic toxicity than the dextro forms. Ropivacaine is said to produce less motor block for the equivalent sensory block to bupivacaine. The dosages are similar.

6. Levobupivacaine. The single levo isomer of bupivacaine which has been shown to have less systemic toxic effects. The sensory block lasts longer than that with bupivacaine used in similar dosages.

Vasoconstrictors

Combined with a LA agent these reduce the risk of systemic toxicity and intraoperative bleeding and prolong the duration of action. Vasopressors are contraindicated in patients with ischaemic heart disease, hypertension or thyrotoxicosis and in those on monoamine oxidase inhibitors. Halothane, a volatile anaesthetic agent, sensitises the myocardium to adrenaline and concomitant use is better avoided. Vasopressors are contraindicated in sites supplied by end arteries. Phenylephrine (0.5%) is a used topically in the nose and is also available combined with lignocaine.

Local anaesthetic uses in ENT surgery

1. Nose. LA used on its own or combined with general anaesthesia.

(a) Modified Moffet's technique. The nasal cavities are sprayed with LA and the patient placed supine with the head extended over the end of the trolley. A 2-ml volume of 5% cocaine is applied to each nasal cavity using a specially angulated cannula. After 10 min the nose is pinched and any remaining solution removed.

(b) Nasal pack. After applying LA to the nasal cavity, ribbon gauze soaked in LA is packed into the nose and left for 10 min. After removal of the pack, two wool applicators soaked in LA are applied, one to the region of the sphenopalatine foramen and the other to the anterior end of the cribriform plate. Additional anaesthesia may be supplied by anterior ethmoidal or maxillary nerve blocks or by infiltration of the columella.

2. Pharynx, larynx and trachea. LA is used for direct laryngoscopy or awake intubation. The oropharynx is anaesthetized by spraying or nebulizing 4% lignocaine, or using a benzocaine lozenge. When using a fibreoptic bronchoscope LA is sprayed as the scope is advanced. Alternatively, the following blocks may be used:

(a) Superior laryngeal nerve.
  - Krause's method – a swab soaked in 4% lignocaine is held, by Krause's forceps, in each piriform fossa for 1 min.
  - Percutaneous – 2 ml of LA is injected where the nerve divides at the greater cornu of the hyoid.

(b) Cricothyroid injection. A 2-ml volume of 4% lignocaine is injected via the cricothyroid ligament after aspiration of air to confirm needle placement. A small intravenous cannula with the needle removed avoids needle stick injury to the posterior tracheal wall during the coughing on injection.

Anaesthesia for tracheostomy is by field infiltration with progressive supplementation. An initial cricothyroid injection can reduce coughing when the trachea is incised.

3. *Ear.* Infiltration may be supplemented by:

(a) Auriculotemporal nerve block – 2 ml of lignocaine is injected anterior to the meatus.
(b) Greater auricular nerve block – 2 ml of lignocaine is injected 2 cm both anterior and posterior to the tip of the mastoid.

Related topic of interest

Anaesthesia – general, p. 14.

BENIGN NECK LUMPS

Classification

(a) Congenital (defined as present at birth): lymphangiomas, dermoids, thyro-glossal cysts.
(b) Developmental: branchial cysts, laryngoceles, pharyngeal pouches.
(c) Tumours of the parapharyngeal space.
(d) Thyroid swellings.
(e) Salivary gland tumours.
(f) Reactive neck lymphadenopathy.
(g) Neck space infection.

The last four groups above are discussed as separate topics elsewhere in the book. This chapter describes congenital, developmental and parapharyngeal-space lumps.

Congenital

Lymphangiomas

There are three types of lymphangioma: simple (thin walled channels), cavernous (dilated lymphatic spaces), and cystic hygroma (cysts of varying sizes). Simple and cavernous lesions arise principally in the lips, cheek and floor of the mouth. Cystic hygromas usually arise in the lower neck. Treatment is by surgical excision. Injection of sclerosants and radiotherapy have been suggested but are not recommended.

Dermoid cysts

These are midline swellings that do not move with swallowing or tongue protrusion. There are three types:

1. Epidermoid cysts, lined only with squamous epithelium.
2. True dermoids lined with squamous epithelium and all other normal skin appendages.
3. Teratoid cysts are lined by respiratory or squamous epithelium and contain ectodermal, endodermal and mesodermal elements, for example teeth, nails or thyroid tissue.

Thyroglossal cysts

These are cysts along the tract of the obliterated thyroglossal duct. They may contain elements of thyroid tissue and may even be the sole source of functioning thyroid tissue. Many experts therefore recommend a ^{99m}Tc or radio iodine (^{131}I) uptake scan prior to excision, although an ultrasound scan is less invasive and will allow confirmation of whether there is a normal gland present. Ninety per cent of thryoglossal cysts are midline and 9% left-sided, occurring between the body of the hyoid bone and the cricoid cartilage. Most occur in childhood (mean age 4 years). They move with swallowing and tongue protrusion as they are ultimately attached on their deep aspect to the larynx. Infection causes the rapid onset of diffuse swelling, pain and tenderness. Thyroglossal cysts should not be incised and drained as this may cause an ugly sinus which is difficult to excise *in toto* and in continuity with the deflated cyst. A long course of antibiotics and repeat aspiration of the cyst, if the child allows, are recommended. The tract may climb anterior or posterior to the body of the hyoid to the tongue base. The body of the hyoid and preferably a wedge of tongue base should therefore be included in the excision of the cyst (Sistrunk's Procedure). Following this procedure the recurrence rate varies from 2% to 8%. If the hyoid body is not removed the recurrence rate rises to 85%.

Developmental

Branchial cysts

Four theories regarding aetiology have been proposed:

1. They arise from elements of squamous epithelium within a lymph node. This is the current consensus view.
2. They arise from remnants of the first pharyngeal pouch.
3. They are remnants of the cervical sinus.
4. They are remnants of the duct connecting the thymus to the third pharyngeal pouch.

Branchial cysts are lined by stratified squamous epithelium and contain lymphoid tissue in their wall. They usually present in young adults, 60% on the left and 60% in males. Most arise along the line of the deep cervical lymph nodes deep to the anterior border of sternomastoid at the junction of its upper third and lower two thirds. Diagnosis is by clinical examination and from fine needle aspiration biopsy. In a patient over the age of 40 years a metastatic node must be excluded. A quarter of branchial cysts become infected and should be managed similarly to an infected thyroglossal cyst. Excision should only be attempted when all inflammation has settled to minimize the risk of rupturing the cyst wall, which may lead to a recurrence or, if wall remnants are left, a fistula.

Laryngocele

Only about 30 occur each year in the UK, 80% in men with a mean age of 55. They arise from the laryngeal saccule, expanding internally to present in the vallecula or externally through the thyrohyoid membrane. In most subjects raising the intralaryngeal pressure causes no expansion of the saccule. In those in whom the saccule expands, perhaps because of a wider than usual true cord to false cord distance (wide neck) or because the false cord is compressed against the saccule to create a one-way valve, coughing, sneezing or trumpet playing may fully develop the laryngocele. They are occasionally associated with a ventricular carcinoma.

An intermittent neck swelling is the usual presentation, perhaps with hoarseness, cough or pain. It is usually impalpable but may become both visible and palpable on performing the Valsalva manoeuvre. Indirect laryngoscopy may reveal fullness of the ipsilateral false cord. Plain anteroposterior and lateral neck radiographs may show an air-filled sac. Laryngoceles may obstruct the larynx, so the safest treatment is excision, which includes the upper half of thyroid cartilage on the side of the laryngocele so that its neck can be ligated.

Tumours of the parapharyngeal space

This space is described in Neck space infection (p. 188).

Parapharyngeal tumours expand either medially, when the tonsil will be displaced towards the midline, or laterally to present in the upper deep cervical region. It is therefore important to exclude a metastatic node as a cause of the swelling. However, the common tumours are:

- Lipomas.
- Parotid deep lobe tumours.
- Neurogenous tumours.
- Carotid aneurysm.

Parotid tumours are the commonest and are discussed elsewhere (see Related topics).

Neurogenous tumours develop from neural crest cells which have differentiated into Schwann cells or sympathicoblasts. Schwann cells give rise to neurofibromas and schwannomas, the sympathicoblasts to ganglioneuromas and chemodectomas (carotid body tumours, glomus vagale and glomus jugulare tumours).

(a) *Neurofibromas* arise from endoneural fibrous connective tissue and are composed of a mass of spindle cells which can entwine nerve fibres, sometimes causing weakness or paralysis of the involved nerve.

(b) *Schwannomas* are benign tumours of the neurolemma or sheath of Schwann and so tend to be encapsulated. Their expansion may compress the involved nerve, giving rise to reduced function, but paralysis is unusual. In the parapharyngeal space a painless neck mass is usually the only sign.

(c) *Chemodectomas* arise from paraganglionic tissue at three common sites in the neck. On the medial side of the carotid bulb are found highly vascular tumours arising from the carotid body cells; these *carotid body tumours* are rare except in high-altitude population centres such as Mexico City. Vagal paragangliomas arise from paraganglionic tissue within the perineurium of the vagus, the *glomus vagale tumour*, which, if it involves the ganglion nodosum just below the jugular foramen, is referred to as a *glomus jugulare*. The cells are not functionally active. Patients present with a slow-growing painless lump in the neck or a mass pushing the tonsil medially, although with the vagal nerve paragangliomas pulsating, tinnitus, syncope, and glossopharyngeal, vagal, accessory and hypoglossal nerve palsies may arise if the tumour expands at the skull base. Carotid body tumours may be pulsatile with an audible bruit. Malignant change rarely, if ever, occurs in chemodectomas of these three sites. Occasional reports of metastases in the literature may be confusing a chemodectoma with a large-cell neuroendocrine carcinoma. Chemodectomas may occur rarely at other sites, particularly the larynx.

A carotid aneurysm may be caused by atheroma, trauma or infection. If expanding or causing transient ischaemic attacks, it can be resected and replaced with a reversed saphenous vein graft.

Investigations

An MRI scan will delineate the position and assess the size and vascularity of the mass. If a carotid body tumour is suspected a digital subtraction angiogram will allow precise definition of the tumour circulation, its principal feeding vessels and the presence of a cross-circulation, all of which must be known prior to surgery. A fine-needle aspiration biopsy, if necessary under CT guidance, may allow a definite diagnosis to be made. Under no circumstance should either a Tru-cut biopsy or a biopsy from within the mouth be attempted because the vascularity of a carotid body tumour may cause a rapidly expanding parapharyngeal haematoma which might occlude the oropharyngeal airway.

Treatment

The mass will as a rule continue to expand so that symptoms may progress. A tissue diagnosis may not be possible. For these reasons, surgery is the treatment of choice for parapharyngeal tumours. The parapharyngeal space can be approached by either a transcervical, transparotid or transmandibular route. The vagus and the hypoglossal nerves are at risk of injury. There is also a small, but definite, risk of stroke from surgery. A significant proportion of young patients will refuse surgery if presented with all the facts. Recent publications have suggested that carotid body tumours may be radiosensitive and radiotherapy may be indicated either as adjuvant treatment or in those unfit or unwilling to have surgery.

Follow-up and aftercare

Review of all parapharyngeal mass patients postoperatively for 5 years, except those who had a lipoma, is indicated. Glossopharyngeal and vagal nerve injury may give rise to aspiration and a hoarse voice, although symptoms gradually settle, especially if an experienced speech therapist is involved in rehabilitation. A vocal cord palsy is treated as discussed elsewhere (see Related topics of interest).

Further reading

Ferlito A, Pesavento G, Recher G *et al.* Assessment and treatment of neurogenic and non-neurogenic tumours of the parapharyngeal space. *Head and Neck Surgery*, 1984; **7**: 32–43.

Jackson CG, Harris PF, Glasscock ME *et al.* Diagnosis and management of paragangliomas of the skull base. *American Journal of Surgery*, 1990; **159**: 389–393.

Wilson J (ed). *Effective Head and Neck Cancer Management. Second Consensus.* British Association of Otolaryngologists, Head and Neck Surgeons, 2000.

Related topics of interest

Neck space infection, p. 188; Vocal cord palsy, p. 354; Salivary gland neoplasms, p. 274; Salivary gland diseases, p. 271.

CALORIC TESTS

Physiology

The semicircular canals are paired sensory structures responsible for the detection of angular acceleration. Each canal possesses a dilation at one end called the ampulla. Within the ampulla exists a saddle-shaped crista upon which sits a gelatinous cupula; the whole membranous canal is filled with endolymph. The inertia of the endolymphatic fluid means that there is a relative difference in the velocity of the canal and the fluid with head movements. This results in fluid being forced through the gap between crista and cupula and a deflection of the stereocilia which causes either an increase or decrease in the resting tonic discharge depending on the direction of deflection. The two labyrinths work in conjunction so that an increase in neural signals from one canal will be associated with a decreased discharge rate from the corresponding canal on the opposite side. As the three canals are mutually at right angles, complex three-dimensional information is provided.

Background

The caloric response can be used to test the integrity of this system and was first described by Robert Barany in 1906 and for which he was awarded a Nobel prize in 1914. He postulated that altering the temperature of the endolymph sets up thermally induced convection currents. This fluid movement leads to stimulation of the stereocilia and consequent nystagmus and vertigo. Caloric testing was further refined in 1942 by Fitzgerald and Hallpike when they described a standardized bithermal caloric test which remains an essential vestibular investigation to this day.

It has become apparent in recent years that thermal convection currents are not the only component in the caloric response. Positional alterations and the presence of a caloric response in microgravity have led to suggestions that a direct thermal effect on the sensory organs may account for as much as one-third of the response, although this in no way reduces the value of the test.

Procedure

The classic bithermal calorics utilize water at 30 and 44°C, kept at these temperatures in two heated tanks about 1 metre above the test couch. The patient reclines on the couch at 30° above the horizontal so as to bring the lateral semicircular canal into the vertical position. After checking that the external canals are clear of wax and debris and that the tympanic membranes are intact, cold water (30°C) is run into the left ear, via a siphon tube and 14G cannula, for 40 seconds. A stopwatch is used to time the period from the start of this manoeuvre to the point at which the nystagmus stops with the patient fixating on a point on the ceiling. This procedure is repeated for the right ear and then for both ears with the warm water (44°C).

A number of variations on this basic theme exist. Cold tap water can be used as a very basic single temperature screening test, and in patients with perforated eardrums air may be used to supply the thermal stimulus. Further refinements can be added by the use of Frenzel's glasses to remove optic fixation or measuring the nystagmus electrically (electronystagmography).

Interpretation

By definition, the direction of the nystagmus is described by its fast phase. Cold stimulation leads to nystagmus with the fast phase to the opposite side, while warm stimulation leads to nystagmus with the fast phase to the same side. This is easily remembered by the mnemonic COWS (cold–opposite, warm–same).

Various formulae exist, based on the recorded times for each part of the standard caloric test, to predict the degree of vestibular activity. The most common abnormalities found are *canal paresis* or *directional preponderance* (or a combination of the two). By the nature of the test a canal paresis or directional preponderance must be greater than 20–25% to be significant.

- Unilateral *canal paresis* denotes that the response of one side to hot and cold stimuli is reduced or absent compared with the opposite side. This finding invariably implies a lesion of the peripheral vestibular system (e.g. horizontal canal or vestibular nerve on that side). Exceptions to this include patients with lesions at the vestibular nerve-root entry-zone of the brainstem (e.g. multiple sclerosis or lateral brainstem infarction), in which there is central pathology and also a canal paresis.
- A *directional preponderance* denotes a non-specific enhancement of nystagmus in one particular direction. It suggests pathology, but is usually non-localizing (may arise from any part of the peripheral or central vestibular system). It may be localizing with some peripheral lesions, when directional preponderance is usually directed away from the diseased ear.

Clinical indications

Caloric testing forms the cornerstone of investigation for any vestibular pathology and is therefore useful in all patients with vertigo. Although MRI scans are now the investigation of choice for an acoustic neuroma, caloric tests may still be of some value, as the tumour usually arises from the superior vestibular nerve and leads to an ipsilateral canal paresis.

Further reading

Luxon LM. Comparison of caloric nystagmus by observation of duration and by electronystagmographic measurement of slow-phase velocity. *British Journal of Audiology*, 1995; **29**: 107–116.
Stahle J. Controversies on the caloric response. *Acta Otolaryngologica*, 1990; **109**: 162–167.

Related topics of interest

CERVICAL LYMPHADENOPATHY

Cervical lymphadenopathy implies disease involving the cervical lymph nodes. In this topic a simple differential of these diseases is presented, but specific details are found elsewhere (see Benign neck lumps, p. 23). The remainder of the chapter is confined to the problem of neck node metastases. A primary carcinoma arising in the upper aerodigestive tract may metastasize to the lymph nodes of the neck. Cervical node status is one of the most important prognostic factors in the head and neck cancer patient. In a patient with positive nodal disease, the usual expected survival rate for any specific primary tumour is reduced by one half. Therefore, control of regional metastatic disease constitutes a significant part of the management of head and neck cancer.

Differential diagnosis

Most cervical masses fall into one of four broad groups:

1. *Congenital* or *developmental* (thyroglossal, branchial and dermoid cysts).
2. *Infectious* (tonsillitis, infectious mononucleosis, tuberculosis, actinomycosis, HIV).
3. *Inflammatory* (sarcoidosis).
4. *Neoplastic* (primary arising from neck structures, metastatic secondaries, haematogenous).

The diagnosis is from the history, examination including endoscopy, radiology and laboratory tests. The specific investigations will be dictated by the differential diagnosis. Fine-needle aspiration (FNA) cytology is probably the single most useful diagnostic procedure if a neoplastic lymph node is suspected. False-negative and, very rarely, false-positive results can occur with FNA, so the information must always be used in conjunction with the clinical findings. An ultra-sound scan (with USS guided FNA) or MRI scan may delineate impalpable nodes. The scans can also reveal the integrity or involvement of the vasculature by a metastatic lymph node. A chest radiograph may show a primary carcinoma or evidence of secondary spread, as well as pulmonary tuberculosis or mediastinal gland enlargement.

Anatomy

The following definitions are recommended for the boundaries of cervical lymph node groups.

- *Level I.* Consists of the submental and submandibular lymph nodes within the triangle bounded by the anterior belly of the digastric, the hyoid bone, the posterior belly of digastric and the body of the mandible.
- *Level II* (upper deep cervical). Consists of lymph nodes located around the upper third of the internal jugular vein and adjacent spinal accessory nerve extending from the level of the carotid bifurcation to the skull base.
- *Level III* (mid deep cervical). Consists of lymph nodes around the middle third of the internal jugular vein extending from the carotid bifurcation superiorly to the cricothyroid notch inferiorly.

- *Level IV* (lower deep cervical). Consists of lymph nodes located around the lower third of the internal jugular vein extending from the cricothyroid notch to the clavicle inferiorly.
- *Level V.* Consists of the posterior triangle nodes which are located between the posterior border of the sternomastoid muscle and the anterior border of trapezius. The supraclavicular nodes are also included in this group.
- *Level VI.* Anterior compartment.

Staging

The staging system in most common use in the UK is that proposed by the International Union against Cancer (UICC), which is based on data developed by the American Joint Committee (AJC) for Cancer Staging.

NX Regional lymph nodes cannot be assessed.
N0 Regional lymph nodes not palpable.
N1 Movable single homolateral node < 3 cm in diameter.
N2 Movable homolateral or bilateral nodes.
    (a) Single ipsilateral node (3–6 cm in diameter).
    (b) Multiple ipsilateral nodes (up to 6 cm).
    (c) Bilateral or contralateral nodes (up to 6 cm).
N3 Nodes > 6 cm in diameter.

Although this system is useful, it has several inherent problems: clinicians will fail to agree on the presence of a palpable lymph node in as many as 30% of cases. In addition, it is generally acknowledged that the number of lymph nodes involved, the lymph node level and the presence of extra-capsular spread (ECS) are the most important prognostic parameters in metastatic disease of the neck. This information is only available after pathological staging (pTNM).

Treatment

The treatment of malignant neck nodes is by either some form of neck dissection or radiotherapy. Broadly speaking, lymph nodes of less than 2 cm diameter can be treated by radical radiotherapy and those greater than this size will be treated by a neck dissection with or without postoperative radiotherapy. The rupture of the lymph node capsule by tumour (ECS) is a bad prognostic sign. Fifty per cent of nodes with a diameter greater than 3 cm exhibit this. Postoperative irradiation to the neck following neck dissection is mandatory in the presence of ECS.

1. N0. The performance of a neck dissection without palpable lymph nodes (prophylactic or elective neck dissection) is considered by some to be of doubtful value. The argument supporting dissection is that some lymph nodes may be invaded by tumour (occult nodes) and still be impalpable. Risk factors for occult nodes are the site, the size and histological grade of the primary tumour. Prophylactic neck dissection has a place in the patient who has a primary tumour with a high incidence of occult nodes (nasopharynx, tonsil, base of tongue, pyriform fossa, supraglottic larynx or oral cavity). There is support for elective treatment of the neck or at least the first echelon nodes in tumours of these primary sites. The treatment can be by selective neck dissection or by irradiation. The modality chosen is usually the same as that used for the primary tumour. For other sites it is argued that no survival benefit is conferred and the morbidity/mortality of the operation outweigh the potential benefit. Many surgeons therefore adopt a wait and watch policy.

2.   *N1.* It is generally accepted that lymph nodes of less than 2 cm diameter can be sterilized by radiotherapy. This has the advantage of avoiding surgery and its morbidity. However, radiotherapy has its own morbidity and can only be used once. Although recurrence after a course of radiotherapy can be treated by neck dissection, the survival after such salvage surgery is poor. The use of radiotherapy also means that valuable prognostic information (pTNM) is not made available. It must be confirmed that the node is metastatic as a high proportion of nodes in this category do not contain tumour and, even if they do, extranodal spread is uncommon. Therefore a modified radical neck dissection is preferred by some surgeons for these patients.

3.   *N2.* Larger nodes (N2a) and multiple ipsilateral nodes (N2b) are best treated by a modified or radical neck dissection because of the high incidence of ECR of the tumour and difficulty in sterilizing even small multiple nodes. Postoperative radiotherapy is indicated if there is ECR or positive margins in the resection specimen. The incidence of further neck recurrence is probably reduced by postoperative radiotherapy, although overall survival is not affected. Patients with a supraglottic carcinoma and bilateral nodes do better than those with cancer of other primary sites at high risk of bilateral neck metastases (base of tongue and hypopharynx). The decision to treat should be taken very carefully as there is a considerable morbidity from a bilateral neck dissection which can be a simultaneous or a staged procedure. Most surgeons advocate either staged bilateral radical neck dissection or, if possible, a modified radical neck dissection on the least invaded side.

4.   *N3.* These nodes used to be referred to as 'fixed', but size is now the criterion for staging. If the tumour invades the internal jugular vein, or the base of skull in the region of the mastoid process, or the brachial plexus, it is almost certainly incurable. Fixation to the skin can be treated by resection of the tumour with involved skin which is replaced with the use of flaps such as a pectoralis major myocutaneous flap. Invasion of the carotid artery can be treated with a bypass procedure performed with the resection, but there is a high operative mortality, and little chance of cure.

Primary of unknown origin

This term is applied to patients with a metastatic carcinoma in cervical lymph nodes with an 'occult primary'. A careful search will usually reveal the primary tumour in the skin or mucosal surfaces of the head and neck, or rarely, in an area below the clavicles, such as the lungs. It is important to search thoroughly for the primary tumour by all available diagnostic methods including history, physical examination, imaging, panendoscopy and selective biopsies from high risk sites (nasopharynx, ipsilateral tonsil excision, base of tongue and pyriform fossa). In approximately 3–11% of cases the primary tumour remains elusive and it is for these that the term 'primary of unknown origin' should be reserved. The prognosis varies from a 30–70% five year survival. The prognosis depends on N Stage and position of the node. Supraclavicular nodes have the worse prognosis, probably because many of these represent distant metastases from non-head and neck sites (e.g. lung or stomach). Patients who have neck dissection and radiation therapy to both sides of the neck and the mucosal surfaces have better neck and local control than those who do not have such extensive treatment. However, this does not seem to translate into prolonged survival. Chemotherapy may have a place in improving this situation.

Palliative therapy

Patients with inoperable neck nodes that have fungated through the skin can be treated with local dressings of kaltocarb and topical metronidazole. These will help prevent colonization by anaerobes and alleviate the odour from tissue necrosis. Death by carotid artery rupture will usually ensue. The patient should always be treated with appropriate doses of opiate analgesia and antiemetics. It is imperative that there is adequate social support and that the patient's family doctor is aware of the situation if the patient is to be cared for in the community.

Further reading

Jones AS, Roland NJ, Field JK, Phillips DE. The level of cervical node metastases: their prognostic relevance and relationship with head and neck squamous carcinoma primary sites. *Clinical Otolaryngology*, 1994; **19**: 63–69.

Snow GB, Annyas AA, Van Slooten EA *et al.* Prognostic factors of neck node metastasis. *Clinical Otolaryngology*, 1982; **7**: 185–192.

Jones AS, Cook JA, Phillips D, Roland NJ. Squamous carcinoma presenting as an enlarged cervical lymph node. *Cancer*, 1993; **72**: 1756–1761.

Related topics of interest

Benign neck lumps, p. 23; Neck dissection, p. 185.

CHOANAL ATRESIA

Congenital choanal atresia is due to the embryological failure of the primitive bucconasal membrane to rupture before birth. This results in the persistence of a bony plate (90%), membrane, or both, obstructing the posterior nares. The condition may be unilateral (most commonly) or bilateral. It occurs in about 1 in 7000 births, and there is a family tendency.

Embryology

The mouth, palate, nose and paranasal sinuses all develop from the cranial portion of the primitive foregut. The nose begins as two epithelial thickenings known as the nasal placodes, which appear above the stomatodeum about the fourth week *in utero*. The placodes deepen to form olfactory pits which lie between the medial and lateral nasal processes. The medial processes fuse to form the frontonasal process. This is compressed to form the nasal septum as the lateral nasal processes approach each other. The nasal septum will then grow posteriorly to divide the two nasal cavities. Each nasal cavity is closed posteriorly by the thinned out posterior wall of the nasal sac, called the bucconasal membrane. This usually breaks down around the sixth week *in utero*. Its persistence is thought to be the cause of choanal atresia.

Clinical features

A unilateral obstruction may be asymptomatic at birth but will later cause unilateral nasal discharge and obstruction. Examination of the nose will show a thick gelatinous secretion on the affected side, and no airway can be demonstrated by holding a cold plated spatula below the nares – only the clear side steaming the surface (mirror test). Older children may allow posterior rhinoscopy to view the occlusion.

Bilateral choanal atresia presents as an emergency at birth. The newborn is a near-obligate nasal breather and the nasal obstruction will therefore produce difficulty in breathing. The alae nasi dilate and the accessory muscles of respiration are used to no avail. There is pallor and cyanosis until the mouth is opened and after a few quick breaths are taken the infant cries. This sequence of events continues. The diagnosis should be suspected immediately and an oral airway inserted to assist respiration.

About half of infants with choanal atresia display other abnormalities, including the CHARGE association. This refers to a problem of multiple congenital anomalies: C, colobama; H, heart disease; A, atresia choanae; R, retarded growth and development; G, genital anomalies; E, ear abnormalities and deafness. In addition, half exhibit facial nerve palsies and one third of cases have laryngotracheal anomalies.

Investigations

The diagnosis can be confirmed by the mirror test or by attempting to pass a catheter through the nose into the nasopharynx. This will not be possible if there is an obstruction. Fibreoptic endoscopy will confirm the diagnosis. If there is still doubt the lesion can be demonstrated radiologically. A CT scan is the method of choice to delineate the nature and thickness of the obstruction.

Management

Cases of unilateral atresia can initially be observed without treatment. In the case of the newborn with bilateral atresia the first priority is to insert and maintain an oral airway. The treatment of choanal atresia is surgical. The challenge is to provide a nasal airway which has an adequate mucosal lining, and to prevent granulation tissue formation and subsequent stenosis. Two approaches are in common use.

1. Transnasal. This is the usual approach in infants. A membranous occlusion may require no more than perforation with a probe. This can also be accomplished with electrocautery or laser. In the more common bony occlusions it will be necessary to perform a trephine and remove the obstruction with a burr or potassium titanyl phosphate (KTP) laser using the operating microscope. A stent should be inserted and a series of dilations of the choana will then be required to maintain an adequate lumen.

2. Transpalatal. This is preferred by some surgeons, particularly when the atresia is unilateral or if a previous transnasal opening has later closed. The palate is incised just in front of the posterior edge of the hard palate. The soft palate is retracted, and the occlusion removed together with part of the vomer and border of the hard palate.

Follow-up and aftercare

Maintenance of the opening following corrective surgery with regular bouginage is now mostly preferred to the use of indwelling tubes. Dilation will probably be necessary every 2 months initially, but this period can be extended as the child grows.

Related topic of interest

Paediatric airway problems, p. 232.

CHOLESTEATOMA

T.H.J. Lesser

A cholesteatoma is a three-dimensional epidermal structure exhibiting independent growth, replacing middle-ear mucosa, resorbing underlying bone and tending to recur after removal. Put more simply, it is 'bad skin in the middle-ear cleft'. The incidence is approximately 10 cases per 100 000 per annum.

Classification

Cholesteatoma can be classified into congenital and acquired types. These are distinct pathological entities.

1. **Congenital cholesteatoma.** Congenital cholesteatoma has been shown by Michaels to be the result of the persistence of a small nidus of epidermoid ectoderm that occurs in the first trimester in the normal fetus and is normally resorbed. It usually manifests itself as an anterior attic pearl behind an intact drum in the first year or so of life. It may present later in childhood with extensive disease in an often cellular mastoid.

2. **Acquired cholesteatoma.** There is no definitive classification of acquired cholesteatoma, but it can be divided into three groups with reference to the tympanic membrane.

(a) Primary acquired cholesteatoma associated with a defect in the *pars flaccida*.

(b) Secondary acquired cholesteatoma associated with a defect in the *pars tensa*.

(c) Tertiary acquired cholesteatoma exists behind an apparently normal eardrum as a result of implantation or previous middle-ear infection.

Aetiology

There are a number of well-established, but unproven, theories regarding the aetiology of cholesteatoma.

1. **Primary acquired cholesteatoma.** This is the most common.

(a) The single most important fact about the skin of the eardrum is that in health it migrates from the centre of the drum outwards along the external ear canal, carrying keratin and wax debris with it. Therefore this skin is self-cleaning. Negative middle-ear pressure tends to pull the pars flaccida into the attic and may form a retraction pocket. Although initially self-cleaning, the epithelium eventually loses its capacity to migrate out of the pocket and is trapped. The pocket fills with epithelial debris, which in turn becomes infected and further expands under tension. As it expands the isthmus tends to narrow, compounding the problem and continuing the cycle.

(b) Direct invasion of migrating squamous epithelium through the pars flaccida may occur, either as papillae through a temporary defect or merely as a change in the direction of migration in the upper part of the tympanic membrane, with skin going in rather than continuing out along the ear canal.

2. Secondary and tertiary acquired cholesteatoma.

(a) Epithelium could migrate around the rim of a *pars tensa* perforation to cause a cholesteatoma.

(b) Acute otitis media may damage the fibrous layers of the *pars tensa* and a piece of squamous epithelium may be implanted should the tympanic membrane rupture. The drum may heal or there may be a permanent defect.

(c) Surgery involving trauma to the tympanic membrane (any middle-ear surgery or even grommet insertion) may occasionally allow squamous epithelium to be directly implanted.

(d) Metaplasia of middle-ear mucosa may occur secondary to episodes of chronic or recurrent acute otitis media.

Pathology

Macroscopically there is a rounded pearly white mass of variable size, often surrounded by friable granulations from infected bone or with polyp formation from infected mucosa. Microscopically, cholesteatoma is a benign keratinizing squamous cell cyst. In the centre are fully differentiated anucleate keratin squames, surrounded by an epithelium several cell layers thick, in turn surrounded by a matrix of inflamed subepithelial connective tissue. The epithelial matrix of acquired cholesteatoma has approximately 15 layers whereas that of congenital cholesteatoma has only about five layers. Electron microscopy shows normal epidermal cells plus Langerhan cells and Merkel cells.

A cholesteatoma invariably enlarges, but little is known as to how this growth is controlled. Infection with bacteria causes an increase in clinical progression. Initially the cyst of skin grows into the area of least resistance, usually into the mastoid antrum and then into the air cells. The epithelium, being naturally migratory, probably accounts for some of the growth, but other changes in the surrounding perimatrix, probably brought on by infection, lead to destruction of the bone locally. These changes include the activation of osteoclasts and the production of lysozymes.

Clinical features

Symptoms depend on the activity of the disease and arise either from the disease itself or from the complications. The disease usually produces a discharge, which may be scanty or just a flaky, waxy deposit, but is often foul and creamy. Deafness may occur – conductive secondary to ossicular erosion, or sensory, probably from toxins involved in chronic inflammation migrating through the round window. Dizziness may indicate a labyrinthine fistula.

The principal signs are an attic crust, a marginal perforation or a pocket of invading keratin debris. Marginal granulations and polyps protruding from the middle-ear cleft indicate osteitis and mucosal hyperplasia, respectively. Behind these may lie a cholesteatoma so that micro-otoscopic removal of an attic crust or aural polypectomy may allow the diagnosis to be made. A positive fistula sign is said to indicate erosion into the labyrinth (see Labyrinthitis, p. 134).

Complications may occur in acute exacerbation of the disease and are either within the temporal bone or intracranial. They are discussed under the topic complications of chronic suppurative otitis media (CSOM).

Investigations

(a) Micro-otoscopy (with the removal of attic crusts and polyps for reasons stated above). If available, examination with a rigid lens otoscope and otophotography should be performed. Angled otoscopes permit examination of the facial recess and sinus tympani.

(b) Pure tone audiometry (with masking).

(c) Radiology. Plain radiographs may indicate the height of the middle fossa dura and site of the sigmoid sinus but usually give little information on disease extent. CT and MRI can both demonstrate the disease and give some idea of its extent. CT reveals a non-enhancing mass-eroding bone, including the ossicles, with sharply defined smooth margins, isodense with CSF. MRI likewise shows a mass with a low intensity T1 weighted signal and a high T2 signal. In practice, it is often difficult on imaging to distinguish between cholesteatoma and pure mucosal disease.

Treatment

Suction clearance may control early disease, but the mainstay of treatment is surgical excision of the disease with reconstruction of the surgical defect and any conductive hearing loss. This usually takes the form of some type of mastoidectomy and tympanoplasty.

Further reading

Ferlito A. A review of the definition, terminology and pathology of aural cholesteatoma. *Journal of Laryngology and Otology*, 1993; **107**: 483–488.

Palva, T. Cholesteatoma surgery today. *Clinics in Otolaryngology*, 1993; **18**: 245–255.

Youngs R. Chronic suppurative otitis media – cholesteatoma. In: *Diseases of the Ear*. 6th edn., 1998: 386–397. Ludman and Wright (eds). Arnold, London.

Related topics of interest

Chronic suppurative otitis media – complications, p. 42; Mastoidectomy, p. 159; Tympanoplasty, p. 341.

CHRONIC SUPPURATIVE OTITIS MEDIA (CSOM)

This can be sub-classified into tubotympanic or safe, and tympanomastoid (atticoantral) or unsafe disease. A classification gaining more prominence is chronic otitis media with or without cholesteatoma. CSOM without cholesteatoma is sometimes referred to as mucosal chronic otitis media and subdivided into active and inactive.

Tubotympanic CSOM

The essential features are a central tympanic membrane perforation and adequate atticoantral drainage. Disease is confined to the mucosa of the anteroinferior portion of the middle ear cleft; the risk of serious complications is minimal. Most perforations arise when an acute perforation occurs during an episode of ASOM and, perhaps because of an inadequate dose, length or inappropriate choice of antibiotic, there is slow resolution. This allows sufficient time for squamous epithelium to migrate over the free edge of the tympanic layers to form a permanent perforation. There is a 1–2% chance of developing a perforation when a ventilation tube is inserted and a 40% chance if a ventilation tube is *in situ* for more than 2 years. The disease is described as quiescent during the first few weeks of a dry ear and inactive when the ear is dry long-term and active when a mucoid or mucopurulent discharge within the middle ear is present. Pathogens gain entry to the middle ear either via the eustachian tube, often triggered by an upper respiratory tract infection, or via the ear canal when contaminated bath, swimming pool or sea water are the most common sources. Chronic mucoid discharge is associated with goblet cell hyperplasia, metaplasia of middle ear mucosa to respiratory type mucosa and poor mucociliary function.

Clinical features

Deafness is proportional to the size of the perforation and not, as is often quoted, the site. An air-bone gap of more than 30 dB is unusual and suggests an ossicular discontinuity. The patient may notice the hearing improves when the ear discharges indicating there is an ossicular discontinuity which has been bridged by mucopus or a polyp. This finding is also common with atticoantral disease. Tinnitus, typically high pitched and vertigo, typically momentary and initiated by sudden head movement are usually associated with a high tone sensorineural hearing loss secondary to toxins reaching the perilymph through the oval or round window.

On examination there is a wet or dry central tympanic membrane perforation. The term 'central' implies there is a rim of tympanic membrane around the perforation and not that the perforation is centrally situated in the tympanic membrane. An infected polyp may protrude through the perforation and there may be signs of the complications of tubotympanic disease.

Complications

- Otitis externa.
- Ossicular erosion, especially the long process of the incus.
- High tone sensorineural hearing loss.
- Vertigo. Typically mild and transient. Intermittent benign paroxysmal positional vertigo has been described. Episodes can also be secondary to acute labyrinthine failure which usually reverses spontaneously but if a permanent paresis occurs it may take several months before compensation is complete.
- Tympanosclerosis.
- Middle ear adhesions.

Intracranial and severe cochleovestibular symptoms are unusual as is a lower motor neurone facial palsy.

Treatment

The principles of treatment are to obtain a dry ear, prevent re-infection and to minimise the disability of any hearing loss. The former is attained by frequent aural toilet, the application of appropriate topical antibiotic ear drops, eradicating any source of intercurrent or chronic upper aerodigestive tract infection and to prevent water entering the external ear canal when swimming or bathing. The current view of the British Association of Otolaryngologists, Head and Neck Surgeons, in contrast to the British National Formulary entry and the Committee on Safety of Medicines, is that the use of aminoglycoside antibiotics is reasonable in the presence of infection of the middle ear and a perforation (or grommet) for a limited period (i.e. until the ear is dry). The decision as to whether surgery in the form of a tympanoplasty or a hearing aid is more appropriate depends on the type and severity of the hearing loss, the hearing in the contralateral ear, the frequency of recurrent infection, the wish to swim and the patients occupation, lifestyle, age and general condition (see Tympanoplasty topic).

Atticoantral CSOM

Also called unsafe, as the ear is at risk of serious complications. It is caused by either cholesteatoma or pure mucosal disease. It has been suggested that some subjects are predisposed to the latter because of a narrow epitympanic space and indeed it has been shown by high definition CT scanning of the petrous temporal bone that as a group these subjects have a gap between the scutum and medial middle ear wall that is significantly narrower than in a matched group without CSOM. In the event of an episode of AOM, inadequate atticoantral drainage causes the mucosa to become chronically inflamed and polypoidal, further compromising drainage. Osteomyelitis of bone lining the polypoidal mucosa is the inevitable result, sometimes causing florid granulation tissue formation. The incidence of intracranial complications in atticoantral CSOM is the same for ears with cholesteatoma or with pure mucosal disease.

Clinical features

Deafness may be a conductive, sensorineural or mixed. The former occurs when an ossicular discontinuity occurs from ossicular erosion by cholesteatoma or chronically inflamed mucosa. Toxin penetration through the round window may be the mechanism of sensorineural loss. Scanty, smelly aural discharge, mild transient vertigo and high pitched tinnitus are typical. Otoscopy may reveal no more than an attic crust which must be removed if cholesteatoma, attic granulations or a perforation are to be revealed. A marginal or attic perforation surrounded by granulation tissue or a polyp is more usual. A sanguinous discharge, otalgia, lower motor neurone facial palsy, a unilateral headache, signs of meningitis or of raised intracranial pressure suggest a serious complication.

Pure tone audiometry varies from normal air conduction if there is limited attic disease to a severe mixed type of hearing loss in extensive disease.

Complications

- Extracranial.
- Intracranial.

Management

The priority is to make the ear safe from intra cranial complications by eradicating disease. If cholesteatoma is not seen on examining the ear, perhaps because of florid granulations, an attempt must be made to dry the ear by means of regular aural toilet, antibiotic ear-drops and systemic antibiotics. The latter should cover anaerobes because they have been found in over 50% of cultures in children with CSOM. A high definition CT scan of the petrous temporal bone will show the extent but not the cause of soft tissue disease, in particular it does not distinguish between cholesteatoma, polypoidal disease or granulation tissue. An unsafe ear without cholesteatoma which continues to discharge despite intensive medical management requires tympanomastoid surgery (see Mastoidectomy topic) as does the presence of cholesteatoma. Exceptions to this rule may arise when the ear is the better or only hearing ear, in very elderly or those medically unfit. Management of attic retraction pockets depends on their stage and in particular on whether they are self cleaning (see Cholesteatoma topic). In cases of lower motor neurone facial paralysis associated with CSOM, urgent surgery to irradicate all inflammatory disease is the priority. Facial nerve decompression is usually unnecessary. CSOM, unlike ASOM, rarely responds rapidly to intravenous antibiotics because the mucosal changes or cholesteatoma are long-standing and surgical delay may compromise facial nerve recovery. As with ASOM, the horizontal portion of the mastoid segment of the facial nerve was implicated as the site of involvement and the facial nerve palsy a neuropraxia which recovered with eradication of the cause.

Further reading

Harker LA, Pignatari SSN. Facial nerve paralysis secondary to chronic otitis media without cholesteatoma. *American Journal of Otolaryngology*, 1992; **13:** 372–374.

Brook I, Burke P. The management of acute, serous and chronic otitis media: the role of anaerobic bacteria. *Journal of Hospital Infection*, 1992; **22** (suppl A): 75–87.

The BAO-HNS Newsletter. 1999; **9:** 1.

Related topics of interest

Acute suppurative otitis media, p. 5; Cholesteatoma, p. 35; Mastoidectomy, p. 159.

CHRONIC SUPPURATIVE OTITIS MEDIA – COMPLICATIONS

Complications of CSOM are associated with a high morbidity and may be life threatening. Cholesteatoma, atticoantral mucosal disease and ASOM (see related topics) cause complications by spread of infection:

(a) *Directly* via the oval or round window to reach the labyrinth, through osteomyelitic bone to reach the dura and lateral sinus or to affect a congenitally dehiscent facial nerve.
(b) *By retrograde propagation* of small foci of thrombophlebitis which may extend through the temporal bone and dura to the major venous sinuses to cause a lateral sinus thrombosis and by further extension a cerebellar or temporal lobe abscess.
(c) *Along the periarteriolar spaces* to cause a temporal or cerebellar lobe abscess.

Browning in a retrospective study has calculated that the risk of a patient with CSOM developing an intracerebral abscess is 1 in 3500.

Classification

1. *Extracranial.*

- Chronic *otitis externa* and meatal stenosis.
- *Ossicular discontinuity* from ossicular erosion.
- *Middle ear adhesions.*
- *Tympanosclerosis* which may spread from the tympanic membrane over the ossicular chain causing ossicular chain fixation.
- *Squamous cell carcinoma* of the middle ear.
- Lower motor neurone *facial nerve palsy.*
- Serous or purulent *labyrinthitis.*
- *Petrositis* and *Gradenigo's syndrome* (signs of ASOM, an ipsilateral abducent nerve palsy and pain in the distribution of the ipsilateral trigeminal nerve).
- *Labyrinthine fistula.*

2. *Intracranial.*

- *Lateral (transverse and sigmoid) sinus thrombosis.* This may extend to involve the superior and inferior petrosal sinus, the cavernous sinus, the sinus confluence, the superior sagittal sinus and the internal jugular vein. There is often a concomitant extradural or subdural abscess which may have precipitated the formation of the thrombus.
- *Meningitis.*
- *Extradural, subdural, intracerebral* (cerebellar and temporal lobe) *abscess.*
- *Otitic hydrocephalus.*

Clinical features

Patients with acute intracranial complications usually present to the neurosurgeons and are most likely to be seen by an ENT surgeon after recovery from the acute episode. Patients with CSOM who present with unilateral or occipital headaches, visual disturbance, vomiting, clumsiness, forgetfulness or drowsiness should have a full neurological examination looking in particular for signs of raised intracranial pressure, meningitis and localizing cerebellar and temporo-parietal lobe signs. A deep throbbing otalgia and serosanguinous discharge may herald malignant change.

Investigations

A high definition CT scan of the petrous temporal bone will show the extent of mastoid disease although it may not distinguish cholesteatoma from mucosal disease. A gadolinium enhanced magnetic resonance scan is now the investigation of choice for the diagnosis of an intracranial venous thrombosis (simple thrombus shows an intermediate signal, vascularized thrombus, granulation tissue and slow flowing blood a high signal, and fast flowing blood no signal) and intracranial abscess (shows a centre of low attenuation with an outer rim of high signal).

Treatment

- High dose intravenous antibiotics to commence after taking a culture swab of the aural discharge.
- Neurosurgeons to manage intracerebral abscess.
- Treatment of initiating otological disorder.

1. Subdural and extradural abscesses require a cortical mastoidectomy to provide adequate exposure before drainage. A lateral sinus thrombosis if not responding to high dose intravenous antibiotics should have a cortical mastoidectomy and the lateral sinus exposed. The diagnosis should be confirmed by needling the sinus. After confirmation some practitioners propose tying the internal jugular vein high up in the neck to prevent infective embolization during evacuation of infected clot. The lateral sinus is opened, the clot evacuated and the sinus obliterated with a temporalis muscle flap reinforced by a bismuth iodoform paraffin paste (BIPP) mastoid pack.

2. A facial palsy secondary to ASOM is invariably a neuropraxia. The nerve does not require decompressing and should recover rapidly with aggressive treatment of the infection. The facial palsy in CSOM is usually secondary to compression from cholesteatoma or granulation tissue. Most otologists advocate an urgent mastoidectomy and decompression of the vertical segment of the facial nerve though this has recently been challenged. If there is an actively discharging ear others would observe for at least 48 hours with the patient on intravenous antibiotics. In this instance the palsy may be a neuropraxia of a dehiscent horizontal segment of the nerve, found in 6% of ears.

3. Labyrithine fistulae may be caused by erosion of bone by cholesteatoma and by osteitis with the formation of granulation tissue. In cholesteatoma the matrix usually becomes apposed to the endosteum within the fistula and a protective walling off does not arise. If a fistula is suspected from clinical signs and operative findings then either: 1) the matrix can be left over the affected portion of the labyrinth and a canal wall down procedure performed leaving an open cavity, or alternatively, 2) the matrix can be peeled off under constant irrigation and the fistula immediately sealed with fascia or muscle as the final manouvre in surgery.

Further reading

Munz M, Farmer JP, Auger L, *et al.* Otitis media and CNS complications. *Journal of Otolaryngology*, 1992; **21**: 224–226.

Herzog JA, Smith PG, Klester GR, Maxwell KS. Management of labyrinthine fistulae secondary to cholesteatoma. *American Journal of Otolaryngology*, 1997; **17**: 410–415.

Related topics of interest

Chronic suppurative otitis media, p. 38; Cholesteatoma, p. 35; Acute suppurative otitis media, p. 5.

CLINICAL ASSESSMENT OF HEARING

Use of clinical tests

It is surprising how often a clinical assessment of hearing is omitted from the routine examination of the otology patient. Voice tests and tuning fork tests are the two main methods, but often only the Weber and Rinne tuning fork tests are performed. Clinical tests can be used to:

- Identify a hearing impairment.
- Determine the nature of a hearing loss (conductive or sensorineural).
- Grade the severity.
- Detect feigning or a non-organic hearing loss.

The main reason that clinical tests of auditory function are overlooked is that they have largely been superseded by more sensitive and reliable audiometric tests. However, audiometry on occasions may be inaccurate or unavailable. Furthermore, exaggerated thresholds may be missed if suspicion is not aroused by clinical testing. Proponents of clinical testing suggest that audiometry may be unnecessary if the hearing is normal or the results would not influence the management.

Masking

Masking is as important in clinical testing as it is in audiometric testing. The non-test ear should always be masked when clinically testing by air conduction, and in theory always when performing tuning fork tests, though this is not always practicable. There are two techniques in common use.

1. The tragal rub.   Occlusion of the auditory canal by putting finger pressure on the tragus with a rubbing motion is the easiest method. Using this technique speech will be attenuated by approximately 50 dB. There is a risk of under-masking if the sound level of speech arriving at the test ear is greater than 70 dB(A) so a Bárány noise box should be used when testing an ear with a severe or profound impairment or when testing bone conduction with tuning forks.

2. Bárány noise box.   This box produces a broad-band noise from a clockwork-driven source. The maximum sound output varies from approximately 90 dB(A) when a box is held at right angles to the ear and 100 dB(A) when held over the ear. These levels are sufficient to mask the non-test ear in all practical circumstances, but the main problem is cross-masking of the test ear. It should be used when a tragal rub does not provide adequate masking.

Voice tests

Difficulties in standardizing the technique and variability of the stimulus provided by the examiner have led to criticisms of this test. The easiest and best method of performing monaural free-field voice testing is by using a whispered voice, conversational voice and then loud voice at 60 cm and then 15 cm. It is usual to start by testing the better hearing ear when there is one. The non-test ear is masked by a tragal rub unless a loud voice is required (use the Bárány noise box). The patient is asked to repeat as accurately as possible what the examiner says. Bisyllable words (e.g. bluebell, cowboy), numbers (e.g. 54, 37, 63) or combinations of numbers and letters (e.g. 4 B 7) can be used depending on the patient's age and understanding. The examiner starts using a whispered voice 60 cm away from the patient, which is the furthest away that is possible when masking the non-test ear. The sound level is increased in steps from a whispered voice at 60 cm, to a whispered voice at 15 cm, to a conversational voice at 60 cm, to a conversational voice at 15 cm, to a loud voice at 60 cm, and finally to a loud voice at 15 cm. The test finishes as soon as the patient repeats 50% of the words correctly at any one voice and distance level.

If a patient can hear a whispered voice 60 cm away from the ear, the pure tone thresholds are likely to be less than 30 dB (normal hearing). Patients who can hear a whisper at 15 cm or a conversational voice at 60 or 15 cm are likely to have thresholds in the range of 30–70 dB hearing level (HL) (mild/moderate impairment). Those patients who can only hear a loud voice are likely to have thresholds greater than 70 dB HL (severe/profound impairment).

Tuning forks

Tuning forks for audiological use are modified to include a finger grip on the stem and an expansion on the base of the stem to allow application to the skull. Ideally a 512- or 256-Hz tuning fork should be used. The duration of the stimulus decreases with increasing frequency, and it is difficult to activate forks with a frequency higher than 512 Hz sufficiently for them to be heard by those with a moderate or severe impairment. Forks with a frequency lower than 256 Hz can make it difficult for the patient to distinguish between hearing the sound and feeling it by vibration. A tuning fork should be set in vibration by a firm strike one-third of the way from the free end of the prong against a firm but elastic object (e.g. elbow or patella). This should produce a relatively pure tone with minimal overtones. It can then be presented by either air or bone conduction. For air conduction it should be held with its acoustic axis (a line joining two points near the tips of the two prongs) in line with and 2–3 cm from the external meatus. For bone conduction the base plate should be placed firmly on the skull, either mastoid process or vertex depending on the test. Although the tuning fork can theoretically be placed at any point on the skull for bone conduction, some points may give less reliable results.

A variety of tuning fork tests were developed to test absolute hearing thresholds (compared with the examiner), to differentiate real from feigned hearing loss, conductive from sensorineural, and cochlear from retrocochlear hearing loss. With the advent of newer and more sensitive forms of investigation, many of these tests are no longer in everyday use. However, a number of tests have stood the test of time and continue in current clinical practice.

The tests are based on two main principles:

1. The inner ear is normally twice as sensitive to sound conducted by air as to that conducted by bone.
2. In the presence of a purely conductive hearing loss, the affected ear is subject to less environmental noise, making it more sensitive to bone-conducted sound.

No single test is diagnostic but all can provide useful information when taken in context. Unfortunately, tuning fork tests are unreliable in children.

Weber test

This test is based on the principle that a conductive loss causes a relative improvement in the ability to hear a bone-conducted sound and the test is of most value in a unilateral hearing loss. The tuning fork is struck and placed on the vertex. The vertex is used as opposed to the forehead as the reliability of the test is thus improved from 72% to 86%. (Further improvements can be achieved by using the upper incisors but these are not always available!) If a conductive loss of 10 dB or more exists, the sound should be heard in the affected ear. If a sensorineural hearing loss is present the sound will generally be heard in the normal ear. In the normal subject or some subjects with a long-standing sensorineural hearing loss, the sound will be heard in the midline.

Rinne test

This test examines each ear individually and is again based on the principle of improved bone conduction perception with a conductive loss. It can be performed in one of two ways. The subject can be asked to compare either the loudness of the tuning fork when presented by air conduction and bone conduction (placed on the ipsilateral mastoid process) or the duration of the sound when presented by both air and bone conduction. The normal response is to hear the sound as louder and longer with air conduction and is referred to as a Rinne positive. A positive response will also occur with a sensorineural hearing loss. A negative response (Rinne negative) will occur if there is a conductive loss of greater than 20 dB or if there is a severe sensorineural hearing loss. The former is referred to as a true-negative Rinne and the latter as a false negative. The two can be distinguished by using a Bárány sound box, in which case the false negative will become positive as the contralateral, minimally attenuated, bone conduction is masked.

Bing test

This test is similar to the Rinne and is based on the improvement in bone conduction perception in the normal subject when the external auditory meatus is occluded. The tuning fork is struck and placed on the subject's mastoid process. After the subject acknowledges hearing the sound, the ipsilateral meatus is occluded by the examiner's finger and the subject is asked if this makes the sound louder or quieter. Occluding the external auditory canal will block out ambient noise, and prevent some of the bone conduction sound, which has emanated into the external auditory canal, from escaping. If the sound becomes louder, the response is positive (and normal). If the sound does not change or becomes quieter, the response is negative, and usually indicates a conductive loss of 10 dB or more.

Stenger test

This test is used to differentiate a real from a feigned hearing loss and is based on the principle that, if two pure tones of equal intensity are presented to both ears at once, the sound will appear to originate in the midline. If the intensity of one side is increased, the sound will appear to originate from that side alone. In practice, the test is commenced by asking the subject to close his or her eyes to help concentrate on the sound. The tester works behind the subject. First a tuning fork is placed 15 cm from the good ear; the subject confirms hearing the sound. A tuning fork is then positioned 5 cm from the bad ear; the subject will deny hearing it. Finally, unknown to the subject, two tuning forks are used simultaneously: one 5 cm from the bad ear and one 15 cm from the good ear. If the hearing loss is real the subject will hear the sound in the good ear and report this. If the hearing loss is feigned, the subject will hear the sound loudest in the bad ear. Unaware that there is a previously audible sound present at the good ear, the subject will deny hearing anything and this suggests the diagnosis.

Further reading

Browning GG. *Clinical Otology and Audiology*. London: Butterworths, 1986; 23–37.
Committee for the consideration of hearing tests. Report of the committee for the consideration of hearing tests. *Journal of Laryngology and Otology*, 1933; **48**: 22–48.
Golabek W, Stephens SDG. Some tuning fork tests revisited. *Clinical Otolaryngology*, 1979; **4**: 421–430.

Related topics of interest

CLINICAL GOVERNANCE AND AUDIT

Clinical governance

In 1997 the government published the first of its white papers on quality within the NHS and introduced the term clinical governance. Clinical governance is defined as 'A framework through which NHS organizations are accountable for continuously improving the quality of their services and safeguarding high standards of care by creating an environment in which excellence in clinical care will flourish'. NHS organizations are presently NHS Trust Boards and the chief executive is ultimately accountable for assuring the quality of services provided by the Trust. The third white paper – 'Clinical governance: Quality in the new NHS' – emphasizes the need for a move to a culture of learning in which education, research, sharing of good practice and multidisciplinary team-work thrives.

The systems embraced by clinical governance include:

- Clinical audit.
- Risk management.
- Evidence-based clinical practice, developing guidelines and protocols.
- Development of clinical leadership skills.
- Continuing education for all clinical staff.
- Audit of consumer feedback.
- Health-needs assessment.
- Managing the clinical performance of colleagues.
- Developing guidelines and protocols.
- Accreditation of hospitals, community providers and primary care practices.
- Continuing professional development for all staff.
- Systems to ensure lessons learnt are implemented.
- A mechanism to ensure all systems are in place and functioning effectively.

Each health organization will be required to set up leadership and accountability arrangements, to carry out a baseline assessment of capability and capacity, to draw up and agree a development plan and clarify reporting arrangements.

New national bodies

1. National Institute for Clinical Excellence (NICE) will set national standards and best practice guidelines.
2. Commission for Health Improvement (CHI) will inspect NHS organizations locally to ensure that clinical governance and the standards set by NICE are being implemented.

   For individual practitioners these changes will mean:

1. Playing a part in the organization's assessment of its present capacity for quality improvement.
2. Working within the team to look at the strengths and weaknesses of the services they deliver and propose ways for improvement.

3. Leading and participating in quality improvement activities in service delivery.
4. Being aware of best practice guidelines from NICE and adopting them as part of clinical audit or individual practice development.
5. Developing ways of involving users and carers in the planning of service improvements.
6. Taking a full part in continuing professional development programmes.

Audit

Audit is defined as the systematic appraisal of the implementation and outcome of any process in the context of prescribed targets and standards.

Clinical audit is the process by which medical staff collectively review, evaluate, and improve their practice. This should include the assessment of patients access to care, the process and outcome of care and financial and administrative efficiency. In the clinical setting the problem with this definition is what to define, for each aspect of medicine, as reasonable targets and standards and this requires research. A working group of the World Health Organization defined audit as a 7-stage procedure, the most vital element being to ensure an improvement (indicating change) in care by reassessing results after the setting of criteria and standards.

The guidelines are:

- Problem identification.
- Setting priorities.
- Determining methodology.
- Setting criteria and standards.
- Comparing performance with standards.
- Designing and implementing remedial action.
- Re-evaluating the quality of care.

The reasons for performing audit are:

- To encourage modification and improvement in clinical practice.
- To allow peer review and support for clinicians.
- It is educational and raises the overall quality of care.

Research and audit

Research and audit are often confused and it is important to clarify the difference. Clinical research tests hypotheses so that they may be accepted as scientific fact or refuted in order to establish what is the best clinical practice. It allows prescribed targets and standards to be defined and may allow a management policy for a specific condition to be drafted. Audit on the other hand seeks to determine whether good practice (the process) has been adopted or whether the prescribed targets and standards gained through research are being met (the outcome). In other words audit tests either process or outcome after research has established that there is a link between them.

Important aspects of clinical audit are:

- Clinical audit meetings should be confidential and involve only clinicians specifically involved in patient care. Anonymity of sensitive data must be secured. In this context it should be remembered that patients, relatives and their legal representative are allowed access to medical but not audit records. Hospital managers are allowed access only to the conclusions of any meeting.
- Each meeting should attempt to provide a specific recommendation which when implemented improves clinical practice.
- Departments should set targets regarding appointments, investigations, admission and outpatient waiting times.
- The use of resources, for example beds, drugs, investigations and duty theatres should be determined and if appropriate, proposals made with the purpose of making them more efficient.
- Treatment policies should be reviewed to minimize morbidity and mortality and maximize quality of life.
- Clinical audit regularly undertaken may provide a basis for a successful medico-legal defence because it can be shown that treatment has been researched and reviewed.

National Audit

This is necessary because each hospital, district and even region has a relatively small number of clinicians performing a proportionately small number of procedures compared to the national total. Type II errors in assessing clinical outcome might be averted.

The National Confidential Enquiry into Perioperative Deaths (NCEPOD)

Perioperative deaths are those which occur within thirty days of a surgical procedure, that is any procedure carried out by a surgeon or gynaecologist, with or without an anaesthetist, involving local, regional or general anaesthesia or sedation.

NCEPOD provides guidelines annually for specific clinical situations with the aim of improving surgical practice. The recommendations come from an independent body with representatives across the surgical speciality fields (the steering group) nominated by an elected body in that speciality (in Otolaryngology it is a British Association of Otolaryngologists and Head and Neck Surgeons [BAO-HNS] proposed representative). The guidelines are issued from information provided mainly by pathologists who supply data regarding perioperative deaths in their hospital. A sample of the reported deaths are reviewed in greater detail by the steering group by sending questionnaires regarding all aspects of the patient's care in the perioperative period to the consultant surgeon and anaesthetist in charge of the patient's care.

Further reading

WHO Working Group. The organization of quality assurance. *Quality assurance in health care.* 1989; **1**: 111–123.

Guidelines to Clinical Audit in Surgical Practice. London: The Royal College of Surgeons of England, March 1989.

Bull AR. Audit and research: complimentary but distinct. 1993; *Annals of the Royal College of Surgeons of England,* **75**: 308–311.

Department of Health. *The new NHS: modern and dependable.* London: The Stationary Office, 1997 (Cm.3807).

Department of Health. *A First Class Service: Quality in the new NHS.* London: Department of Health, 1998 (Health Service Circular: HSC (98) 113).

Department of Health. *Clinical governance: Quality in the new NHS.* London: Department of Health, 1999 (Health Service Circular: HSC (99) 065).

COCHLEAR IMPLANTS

S.R. Saeed

Over the last decade cochlear implantation has evolved to become an established means of auditory rehabilitation in selected adults and children with severe or profound hearing loss. The device aims to provide perception of sound by attempting to emulate the transducer function of the cochlea, thereby stimulating residual auditory neural tissue. In appropriately selected individuals, the original premise that cochlear implantation would allow recognition of environmental sound and serve as an adjunct to lip-reading has been realized. In reality, many individuals have derived greater benefit including the ability to understand speech with little or no lip-reading.

History

The first report of cochlear implantation was from Djourno and colleagues in 1957 who described the insertion of a device into two totally deaf individuals. Paralleled by developments in pacemaker technology, this stimulated considerable interest in the 1960s and 1970s among several investigators: the House group in Los Angeles, USA, Michelson and colleagues in San Francisco, USA, Clark and colleagues in Melbourne, Australia, Hochmair-Desoyer's team in Austria and Chouard and colleagues in France. Not surprisingly, many of the original and current commercially available devices bear their origins in these pioneering research programmes (3M and Clarion devices from California, USA, Nucleus devices from Australia and Med-El devices from Austria). The success of these early implant programmes generated considerable interest in the UK: the first single channel device was implanted in London by Fraser in 1984 with the first multichannel device being inserted by Ramsden in Manchester in 1988. Initially, implant programmes in the UK were funded through research and charitable sources, but the MRC report by Summerfield and Marshall (1995) based on a multicentre pilot study, in effect procured central funding for cochlear implantation.

Implant design

Current cochlear implants consist of two parts: an external component and a surgically implanted internal component. The external part comprises a microphone, speech processor and transmitter coil. The microphone unit is hooked behind the ear in a manner not dissimilar to a conventional behind-the-ear hearing aid. Sound received by the microphone is converted into electrical energy, which is conveyed to the speech processor. This body worn component utilizes various speech strategies (see below) and sends the processed signal to the transmitting coil which is held on the scalp behind the ear by a magnet in the coil and the implanted part of the device. The transmitter coil transfers the processed information to the internal implanted receiver–stimulator package by transcutaneous induction. From the receiver–stimulator package, information is conveyed to the electrode array which is implanted within the cochlea: the current hypothesis is that the implanted electrodes stimulate the spiral ganglion cells of the auditory nerve directly. Depending on the manufacturer, the number of active electrodes varies from 12 to 24 (multichannel devices). Modified electrode arrays are available for use in the partially ossified cochlea: compressed arrays carrying a smaller number of electrodes or double electrode arrays for insertion into the basal and middle cochlear turns independently. The implanted component of the device needs to be constructed from biocompatible materials with high tensile strength and resistance to corrosion. The electrodes themselves are made of a platinum-iridium alloy housed in silicone with either a ceramic or silicone casing for the receiver package. At the time of writing, the cost of the implant hardware in the UK is around £15 000.

Speech coding strategies

A speech signal has two main components: spectral (pitch) information and temporal (loudness and change in loudness) information. Various speech coding strategies have evolved over the last 20 years in an attempt to emulate and present this information to the auditory nerve. The original strategies based on extracting vowel and fundamental formant information are now obsolete. Current devices digitize the input and utilize band pass filters to divide the signal into frequency specific components. This information is presented in a pulsatile waveform to the individual channels of the electrode array. This reduces cross-interaction between channels thereby enhancing spectral information. By stimulating a smaller number of the available electrodes with the signal components that have the highest amplitude the overall rate of stimulation increases, enhancing temporal information. The implementation of the principles of the speech strategies differs between manufacturers and continues to evolve. In terms of outcomes, the current strategies for multichannel implantation from the different manufacturers are all capable of providing comparable results.

Neural plasticity

This is the ability of the central nervous system to be programmed to learn a task. In cochlear implantation two components are of paramount importance: changes in the brainstem auditory nuclei and the auditory cortex in response to sound and also the neural plasticity of speech articulation. Auditory plasticity, and with it the ability to listen, is lost by the age of 8 years whilst the ability to develop good speech articulation only occurs if speech sounds are heard by the age of 3 years. On this basis, hearing impaired individuals are classified as postlingual (speech acquired before becoming deaf) or prelingual (become deaf before acquiring speech). In addition, a third group are those children that lose their hearing around the time of speech development (perilingual). Postlingual adults and children may be considered for implantation. In pre- and perilingual children the timing of cochlear implantation is critical taking into account the issues of neural plasticity. Profoundly deaf prelingual adolescents and adults, however, are unlikely to derive benefit from cochlear implantation as the neural plasticity required to make sense of the auditory stimulation from an implant has already been lost.

Candidacy

The process of selecting appropriate individuals for implantation is of critical importance for a successful outcome and is task that involves all the members of the implant team. The selection criteria continue to evolve and may be considered under the following headings:

1. Age. There is no upper age limit as long as the potential recipient is in good health. A family history of longevity may also be taken into consideration. The initial controversy surrounding implantation in children has abated and successful implantation has been undertaken in selected children below the age of 18 months.

2. Cause of the deafness. Implantation is indicated in deafness due to cochlear pathology: central and auditory nerve causes are a contraindication. Within the cochlea, different aetiologies have a greater or lesser effect on the spiral ganglion cell population. In addition, secondary changes in the cochlea such as fibrosis and ossification (such as after meningitis) need to be recognized as surgery may require a cochlear drill-out or use of a modified electrode array as described above.

3. Duration of severe or profound deafness. In postlingually deafened adults, the duration of severe or profound deafness is recognized as a prognostic indicator with respect to outcome, with those individuals deafened for more than 20 years tending to fare less well. With regards to children and adolescents, the relationship between the onset of deafness and speech development is of critical importance.

4. Audiometric and vestibular assessment. Selected individuals that derive little or no benefit from a trial of conventional hearing aids may be considered for cochlear implantation. The audiological evaluation includes aided and unaided pure tone audiometry and speech audiometry. In children, particularly those with congenital deafness, electrical response audiometry is utilized to confirm the presence of a profound hearing loss and to act as guide as to which ear to implant. The original criteria for implantation were pure tone thresholds greater than 100 dBHL at 2 kHz and above with speech discrimination scores less than 10%. More recently, with the observation that many implanted individuals seem to fare better than marginal hearing aid users several centres now use a 30% speech score as the ceiling for consideration for implantation.

Loss of vestibular function may accompany the hearing loss, particularly after meningitis. Central compensation occurs more readily in children than adults and the latter will require a caloric test to establish the presence or absence of labyrinthine function. If implantation is to be undertaken in the ear with better or only vestibular function then appropriate preoperative counselling needs to be discussed with the patient.

5. Otological examination. Active chronic suppurative otitis media remains a contraindication to implantation. Surgery to render the ear disease free must be undertaken as a prelude to insertion of the device. This is usually staged with obliteration and blind-sac closure of an open mastoid cavity if present. At the time of implantation, the tympanomastoid cleft can be evaluated for the presence of any infection or cholesteatoma and surgery can proceed if the ear is disease free.

6. General medical history. The principle of assessment of the patient's general health prior to elective surgery under general anaesthesia applies as for any other planned otological surgery. In the presence of cardiovascular or respiratory disease, a decision has to be reached in terms of the risks of surgery against the benefits of implantation. In addition, the severity of other disabilities such as blindness and locomotor dysfunction also require careful consideration.

7. Radiological assessment. This is a mandatory part of the evaluation process. Imaging aims to firstly establish the presence of a normal cochlea (not always the case in congenital deafness) and to establish cochlear patency. In addition, appropriate radiology gives information about the internal auditory meatus (the narrow meatus with normal facial function may only contain a facial nerve) and provides general information about the temporal bone anatomy such as pneumatization, soft tissue opacification of the tympanomastoid cleft and the anatomy of the jugular bulb. Radiology may also demonstrate the aetiology in 'idiopathic cases' such as the large vestibular aqueduct syndrome or previously undiagnosed cochlear otosclerosis. Two imaging modalities are utilized. The standard examination is a high resolution CT scan. However, CT scanning may fail to demonstrate cochlear fibrosis and therefore in post-meningitic deafness T2 weighted MR imaging is the investigation of choice. This may also be considered the case in deafness due to otosclerosis, autoimmune hearing loss and labyrinthitis due to causes other than meningitis. In selected cases both types of imaging will be required in order to fully assess the feasibility of inserting the electrode array.

8. Psychological profile and expectations. The expectations of the potential adult recipient need to be realistic: the implant does not restore hearing in the natural sense and the patient needs to understand this. In addition the individual needs to be motivated for the intensive rehabilitation that will be required to maximize the potential from the device. In children the expectations and motivation of the immediate family are also of critical importance. In particular, rehabilitation requires numerous visits to the implant centre possibly over several years and the family need to commit themselves and the child to this process.

Surgery

Surgery is usually undertaken under general anaesthesia after informed consent with particular reference to the facial nerve and chorda tympani. The author routinely uses a facial nerve monitor and parenteral antibiotics are given at the start of surgery with two further doses postoperatively. Two types of skin incision are commonly used: the extended endaural and modified post aural. The musculoperiosteal flap is usually raised separately. A cortical mastoidectomy with undermined margins is undertaken and a bed drilled in the skull for the receiver–stimulator package. The facial recess is approached via a posterior tympanotomy preserving a bridge of bone between the tympanotomy and the fossa incudis. The tympanotomy should allow visualization of the incudostapedial joint and the round window niche to allow correct placement of the cochleotomy. The opening into the scala tympani is made just in front of and above the round window niche. Some surgeons prefer to enter the basal turn via the round window itself. An attempt is made to initially preserve the endosteum of the scala tympani and to open into the basal turn with a needle rather than the drill, thereby reducing the risk of trauma to the spiral lamina and remaining neural elements. The electrode array is guided into the cochlea and advanced using a claw designed for this purpose. An attempt is made to insert the array as far into the cochlear duct without damaging the array. The receiver package is then secured in its bed either with ties or bone cement. The proximal electrode array lies under the undermined margins and may also be secured with ties, clips or bone cement. A muscle plug is used to seal the cochleotomy and the posterior tympanotomy conferring further stability. The wound is closed in the conventional manner and a mastoid dressing and pressure bandage applied for 48 h. A plain transorbital X-ray is undertaken the day after surgery to confirm the position of the electrode array in the cochlea. The patient is usually fit for discharge on the third day post operation and the sutures removed at 1 week.

Rehabilitation

The initial 'switch on' of the device usually occurs after about 4 weeks when all the postoperative scalp swelling has settled and the wound is fully healed. For several weeks after this, an intensive programme of auditory and speech training takes place with fine tuning of the speech processing map for the particular individual. In children considerable support from their teachers is required with close co-operation between the implant team and the educationalists. The rehabilitation process continues for several months for adults and years for children. The full benefit of the implant is not usually realised for at least 6 months and may take 12–18 months when the learning curve flattens and the recipient adjust to the new auditory stimulus.

Outcomes

Numerous tests have been developed to evaluate the outcome of implantation in a given individual. In adults, open set tests are commonly used. Such tests assess the ability to distinguish speech without any contextual clues or lip reading. The majority of adults report identification of environmental sound and a marked improvement in their lip reading skills. A sizeable proportion are able to track speech without lip-reading and a smaller number can, in ideal conditions converse almost normally or use the telephone, particularly when listening to familiar voices. The outcomes in children are dependant on their language status at the time that the hearing was lost and to a degree on the age at implantation. In one series almost all the postlingually deafened children developed open set listening with good speech intelligibility. Of the prelingually deafened children around one half developed open set listening with good or average speech intelligibility. It is not surprising, therefore, to see children implanted at the age of 2 or 3 years entering mainstream education at the age of 5 or 6 years.

Complications

1.   Surgical complications.   Surgical complications in cochlear implantation are in fact relatively uncommon. This is probably because surgeons undertaking this type of work already have a considerable otological experience and international implant workshops are readily available for those embarking on this type of surgery. Injury to the facial nerve is rare whilst chorda tympani trauma is probably under-reported. Damage to the electrode array and electrode misplacement have been reported in most large series. One of the most serious complications is ischaemia or sepsis in the scalp flap with loss of flap viability around the receiver package. This situation is difficult to salvage and may result in device extrusion and subsequent need to remove the device. With experience and meticulous attention to incision placement and soft tissue handling major scalp complications can be avoided.

2. Device complications. Device malfunction is categorized as a *soft failure* if there is deviation from the specification without total loss of function (such as an electrode fault that can be programmed out) or as a *hard failure* if the implant ceases to function, necessitating re-implantation. Such events have been reported by all the implant manufacturers and tend to occur early in the life of the device. With continuing research and development device failure has become less common and by way of example, the cumulative survival for devices from one of the manufacturers is greater than 98% after 5 years.

3. Non-auditory stimulation. Undesirable effects of electrical stimulation of the inner ear include pain in the ear, scalp or throat, intrusive tinnitus and facial nerve stimulation. All are uncommon and the offending electrode or electrodes can usually be programmed out. Facial nerve stimulation is a particular feature in those individuals deafened by otosclerosis or temporal bone fractures and it is postulated that the fracture line or otospongiotic focus allows current escape and stimulation of the intralabyrinthine segment of the facial nerve.

Future developments

Cochlear implantation is a fertile area for research and development both by implant teams and the manufacturers. Current clinic studies include bilateral implantation, implantation in marginal hearing aid users, cochlear implantation in patients with bilateral vestibular schwannomas and evaluation of music perception. Hardware developments include modiolus hugging electrode arrays, magnetless coupling mechanisms and refinements in speech processing strategies. The ultimate goal is the totally implantable device which is probably only a few years away.

Further reading

Various authors. *The American Journal of Otology.* 1997; **18** (Suppl 6): 1–170.
Gibson WPR. Cochlear implants. In: Booth JB (Ed). *Scott-Brown's Otolaryngology.* Oxford: Butterworth-Heinemann, 1997; pp. 1–25.

CONGENITAL HEARING DISORDERS

We define the term congenital as existing at birth. Congenital deafness may be sensorineural, conductive or mixed and may occur in isolation or with other congenital abnormalities (the syndromes). Sensorineural deafness may be a hereditary degenerative deafness where there is progressive loss of hearing, typically in late childhood in subjects with a previously normal cochlea in both structure and function (*the abiotrophies*). Recessive genes account for 80% of hereditary deafness. Most of these are non-syndromic and many are abiotrophies.

There are a multitude of syndromes associated with congenital deafness. Below are those we consider to be the most important:

Autosomal recessive

1.   *Pendred's syndrome.*   Sensorineural hearing loss (SNHL) and a thyroid goitre.

2.   *Usher's syndrome.*   Retinitis pigmentosa and SNHL.

3.   *Jervell and Lange-Nielson syndrome.*   Prolonged electrocardiographic Q-T interval and SNHL.

4.   *Refsum's disease.*   Retinitis pigmentosa, cerebellar ataxia, peripheral neuropathy and SNHL.

5.   *Branchio-oto-renal syndrome.*   Branchial arch anomalies, renal dysplasia and a mixed type of hearing loss.

Autosomal dominant

1.   *Waardenburg's syndrome.*   Telecanthus, pigment disorder (20% have a white forelock and 45% heterochromia iridis) with SNHL.

2.   *Treacher-Collins syndrome.*   Hypoplasia of the malar bones, maxilla and mandible. There may be microtia or multiple, external and inner ear abnormalities.

3.   *Pierre-Robin syndrome.*   Hypoplastic mandible, cleft palate, glossoptosis. There may be external, middle or internal ear deformities.

4.   *Crouzon's disease.*   Hypoplastic mandible and maxilla, parrot beak nose, craniostenosis and exophthalmos associated with external and middle ear abnormalities.

5.   *Apert's syndrome.*   Congenital fixation of the stapes footplate, acrocephaly, syndactyly, cleft palate, saddle nose, maxillary hypoplasia.

The dysplasias

The dysplasias describe four congenital abnormalities of the cochlea and often occur as a component of the hearing syndromes. They comprise:

1.   *Michel's deformity.*   The most severe 'dysplasia' (more correctly this is an aplasia) with agenesis of the labyrinth and total sensorineural deafness.

2. *Mondini's dysplasia.* Only the basal coil of the cochlea is present and the semicircular canals may be absent. There are islands of residual hearing, especially in the high tones.

3. *Bing-Siebenman dysplasia.* The bony labyrinth is normal, but there is maldevelopment of the membranous labyrinth.

4. *Scheibe dysplasia.* The bony labyrinth is normal, but the stria vascularis has alternating regions of aplasia and hypoplasia. There are few hair cells and the saccule is collapsed, hence its synonym cochleosaccular dysgenesis. Hearing loss is severe.

Congenital conductive hearing loss

The external ear canal develops from the first branchial cleft lying between the first and second branchial arches. These arches form the pinna (mesoderm and ectoderm), bony labyrinth (mesoderm), membranous labyrinth (ectoderm) and, from the dorsal end of cartilage within each arch, the ossicles (mesoderm). The ventral arch cartilage forms the mandible (1st arch) and the hyoid bone (2nd arch). Anomalies of structures associated with these arches gives rise to multiple deformities, for example Treacher-Collins and Pierre-Robin syndromes. The external and middle ear anomalies are classified into three groups:

1. *Minor aplasia.* The external auditory meatus is narrow, the tympanic membrane functional, the pinna either normal or with a minor deformity and there may be ossicular fixation, usually of the stapes. Stapes surgery is difficult because of limited access and there is an increased risk of a perilymph gusher so that a small fenestra technique is recommended should stapedectomy be attempted.

2. *Major aplasia.* There is usually microtia with external ear canal atresia and fixation of an abnormal malleus and incus. The stapes is usually functionally normal.

3. *Major aplasia/atresia.* The external ear may be atretic, the tympanic cavity small, mastoid pneumatization absent and there is a significant risk of one of the cochlear dyplasias.

Classification of congenital sensorineural deafness

1. *Hereditary*
(a) Deafness present at birth: Deafness alone; syndromes associated with deafness.
(b) Deafness appearing in childhood: Deafness alone, syndromes associated with deafness.

2. *Secondary to intrauterine disease*
(a) Infections: rubella, cytomegalovirus, toxoplasmosis, congenital syphilis.
(b) Ototoxic drugs (see ototoxicity chapter).
(c) Metabolic disorders: e.g. maternal diabetes mellitus.
(d) Perinatal disorders: e.g. hypoxia, hyperbilirubinaemia, premature delivery, low birth weight.

Classification of congenital conductive hearing loss

1. Hereditary abnormal external or middle ear.

(a) Present at birth: e.g. Apert's syndrome, Crouzons disease, Treacher-Collins syndrome, Pierre-Robin syndrome.

(b) Appearing in childhood: e.g. osteogenesis imperfecta, otosclerosis.

2. Congenital disorders predisposing to glue ear.
Cystic fibrosis, cleft palate, Down's syndrome, Kartageners syndrome.

3. Miscellaneous conditions.
Congenital cholesteatoma, Fibrous dysplasia, Goldenhar's syndrome.

Management

The congenital hearing loss may be suspected at birth because of the family history. These babies and those suspected of having one of the syndromes or dysplasias should be referred to a paediatric otologist or audiologist who will be able to investigate the suspected hearing loss and institute, depending on the cause, appropriate surgery or/and rehabilitation.

Recent developments

There have been significant advances in the genetic basis of hearing loss. Many non-syndromic genes are now mapped as are several genes coding for syndromic deafness. The Jervell and Lange-Nielsen gene has been mapped to the short arm of chromosome 11, Waardenburg syndrome type 1 to the long arm of chromosome 2 and the branchio-oto-renal gene, a homologue of the Drosophilia absent eye gene, has been mapped to the long arm of chromosome 8. Mapping genes of non-syndromic deafness is difficult and relies on finding large families who have a significant number bearing the trait. Easily identifiable regions of chromosomes (markers) are inherited and the ability to map a non-syndromic gene depends on the proximity of this gene to a marker so that the two are inherited together and in this way a linkage map is generated.

Mapping a gene gives rise to the possibility of gene transfer. Presently a safe, efficient vector to deliver the gene to a spiral ganglion hair cell and which produces long term transduction and a minimal immune response is still being researched. Ideally the transgene insert will include an inducible promoter that will allow turning gene expression on and off according to need. The introduction of a correct, non-mutated copy of a mutated gene coding for a deafness genotype has recently been shown to correct the phenotype so that when hair cell specific vectors are available, it may be possible to extend gene therapy to the abiotrophies. Mutant genes coding for deafness at birth will be more difficult to resolve and will necessitate fetal gene therapy.

Further reading

Lusting LR and Tunnel DE. Sensorineural hearing loss in children. *Current Opinion in Otolaryngology & Head and Neck Surgery*, 1998; **6**: 360–367.

Morrell RJ. Recent progress in hereditary hearing loss. *Current Opinion in Otolaryngology & Head and Neck Surgery*, 1999; **7**: 259–265.

Related topics of interest

Ototoxicity, p. 228; Paediatric hearing assessment, p. 239; Hearing aids, p. 117; Cochlear implants, p. 53.

COSMETIC SURGERY

This chapter is confined to a description of rhinoplasty, pinnaplasty, facial reanimation, hair transplantation and rhytidectomy.

Rhinoplasty

Indications

1. Cosmetic: dorsal hump, dorsal saddle, too wide or too narrow dorsum, under- or overprojected tip, polly beak.
2. Functional: nasal obstruction, snoring, sleep apnoea.

Much is written about the ideal nasal size and shape. This however depends on the dimensions of the upper, mid and lower thirds of the face, the thickness of the nasal skin and the race of the patient. There is no singly perfect shape. It is not disputed however that a nose should be straight and have a uniform dorsal width from nasion to the tip. The nasolabial angle should be about 90° in males and 110° in females. It is important that the patient states specifically what they dislike about their nasal shape and for the surgeon to state exactly what deformities he is aiming to correct, so the patient will have a realistic expectation of the likely operative result. It is often the case that it is not possible to make an ugly nose pretty, but it is usually possible to correct specific defects so that the nose no longer brings attention to the face.

Technique

Most rhinoplasty surgery consists of a basic technique comprising nasal dehumping, medial and lateral osteotomies with in-fracture and excision of a cephalic rim of lower lateral cartilage if the tip requires cephalic rotation. A dilemma in rhinoplasty surgery is what graft to use when augmentation is necessary. Again there is no ideal graft that fits all scenarios. Cartilaginous augmentation by manoeuvring quadrate cartilage into a new position or using conchal cartilage with perichondrium attached, bony dorsal augmentation using a rib graft (not a straight graft but it can be osteotomized), iliac crest (the bone here is cancellous) or a silastic implant will cover most situations. In the USA there is a current vogue for external rhinoplasty which has the advantage of visualizing directly the osteocartilaginous vault during surgery.

Pinnaplasty

Most surgeons wait until the patient is at least 3-years-old so that the ear is not too small to manipulate and for the full deformity (e.g. there may be an overlarge conchal bowl in addition to an absent antihelix) to become apparent. Ideally, surgery should be performed before infant school to prevent ridicule.

The two common techniques are:

1. Anterior conchal scoring technique described by Stenstrom allowing the cartilage to curl back to form an antihelix without suturing.
2. Mustarde technique in which the antihelix is folded and kept in position with mattress sutures.

Most surgeons will have their own modification of one of these techniques which works well for them (e.g. thinning the region of the antihelix fold in the Mustarde technique with a diamond drill to reduce cartilage tension and to allow a more natural curve).

An important and often neglected portion of the procedure is the pressure dressing. Cotton wool should support the post-auricular region and fill the conchal bowl, and a firm head dressing applied in such a way that it will not slip until it is removed 7–14 days later. The only indication to remove the dressing is increasing aural pain, which usually indicates that a subperichondrial haematoma has formed due to inadequate pressure. It is unusual for the head dressing to be too tight and then the main symptom will be a persistent headache, the operated ear being splinted and protected. Many surgeons state that it is better not to apply a head dressing than apply one which is inadequate, as the trauma to the ear from repeated redressing will predispose to infection or haematoma.

Facial reanimation

Surgery to produce improved facial symmetry after a facial nerve palsy should not be undertaken until the surgeon is sure there will be no spontaneous improvement. This may be immediate if trauma, either external or iatrogenic, has caused an immediate and total palsy suggesting nerve transection. One year post onset is arbitrarily taken as the minimum time to allow the nerve to recover maximum function after injury or following attempted reinnervation.

Facial nerve grafting

The reinnervation procedure chosen will depend on the site of injury and the surgeon's personal preference. Direct apposition of the nerve ending using monofilament 9-0 nylon suture material should be attempted only if it is possible to avoid tension on the anastomosis. Otherwise, a cable graft using sural or great auricular nerve should be attempted. For more proximal injuries such as those occurring after acoustic neuroma surgery, hypoglossal to facial or accessory to facial nerve anastomosis are the options. The latter uses the larger branch to trapezius muscle with little loss of shoulder movement or strength. When only half the width of the hypoglossal nerve is anastomosed to the facial trunk, in order to preserve tongue movement, slightly less satisfactory facial tone occurs. Reliable results are obtained only if anastomosis is attempted within one year of the onset of a palsy whereas the standard procedure is reliable when used up to two years after facial palsy.

Dynamic and static suspension

Dynamic suspension comprises transposition of the temporalis muscle to the submucosa or the orbicularis oris muscle in close proximity to the angle of the mouth. It improves the symmetry of the face at rest and on voluntary smiling in those with a permanent facial paralysis but does not improve lagophthalmos. It can be complimentary to facial nerve cable grafting or hypoglossal-facial anastomosis. The technique comprises placing the muscle sling lateral to the fascia overlying the muscles of facial expression to avoid the underlying facial nerve twigs. In some centres only the middle section of the muscle is transposed, Gore-Tex being used when necessary to lengthen the sling. Sterile 1 mm thick Gore-Tex Soft Tissue Patch can be used for static suspension in those unsuitable for dynamic suspension. The material is pre-stretched and so postoperative sagging is unusual in contradistinction to fascia lata. The material is attached to the zygomatic arch and the orbicularis muscle to elevate the mid-facial and perioral region. Most series have reported a high rate of extrusion and infection compared to fascia lata.

Eyelid procedures

A gold weight implant positioned over the tarsal plate and centred at the junction of the medial and middle third of the upper eyelid has been used for more than thirty years to rehabilitate the eyelid following facial nerve paralysis. Implants of different weights are taped to the upper lid preoperatively to determine the correct weight to just allow closure without ptosis. The main complications are infection and haematoma in the early postoperative period and extrusion, which can occur early or several years after implanting. To minimize extrusion rates it is recommended a drill hole is fashioned through the implant and this used to attach it to the tarsal plate by a nylon or prolene suture.

Hair transplantation

Modern techniques such as minigraft, micrograft, scalp expanders, scalp extenders and flaps now allow the creation of a virtually undetectable hairline and yield results not possible just five years ago.

The commonest form of hair loss is androgenic alopecia (AA) which may present as male or female pattern AA or diffuse AA. Most patients with AA are candidates for some form of hair replacement procedure. A small percentage of patients who develop excessive alopecia including the fringe areas, may not be suitable for any form of surgery. Male pattern alopecia is progressive and this may compromise long term results.

Micrografts are single hair grafts, usually placed along the frontal hair line to give a natural feathered appearance. They are placed into wounds created by needles or specifically designed small knife blades to create a 1 cm zone of single hair grafts.

Minigrafts (3–5 hairs per graft) are placed into holes created by a punch or laser, or an incisional slit. Grafts are harvested from the dominant fringe using special multiblade knives which allow the harvesting of multiple strips of hair-bearing scalp simultaneously. The strips are then divided into micro or minigrafts. Up to 1000 grafts may be taken in a single session. Several sessions of mini and micrografts 3 or 4 months apart may be required to achieve a satisfactory result.

Rhytidectomy

The original facelifts were the equivalent of modern minilifts in which an ellipse of skin is excised at or in the hairline and the tension of closure used to pull the facial skin taught.

Anterior subcutaneous elevation in a plane superficial to the fascia of the muscles of facial expression to avoid injuring the facial nerve became widespread in the 1970s, allowing elevation up to the midline. This technique had the disadvantage of occasionally causing skin necrosis or a wide scar due to increased skin tension on the suture line. In the 1970s a superficial muscle and aponeurotic system (SMAS) was described and most modern facelifts involve elevating the SMAS and fat to provide a more effective and longer lasting result. The technique has been further developed to the present day multi-directional facelift, subperiosteal facelift, deep plane facelift and the composite and extended SMAS facelift, the details of which may be found in operative texts.

Further reading

Kunihiro T, Kanzaki J, O-Uchi. Hypoglossal-facial nerve anastomosis. *Acta Otolaryngologica*, 1991; **487**: 80–84.

Ebersold MJ, Quast LM. Long-term results of spinal accessory nerve–facial nerve anastomosis. *Journal of Neurosurgery*, 1992; **77**: 51–54.

May M, Drucker C. Temporalis muscle for facial reanimation: A 13-year experience with 224 procedures. *Archives of Otolaryngology Head and Neck Surgery*, 1993; **119**: 378–382.

Pickford MA, Scamp T, Harrison DH. Morbidity after gold weight insertion into the upper eyelid in facial palsy. *British Journal of Plastic Surgery*, 1992; **45**: 460–464.

Campbell AC and Shumrick KA. Rhytidectomy: past, present and future. *Current Opinion in Otolaryngology and Head and Neck Surgery*, 1997; **5**: 234–242.

Related topics of interest

Nasal trauma, p. 177; Facial nerve palsy, p. 92; Reconstructive surgery, p. 267.

DAY CASE ENT SURGERY

Definition

An ENT surgical day case patient is one admitted for operation on a planned non-resident basis but who requires facilities for recovery. Full admission procedures and records are required, which therefore excludes those operations and procedures undertaken in the outpatient or accident and emergency department.

Patient selection

The patient may be admitted into either a self-contained day surgery unit with its own admission suites, wards, theatres and recovery area, or less desirably a day case ward or unsatisfactorily a general ward. In a general ward booked admissions may be blocked by emergency admissions; this is an expensive option because the ward is not closed at night or at the weekend.

An adult must be available to supervise the patient during the evening and first night. A telephone must be accessible so that the hospital can be contacted in an emergency. The home should be within a 20-min drive of the hospital if the patient is at risk of a primary haemorrhage, for example after adenoidectomy or submucosal diathermy. The patient must be taken home by an adult in a car or taxi on discharge. No mechanical device should be used nor cooking undertaken, and legal documents should not be signed during the first 24-h postoperative period, when alcohol is also forbidden. Driving is not advised within 48 h of a general anaesthetic. Operations likely to take longer than 60 min are unsuitable because of the slow speed of recovery from general anaesthetic, and patients should normally be of ASA I or ASA II status (the American Society of Anesthesiologists classification of physical status: class 1, the patient has no organic, physiological, biochemical or psychiatric disturbance and the pathological process for which surgery is to be performed is localized; or class 2, mild-to-moderate systemic disturbance caused either by the condition to be treated surgically or other pathophysiological processes, for example non-insulin-dependent diabetes mellitus or essential hypertension). As a rule an upper age limit of 75 is recommended although older patients with a low biological age should be considered. Patients with a body mass index (BMI) greater than 35 are unsuitable. Every day surgery unit should produce, by collaboration between anaesthetists and physicians, guidelines for surgeons regarding medical suitability for day case surgery. An example of a guideline sheet is shown in appendix 1 and can be modified according to the preferences of each unit.

Paediatric surgery

Special facilities for children are required. They should have their own designated area away from adult patients, with its own play area and parental waiting area. A preadmission visit allows familiarization. It is permissible to have a children-only operation day in a day surgery unit or day case ward if the required facilities are present. The children's area should be staffed by paediatric-trained nurses.

Advantages

- Lower costs.
- Reduced in-patient theatre workload.
- Increased efficiency.
- Reduced disruption to life.
- Early mobilization.
- Less psychological preparation required.
- Anaesthetic administered allows rapid recovery.

Disadvantages

- Limited care available to the patient after discharge.
- In-patient admission, if needed, must be arranged at short notice.

Appropriate Procedures

1. Ear.   Excision of accessory auricles, skin tags, preauricular sinuses. Removal of impacted wax or foreign bodies. Wedge excision biopsy of pinna lesion, myringotomy with or without grommet insertion, aural polypectomy.

2. Nose.   Reduction of nasal fractures, limited functional endoscopic sinus surgery, limited intranasal polypectomy, electrocautery of the nasal septum, submucosal diathermy of the inferior turbinate, septoplasty, submucosal resection of the nasal septum, bilateral antral puncture.

3. Head and neck.   Adenoidectomy, tonsillectomy (controversial), examination under anaesthetic (EUA) and biopsy of the laryngopharynx and oesophagus provided there is no risk to the airway. Selected patients requiring laser therapy, for example vocal cord polypectomy or nodule excision and laser excision of small tongue lesions. Other indications include the division of tongue tie and lymph node excision biopsy.

Further reading

Report of the Working Party on Guidelines for Daycase Surgery. Revised edition. London: The Royal College of Surgeons of England, 1992.

Appendix 1

Selection criteria

All patients should be ASA I or II and ambulant. Surgery time should be less than 1 h.

Social circumstance	No escort home	Unsuitable
	No adult overnight	
	Lives >1 h away	
Age	60–75 years but fit; ECG satisfactory	Suitable
	<12 months	Unsuitable
CVS	MI less than 3 years ago	Unsuitable
	Unstable angina	
	Symptomatic heart disease	

	Ventricular arrhythmia	
	Pacemaker due to 2nd or 3rd degree heart block	
	Stable angina or controlled atrial fibrillation with satisfactory ECG and serum urea and electrolytes	Suitable
Hypertension	BP < 170/100	Suitable
	BP > 175/105	Unsuitable
Respiratory disease	COAD or emphysema but:	
	(i) able to climb two flights of stairs	Suitable
	(ii) unable to climb two flights of stairs	Unsuitable
Asthma	Well controlled on inhalers	Suitable
	Previously hospitalized or taking systemic steroids	Unsuitable
Diabetes	Insulin dependant	Unsuitable
	NIDDM and BM stix <11 and ECG satisfactory	Suitable but instruct no medication on day of surgery
Neurological disease	Restriction of normal activity or CVA within past 1 year	Unsuitable
	Not restricting normal activity	Suitable
Epilepsy	Poorly controlled	Unsuitable
	Well controlled (no seizures during previous 1 year)	Suitable
Hiatus hernia	Consider H2 blockers before surgery	Suitable
Bleeding disorder		Unsuitable
Drug history	Systemic steroids within previous 3 months or cardiac drugs other than antihypertensives or taking MAO drugs	Refer for assessment
	Diuretics but satisfactory ECG and serum urea and electrolytes	Suitable
Anaesthetic problem	Difficult intubation	
	Malignant hyperpyrexia	Refer for assessment
	ITU admission	
	Blood relative died or had any of above	
	Minor (e.g. nausea or very slow to arouse)	Suitable

EPIGLOTTITIS

Acute epiglottitis is an uncommon but dangerous bacterial infection of the throat. There is an acute inflammation of the larynx which affects all the supraglottis, but predominantly the loose connective tissue of the epiglottis.

Aetiology

Haemophilus influenzae type B (HIB) is the usual causative organism, but this is not invariable. β-Haemolytic streptococci, pneumococci and staphylococci have also been isolated, especially in adult cases. Quite why the infection has a predilection for the epiglottis is not clear. Epiglottitis is usually seen in children between the ages of 2 and 6 years, with a peak incidence between the ages of 3 and 4. It may also occur in adults. In children under the age of 2 years *Haemophilus* tends to cause meningitis. It has been suggested that previous contact with *H. influenzae* in early childhood may later be followed by a type III Arthus hypersensitivity reaction which would account for the rapid onset of epiglottitis.

Prophylaxis

In recent years efforts have been focused on the prevention of HIB infections. There seems to have been a decline in new cases over the last few years, which may be attributed to the new conjugated HIB vaccine approved for administration to 2-month-old infants.

Clinical features

The disease may present at any time of the year but is more common in winter. Initially the child usually complains of a sore throat and pain when swallowing. The inflammation and oedema will rapidly progress to cause muffling of the voice and respiratory obstruction. Inspiratory stridor then occurs. A critically ill, breathless child may then present to the casualty department having a toxic, flushed appearance and a high temperature (38–40°C). The child will usually sit up and lean forward dribbling saliva. The provisional diagnosis is made on the history and the examination of the child. Attempts to depress the tongue or indirect laryngoscopy should not be undertaken to confirm the diagnosis as this can precipitate laryngospasm. This can also occur if the child becomes distressed and starts to cry, so nothing that may be frightening should be allowed.

Investigations

Maintenance of the patient's airway is the primary consideration, and all investigations should be delayed until this is secure. In the early case a lateral soft-tissue neck radiograph may confirm a swollen epiglottis but is not essential and may be dangerous. The taking of a radiograph should never be done if epiglottitis is suspected and there are already signs of respiratory difficulty. Furthermore, no child should be sent for a radiograph without the continuous presence of someone skilled in paediatric intubation.

Treatment

The first requirement of treatment is to safeguard the airway. An experienced paediatric anaesthetist and otolaryngologist should be in attendance. The child is allowed to remain in an upright posture as sudden changes in position, especially lying down, may result in airway obstruction. Intravenous access is not attempted and the child should be moved to a quiet induction area with adjacent operating facilities. A gentle inhalation induction using sevoflurane and oxygen is preferred. The oxygen saturation is closely monitored with pulse oximetry. A parent should be present and at all times the child is talked to and reassured. When the child is asleep, the parent is shown from the room. Direct laryngoscopy should be performed to establish the diagnosis and to pass an endotracheal tube. Oedematous aryepiglottic folds and a cherry red epiglottis are characteristic signs of the disease. An appropriately sized orotracheal tube is inserted to immediately restore the airway. This should then be replaced with a nasotracheal tube as they are more readily tolerated and more securely fixed. There may be difficulty establishing an endotracheal airway, and if intubation fails a rigid bronchoscope should be inserted immediately and subsequently replaced with an endotracheal tube. Rarely, a tracheostomy may be necessary.

Once an airway has been established swabs are taken from the epiglottis and a blood culture is performed. An intravenous line is inserted for fluid replacement and antibiotic therapy. The current choice of antibiotic is chloramphenicol (100 mg per kg body weight per 24 hours) as up to 30% of *Haemophilus* strains are resistant to ampicillin. Because of the side effects of chloramphenicol, third generation cephalosporins are an alternative. A nasogastric tube should be inserted for feeding. The sedated child is transferred to a paediatric intensive care unit for rehydration, antibiotics and humidified inspired gases.

Follow-up and aftercare

There is usually a prompt response to treatment with fluid replacement and antibiotics. As the epiglottic oedema settles an increasing leak around the endotracheal tube is expected. Once the child is afebrile and appears well, extubation can be considered. This is usually possible within 48 hours. Some surgeons advocate the use of corticosteriods before decannulation to help reduce oedema caused by the tube.

Further reading

Hugosson S, *et al.* Acute epiglottitis – aetiology, epidemiology and outcome in a population before large scale *Haemophilus influenzae* type b vaccination. *Clinical Otolaryngology*, 1994; **19**: 441–445.

Kessler A, Westmore RF, Marsh R. Childhood epiglottitis in recent years. *International Journal of Otolaryngology*, 1993; **25**: 155–162.

Pascucci RC. Paediatric intensive care. In: Gregory GA (ed.) *Paediatric Anaesthesia*, 2nd edn. New York: Churchill Livingstone, 1989; 1327–1337.

Related topics of interest

Paediatric airway problems, p. 232; Paediatric endoscopy, p. 237.

EPISTAXIS

Aetiology

1. Local causes
- Idiopathic (85%).
- Traumatic (fractures, foreign body, nose picking).
- Inflammatory (rhinitis, sinusitis).
- Neoplastic (tumours of the nose, sinuses and nasopharynx).
- Environmental (high altitude, air conditioning).
- Endocrine (menstruation, pregnancy).
- Iatrogenic (surgery, steroid nasal sprays).

2. General causes
- Anticoagulants (warfarin, aspirin).
- Diseases of the blood (haemophilia, leukaemia).
- Familial haemorrhagic telangiectasia (Osler–Rendu–Weber).
- Hypertension.
- Raised venous pressure (whooping cough, pneumonia).

Blood vessels involved

The upper parts of the nose are supplied by branches from the internal carotid artery (anterior and posterior ethmoidal arteries) and the rest from branches of the external carotid artery (greater palatine, sphenopalatine, superior labial). Little's area (Kiesselbach's plexus) is the commonest site of bleeding, which may be more to do with its comparatively exposed position in the anterior part of the septum than the fact that this is where the vessels anastamose.

Clinical assessment

Always make sure that the patient is not in shock, especially when bleeding is brisk, but the instigation of immediate resuscitation is not usually necessary. It is important that nursing support is available in this situation to assist with management of the patient. Protect the patient's clothing and your own with an apron, and wear gloves. Take a full history and on examination try to localize the area from which bleeding is arising and any specific bleeding points. If the bleeding has been significant start an intravenous infusion. Investigations should include a full blood count (FBC) (check Hb, white cell count and platelets), clotting studies and blood for group and cross-match if necessary.

Management

The aims are to arrest the haemorrhage and to treat the underlying cause. The bleeding is usually stopped by one of the following methods:

- Pressure on the nostrils (can be supplemented with ice-cold packs and sucking ice cubes).

- Local cautery (chemical or electrocoagulation).
- Anterior nasal packing (paraffin gauze, BIPP, merocel).
- Packing of the postnasal space (gauze, Foley's catheter, Brighton balloon).

Calm reassurance coupled with sedation (i.v. diazepam) will relieve the patient's anxiety. If nasal packing is required, systemic antibiotics should be given to prevent otitis media from Eustachian tube blockage, and sinusitis. Examination under general anaesthetic may become necessary if the above measures fail to allow better identification of the bleeding site and more effective cautery and packing. Further surgery is indicated only on the rare occasion when haemorrhage is not controlled by packing and cautery, or if a severe epistaxis recurs.

Surgical intervention

1. *Submucosal resection*

2. *Endoscopic approach.* For exposure and ligation of the sphenopalatine artery.

3. *Ligation or clipping of the maxillary artery in the pterygomaxillary fossa.* A Caldwell Luc incision is made, the antrum entered and a window made in the posterior wall of the sinus. The artery is encountered in the pterygopalatine fossa and teased away from the fat pad. Each tortuous branch is clipped in turn.

4. *Anterior ethmoid artery clipping* is required for uncontrollable bleeding from the upper part of the nose, above the middle turbinate. The approach to the anterior ethmoidal artery is via a medial orbital incision with lateral displacement of the upper orbital contents. The artery is surrounded by periosteum about 2.5 cm deep to the orbital rim just above the level of the medial canthus and is readily controlled by clipping.

5. *External carotid artery ligation* Ligation of the external carotid in the neck may be needed if maxillary artery clipping is unsuccessful.

6. *Embolization of vessels under radiographic control* with gel sponge or beads is advocated in some centres, but because of the risks involved (e.g. cerebrovascular embolus) has not been fully accepted.

Hereditary haemorrhagic telangiectasia

A specific problem in the management of epistaxis (and favourite examination topic) includes hereditary haemorrhagic telangiectasia or Rendu–Osler–Weber disease. Patients with this are easily recognized by red spots on the lips and the mucous membrane of the mouth, especially the tongue, as well as telangiectases on the face and nose. The condition may be complicated by the presence of lesions in the gut, which may bleed, or arteriovenous malformations in the lungs. In addition to repeated local treatment, other therapies include oestrogens, radiotherapy, sclerosants, lining mucosa with placenta or split skin grafts and laser therapy (argon or Nd-YAG).

Follow-up and aftercare

This depends on the cause and severity of the bleeding, but all patients who have required admission and treatment in hospital should be reviewed in the outpatient department. The patient is asked if there has been any further bleeding and their haemoglobin levels checked before discharge.

Further reading

McGarry. Endoscopic ligation of the sphenopalatine artery. *Clinical Otolaryngology.*

Related topic of interest

Examination of the nose, p. 84.

EVIDENCE BASED MEDICINE

P.J. Bradley

Definition

The term 'evidence based medicine' (EBM) was first used in the 1980s at McMaster University in Canada. During the 1990s it was defined as: 'medical practice in which clinical problems are addressed by formulating clearly defined questions, finding and evaluating all relevant research evidence, and reaching a conclusion about which option would have the greatest liklehood of effectiveness'.

Problems

There are many reasons cited for the reluctance to embrace EBM into daily clinical practice:

1. the size and complexity of the research required;
2. difficulties in developing evidence-based clinical policy;
3. difficulties in applying evidence due to:
   - poor access to best evidence and the need for validated guidelines;
   - organizational barriers;
   - poor continuing educational programmes;
   - Poor compliance to treatments by patients.
   - The heterogeneity of the patient population.

The first two points concern the equipping of clinicans and managers with critical appraisal skills, to assess the research evidence, as well as taking note of systemic reviews that have been performed by institutions such as the Cochrane Centre and through the medium of well drawn-up guidelines. Access to evidence is improving with the recognition for the need of a 'chief knowledge officer' to disseminate information to the rest of the organization. Apart from the barriers identified, there is also the need for changes in clinical behaviour that are necessary to ensure the successful implementation of guidelines. A veriety of interventions are required, leading to a behavioural change in those required to follow a different way of working. A change in behaviour can be reinforced by providing incentives to work in a different way. Incentives such as financial reward, resource allocation, education, and training, performance feedback and empowerment have all been shown to be effective but need resourcing. As with the pocess of obtaining the commitment of stakeholders, patients and employers, incentives that are locally negotiated and agreed are more likely to succeed than those imposed from above.

Clinical governance

The introduction of Clinical Governance with the expectation that the use of guidelines and audit will improve patient care. The National Services Frameworks will rationalize this process in the UK through the National Institute for Clinical Excellence (NICE) with external monitoring being provided by the Commission for Health Improvement (CHI). The BAO-HNS will work with these groups and will welcome the additional contribution being made by the National Otolaryngological

Trials Office (NOTO) in Newcastle and by the Cochrane ENT Working Group in Oxford.

Clinical evidence

EBM is the conscientious, explicit and judicious use of current evidence in making decisions about the care of individual patients. Its practise requires the integration of individual clinical expertise with the best available clinical evidence from systematic research. The best available clinical evidence refers to clinically relevant research, which may be from basic sciences, but in particular from patient centred research into the accuracy and precision of diagnostic tests, the power of prognostic factors, and the efficacy and safety of therapeutic, rehabilative and preventa-tive regimens. The levels of evidence are classified as 1–4, with level 1a being evidence obtained from meta-analysis of randomized controlled trials (the gold standard) to level 4 which is the evidence obtained from expert committee reports or opinions and/or clinical experience of respected authorities.

Interpretation

In essence, therefore, EBM is simply a method for identifying and interpreting the relevant research data to help with the questions faced in our clinical lives. The steps comprise:

- rephrasing our problems or information needs into answerable questions;
- efficiently tracking down the best evidence with which to answer them;
- being able to appraise the evidence we find for validity and usefulness;
- applying the evidence to pure practice;
- evaluating our own resulting performance.

The feedback loop implied by the last two points indicates the relationship between audit and EBM; EBM includes audit as well as consideration of the external evidence.

EBM divides clinical questions into a number of types.

- Prognosis questions – outcomes, with no direct comparison of treatments.
- Diagnostic test questions – the accuracy of diagnostic or prognostic tests.
- Treatment questions – ask what the efficacy of a specific treatment is commonly compared to placebo.
- Harm and aetiology questions – the risk of harm arising out of treatments or interventions or about the association between a factor and a medical condition (smoking and lung cancer).

Regardless of the type of question asked, the steps in answering them are the same.

1. What is the evidence?
2. Is the evidence valid?
3. Is the evidence important?
4. Should we change our practice because of the new evidence. If so how?

Problems

Surgeons have been severely criticized for their failure to apply EBM in the past, particularly their failure to conduct randomized control trials (RCTs).

There are several reasons for not performing RCTs in surgery. First history. Once a treatment is accepted as the standard for the management of a given condition, it is difficult to achieve the level of uncertainty ('equipoise') about its benefit required to persuade clinicians to test it again against a placebo. In many cases, the benefits of the treatment are so great and obvious that such a trial would be clearly unethical. This situation is not confined only to surgery: old drugs such as morphine, asprin and digoxin are also difficult to randomise against a placebo.

The second obstacle to trials of operations is the difficulty that arises when attempting to compare surgical against non-surgical treatments. Medical management of appendicitis against surgical appendicectomy. Finally, there are important practical difficulties in performing RCTs of surgical operations that do not exist with most medical treatments. It is difficult to blind patients and staff to the operation performed, though this can sometimes be done with an imaginative trial protocol.

Conclusion

A review of the published literature during 1990–1994 in five major general otolaryngological journals, one UK and the other four USA based, suggested that there is poor evidence base for our specialty if one regards randomized controlled trials as the gold standard. Studies more recently do not justify a major revision of the hierarchy of evidence, but they do support a flexible approach in which a randomized controlled trials and observational studies have complementary roles. High quality observational studies may extend evidence over a wider population and are likely to be dominant in the identification of harms and when randomized controlled trials would be unethical or impractical.

Further reading

Patterson JV, Stewart-Brown SL. What are general practitioners' attitudes towards evidence-based medicine, and are these changing? *Journal of Clinical Excellence*, 1999; **1:** 27–34.

Haynes B, Haines A. Barriers and bridges to evidence based clinical practice. *British Medical Journal*, 1998; **317:** 273–276.

Bradley PJ. Clinical guidelines for otorhinolaryngology. *Clinical Otolaryngology*, 1997; **22:** 483–484.

Sackett DL, Richardson WS, Rosenberg W, Haynes RB. Evidence-based medicine: how to practise and teach EBM. Edinburgh: Churchill Livingstone, 1997.

Evidence-Based Medicine Working Group. Evidence medicine: a new approach to teaching the practice of medicine. *JAMA*, 1992; **268:** 2420–2425.

Maran AGD, Moloney NC, Armstrong MWJ, Ah-See K. Is there evidence base for the practice of ENT surgery? *Clinical Otolaryngology*, 1997; **22:** 152–157.

Barton S. Which clinical studies provide the best evidence? *British Medical Journal*, 2000; **321:** 255–256.

EVOKED RESPONSE AUDIOMETRY

In response to sound stimulation, electrical signals are produced by various parts of the auditory system from cochlea to cortex. Evoked response audiometry (also called electric response audiometry) is a technique designed to measure these signals. No conscious response is required from the patient, so the tests are less open to the bias in results which arise in those tests requiring patient cooperation. However, the tests are not truly objective as a tester will have to interpret the complex tracings obtained from the procedure. In practical terms three main responses can be recorded:

- Electrocochleogram.
- Brainstem electrical response.
- Cortical electrical response.

Electrocochleography

Electrocochleography (ECochG) aims to measure the signal produced by the cochlea and cochlear nerve in response to acoustic stimulation.

Technique

The patient lies comfortably in a soundproof room. A ground electrode is attached to the patient's forehead and a reference electrode to the ipsilateral mastoid. The active electrode is usually a trans-tympanic needle placed on the promontory (canal electrodes may be used but give a less satisfactory signal) after preparation with local anaesthetic. The test signal can be produced using a loudspeaker or headphones (especially if acoustic conditions are less than ideal). As the amplitude of the evoked electrical response is small relative to the body's background electrical noise, a variety of filters and an averaging computer are used. Wideband clicks and high-frequency tone bursts are the usual stimulating test signals.

Physiology

The signal recorded by ECochG is described as a compound action potential. It is diphasic at threshold and has a signal latency which decreases with increasing signal intensity and is made up of three parts:

1. ***The cochlear microphonic.*** This signal is produced by the hair cells and resembles the pattern of the basilar membrane vibration. It has no threshold and increases in amplitude with the stimulus intensity. Its polarity follows that of the test signal.

2. ***The summating potential.*** This complex potential is derived from a variety of sources but in essence is an alteration of the electrical potential baseline (usually negative) in response to a sound stimulus. It is also produced by cochlear hair cells and does not adapt in response to high stimulation rates.

3. **The action potential.** This is the depolarization of the cochlear nerve and is similar in many respects to any neural depolarization. It has a threshold, is independent of signal polarity and exhibits adaptation.

Clinical indications

High-resolution computerized axial tomography and MRI have superseded many older otological investigative techniques and consequently removed many of the indications for EcochG, particularly the search for an acoustic neuroma. In current practice ECochG may be used for:

1. **Threshold testing.** ECochG is the most accurate of the electrical response audiometric techniques for threshold testing and can predict to within 5–10 dB of the psychoacoustic threshold at 3–4 kHz. Unfortunately, it gives little low-frequency information (< 1 kHz) but has the advantage of being a mon-aural test technique and is relatively resistant to minor muscular contractions which would preclude brainstem response audiometry and is unaffected by general anaesthetic. It is therefore particularly useful in very young children or those with neurological disorders.

2. **Investigation of suspected Menière's disease.** Typically there is an increase in the summating potential with a normal action potential in the affected ear.

3. **Intraoperative monitoring during surgery around the inner ear and internal meatus.**

Brainstem electrical response audiometry

Brainstem electrical response audiometry (BERA) records the signals produced in the brain stem detected by electrodes placed over the mastoid, forehead and vertex.

Technique

The patient reclines on a bed or couch. The electrodes are surface electrodes. The active electrode is attached to the vertex, the reference electrode to the ipsilateral (test ear) mastoid process and the ground electrode to the contralateral mastoid process. The hardware and test signals used (wideband clicks and high-frequency tone bursts) are identical to those used for EcochG, but the filter and time window settings are altered. The signals are usually presented using headphones to allow monaural testing. As the evoked responses are so small they are easily masked by other neuro-muscular signals. It is therefore important that the patient stays as still as possible and, because of their size, several thousand responses are analysed as opposed to hundreds in ECochG. The results are analysed by looking at the absolute values for various wave latencies, the so-called I–V latency, and comparing results between the two ears. The accuracy of the I–V latency has been improved by combining ECochG with BERA to aid the detection of wave I.

Physiology

The signal recorded by BERA is made up of a five-wave complex, which is thought to represent successive synapses in the auditory pathway as follows (Jewett classification):

Wave	Site of generation	Latency (msec)
I	Cochlear nerve	2.0
II	Cochlear nucleus	3.0
III	Superior olive	4.7
IV	Lateral lemniscus	5.3
V	Inferior colliculus	5.9

These potentials are very small and rarely reach more than 1 mV (potentials of 10 mV may be obtained in electrocochleography).

Clinical indications

1. **Acoustic neuroma.** One of the main indications for BERA is to exclude an acoustic neuroma (or other brainstem tumour) in patients with asymmetrical hearing loss. In this case the I–V interval in the affected ear should be prolonged by more than 0.4 msec when compared with the normal ear. However, useful results are virtually impossible if the affected ear has very poor thresholds (> 70 dB), and gadolinium-enhanced MRI is a more sensitive and specific test for this condition.

2. **Threshold testing.** This is particularly useful in children as it is non-invasive and not influenced by anaesthetic, but it is not frequency specific.

3. **Brainstem lesions.** BERA can be used to define the site of a brainstem lesion depending on the presence or absence of successive waves. Unusual results may indicate multiple sclerosis.

4. **Intraoperative testing.** The technique may be used as a monitor during tumour surgery designed to preserve hearing.

Cortical electrical response audiometry

The cortical ERA (vertex or V potential) is a relatively late phenomenon and can be detected as a bi- or triphasic wave commencing after 50 msec and continuing beyond 200 msec. It is too late to be considered a primary cortical response and almost certainly represents a secondary, perceptual cortical phenomenon; as such its presence can be associated with clinical hearing. Unfortunately, it is strongly influenced by the patient's conscious level and attendance to the stimulus and so is only of value in the cooperative patient. If feasible it offers excellent frequency specificity.

Technique

The patient sits comfortably in a chair, staying both still and awake, as movement and consciousness level can easily influence the response. Surface electrodes are placed, with active on the vertex, reference on either mastoid process and ground on the forehead. Tone bursts are the preferred test stimuli and are presented by headphones. Fewer than 100 responses need be sampled to achieve a useful result. Threshold is taken as the point at which the V-potential disappears.

Clinical indications

1. *Threshold testing.* In medicolegal cases this is restricted to 1, 2 and 3 kHz; any more would be too time-consuming.

2. *Central deafness.* In rare patients ECochG and BERA are normal but the V-potential is absent.

Further reading

Ballantyne D. *Handbook of Audiological Techniques.* London: Butterworth-Heinemann, 1990.
Hyde ML. Auditory evoked potentials. *Current Opinion in Otolaryngology and Head and Neck Surgery,* 1994; **2:** 177–185.

Related topics of interest

EXAMINATION OF THE EAR

There is absolutely no doubt that you will be asked to assess an ear at some point during the course of any ENT examination. Time taken in practising your technique is therefore well spent. It is not just a question of spotting the particular clinical signs or disease process. The examiner will want to establish that you have an orderly and thorough technique, and that you are able to present your findings accurately and clearly. You will be asked how you would manage the patient, so be thinking about this as you present your examination findings.

Introduce yourself to the patient before starting the examination. Ask which is the better hearing ear. Always begin the examination with the better ear and never touch the patient before asking if there is any tenderness. The ear should be examined with either reflected light from a head mirror or an electric powered head light. When using a head mirror, position the patient to one side of an electric lamp with the light source slightly above the level of the ear. The patient should be seated sideways to the surgeon, who sits opposite the ear to be examined and reflects light on to it.

The pinna

Examine the pinna in front and behind for signs of inflammation or skin lesions. The mastoid process should be carefully examined for scars, redness or tenderness. Be particularly careful not to miss a fading postauricular or endaural scar. Note any discharge from the external auditory meatus as well as any inflammation of the skin. Select a suitably sized speculum for insertion into the external canal. Common examination subjects include congenital lesions of the pinna, cauliflower ears, perichondritis and surgical scars.

The external auditory canal

To examine the external auditory canal, pull the pinna upwards, outwards and backwards. In infants, owing to non-development of the bony external meatus, the pinna has to be drawn downwards and backwards. Introduce the otoscope speculum just past the hairs of the outer canal, but avoid contact with the sensitive bony part of the canal. A good view of the tympanic membrane should then be possible. Common examination subjects include canal stenosis and exostoses.

The tympanic membrane

Look for the prominent lateral process and handle of the malleus. Examine all quadrants of the membrane. The long process of the incus is frequently observed behind and parallel to the handle of the malleus and it is sometimes possible to see it articulate with the head of the stapes.

If there is a perforation note its position, size and whether it is central or marginal. If you do discover a perforation then make sure you can describe what you see looking through it, for example the promontory, round window, incudostapedial joint, dehiscent Fallopian canal or some tympanosclerosis may be visible. A Siegle speculum or otoscope with a pneumatic attachment should be used to assess the mobility of the membrane. Immobility may be due to fluid in the middle ear, a perforation or tympanosclerosis. If the patient has had mastoid surgery determine the type of cavity, assess access (meatoplasty size and height of the facial ridge) and decide if the cavity is healthy or not. Perform a fistula test by applying tragal pressure or preferably use the pneumatic otoscope. Look for conjugate deviation of the eyes away from the examined side and then (whilst maintaining pressure) nystagmus in the direction of the diseased side. Remember to tell the patient what you are doing beforehand.

Hearing tests

Perform free field speech tests by asking the patient to repeat words spoken with a whispered voice, conversation voice and shouted voice at 60 cm from the ear. The non-test ear is masked either by using a Bàràny noise box or by pressing the tragus backwards and rotating it with the index finger. The patient sits side on to the surgeon so that lip reading is not possible.

Use double figure numbers or bisyllable words as the words the patient is asked to repeat should not be easy to guess. The Rinne and Weber tuning fork tests, using a 512 kHz fork, should then be performed to help differentiate between a conductive and sensorineural hearing loss.

Other tests

The postnasal space should be examined to exclude a lesion and if possible to obtain a view of the Eustachian tube orifice. The cranial nerves should be formally examined if there is active ear disease. In a short case examiners will sometimes stipulate that they are only interested in facial nerve function, and this should always be routinely tested in examination of the ear.

Summary of examination of the ear

1. Introduce yourself to the patient.
2. Position the patient.
3. Ascertain which is the better ear and start with this.
4. Inspect the pinna, mastoid and external auditory meatus.
5. Pneumatic otoscopic examination of the tympanic membrane.
6. Fistula test.
7. Free field voice tests.
8. Tuning fork tests.
9. Facial nerve.
10. Postnasal space.

Related topics of interest

Clinical assessment of hearing, p. 45; Examination of the nose, p. 84; Examination of the throat, p. 86.

EXAMINATION OF THE NOSE

The diagnosis in nasal disease is often obvious after an accurate history has been taken. The essential symptoms are nasal obstruction, sneezing, rhinorrhoea, postnasal drip, headache and facial pains, abnormal sense of smell, epistaxis, snoring and cosmetic deformity. A previous history of trauma or allergy may also be relevant. Nasal disease is common, signs can be elicited quickly and management of the common diseases makes good discussion. Common findings are septal deviation, hypertrophied turbinates, septal perforation and nasal polyps. It is therefore essential that you are familiar with the aetiology, relevant investigations and treatments of these conditions. There may be a combination of signs (for example, a deviated septum and nasal polyps) so be thorough with your examination.

Position of the patient

Introduce yourself to the patient and sit opposite with an electric lamp at eye level over the patient's left shoulder. Sit with your knees together and to the right side of the patient's legs. This is more elegant than sitting with your legs astride the patient's.

Inspection of the external nose

Examine the nose in relation to the rest of the patient's face. Pay particular attention to its size and shape: the convexity or concavity of the dorsum, the width or projection of the tip, the deviation of the nose, the shape of the columella and nares. The thickness of the skin may be relevant if cosmetic surgery is contemplated. Look for swelling, bruising, erythema or for ulceration of the skin. An old examination favourite is a patient with the lupus pernio rash of sarcoid on their nose, with a septal perforation. Turn the patient's head to the left and then to the right to check the profile. Be especially vigilant to look for a fading lateral rhinotomy scar or hidden bicoronal incision wound behind the hairline. Lift the tip of the nose with the thumb to obtain a view of the nasal vestibules. The patency of the nasal airway is assessed by occluding each nostril in turn with the tip of the thumb and asking the patient to sniff or alternatively watching the shiny surface of a Lack tongue depressor held under the nose cloud over as the patient exhales.

The nasal cavity

Anterior rhinoscopy is carried out using a Thudichum speculum. Gently introduce this into the nose remembering that the nasal mucosa is very sensitive. If a lesion is immediately obvious, for example nasal polyps or a nasal tumour, note the position in relation to the turbinates and septum. Do not assume that they will be the only abnormality, be thorough in the rest of your examination. Assess the mucosa; note its colour, vascularity and crusting. Examine the septum for its position in relation to the nasal airways; is it deviated to one side or is it dislocated off the maxillary crest? Examine the mucoperichondrium for its colour and vascularity. Note any lesions or perforation of the septum. Examine the lateral nasal wall and evaluate the size and colour of the inferior turbinate. If a better view is needed the nasal mucosa can be shrunk using a local anaesthetic/vasoconstrictor (e.g. 5 or 10% cocaine hydrochloride or phenylephedrine with lignocaine). In clinical practice a 0–4-mm 0° or 30° nasendoscope can be used. This will allow an inspection of the lateral nasal wall and the anatomy (and any pathology) of the middle meatus.

Oral examination

Inspect and percuss the upper teeth. The floor of the maxillary sinus lies over the alveolar process of the maxilla and the roots of the second premolar and first molar teeth. Assess movement of the soft palate and if there is a bifid uvula be aware that this may signify a submucous cleft.

The nasopharynx

Explain to the patient what you are about to do. This is a difficult procedure and needs practice. Warm a small postnasal mirror and pass it through the mouth while gently holding the tongue down with a tongue depressor. Some patients have too strong a gag reflex to allow adequate examination. Report the problem to the examiner and suggest that in normal circumstances you would proceed to use a flexible fibreoptic nasendoscopy after applying topical anaesthetic and decongestant to the nasal airway. Inspect the posterior end of the septum, the posterior choanae, through which the posterior ends of the inferior turbinates may be visible. In the lateral wall the tubal ridges of the pharyngeal ends of the Eustachian tubes can be seen. The fossae of Rosenmüller lie immediately above the tubal orifices and can be the site of a nasopharyngeal carcinoma.

The neck

Inspect and palpate the neck and look for the presence of lymphadenopathy. The lymphatic drainage from the anterior part of the nose is to the submandibular nodes and upper deep cervical nodes. Drainage from the posterior part is to the middle deep cervical nodes.

Summary of examination of the nose

1. Introduce yourself.
2. Position the patient.
3. Inspect the external nose.
4. Examine the nasal tip and vestibule and assess the nasal airways.
5. Anterior rhinoscopy with a Thudichum speculum.
6. Oral examination.
7. Postnasal space examination.
8. Neck.

Related topics of interest

Examination of the ear, p. 82; Examination of the throat, p. 86; Nasal polyps, p. 174; Nasopharyngeal tumours, p. 180.

EXAMINATION OF THE THROAT

The symptoms associated with throat disease include hoarseness, dysphagia, sore throat, lump in the throat, referred otalgia, cough, lump in the neck and weight loss. Throat is a vague term, unfortunately applied indifferently by some examiners to the pharynx and larynx. The technique outlined in this topic is ideal for a long case but may need to be modified for a short case. Listen carefully to the examiner and do what is asked. Unless clearly stipulated, do not assume that the examiner merely wants an indirect laryngoscopy performed. On the other hand, do not irritate the examiner by examining parts of the patient that have not been mentioned. However, if in doubt it is better to be thorough. There are a few scenarios:

- *Examine the patient's throat*: systematically examine the patient's pharynx and larynx as you would any patient in clinic who complained of the aforementioned symptoms.
- *Examine the mouth*: inspect and examine the oral cavity.
- *Examine the patient's neck*: inspect and palpate the neck.

Common findings are patients with vocal cord paralysis, vocal cord oedema, vocal cord polyps, vocal cord nodules, laryngeal papillomas, occasionally patients with a neoplasm and laryngectomy patients.

Position of the patient

A head mirror to reflect light from a bulls eye lamp, or an electric head light can be used. If a head mirror is used, the patient should sit opposite the surgeon with an electric lamp positioned at eye level over the left shoulder. The surgeon should sit with knees together and legs to the right side of the patient's. Ask edentulous patients to remove their dentures. Expose the whole of the neck up to and including the clavicles. Remove any neck scarf which may hide a wound or stoma.

The oral cavity

Inspect the lips for perioral lesions. Ask the patient if there is any tenderness in the mouth. Take two metal tongue depressors and insert them to retract the buccal mucosa on each side. Ask the patient to protrude the tongue and move it from side to side and then up to the palate and down. This should allow an inspection of the dorsal and ventral surfaces of the tongue, the tongue's lateral borders and the floor of the mouth; it also tests hypoglossal nerve function. The two tongue depressors are then used so that the buccal mucosa, teeth and alveolar ridges and the opening of the parotid ducts (opposite the upper second molar) can be examined. Then dispense with one of the tongue depressors and use the other to depress the tongue. Check over the palate, the tonsils and the posterior pharyngeal wall. Ask the patient to say 'aah' and check movement of the palate. Remove the tongue depressor and put a glove on. Bimanually palpate the floor of the mouth overlying the submandibular duct for calculi or masses. Palpate the base of tongue, as a tumour in this site may not be visible but easily palpable.

Postnasal space examination

Explain to the patient what you are about to do. Warm a postnasal mirror and pass it through the mouth while gently holding the tongue down with a tongue depressor. Ask the patient to breath gently through the nose. Look for any obvious lesion, but be particularly vigilant on inspection of the laterally placed Eustachian tube elevations, above which lie the fossae of Rosenmüller, the usual site of origin of nasopharyngeal carcinoma. In clinical practice the PNS can be examined by using a 2.7 mm 30° rigid or flexible nasendoscope.

Indirect laryngoscopy

Explain to the patient what you are about to do. Warm a laryngeal mirror and check its temperature on the back of your hand. Ask the patient to protrude the tongue and gently grasp it with a swab held in the left hand. The patient should then be requested to breathe normally through the mouth as the mirror is introduced gently up to the soft palate. If the patient nose breathes and arches up the tongue, obstructing the view, it is possible to obtain some improvement by asking the patient to quietly make a 'hah' noise breathing in and out. Inspect the base of the tongue, the vallecula and the upper part of the epiglottis. Examine the posterior pharyngeal wall, and then both sides of the epiglottis, the aryepiglottic folds, the pyriform fossae, the arytenoids, the ventricular folds and the vocal cords. Note any inflammation, ulceration or exophytic lesion. The movements of the vocal cords are studied by asking the patient to say 'ee' followed by a deep breath and 'ee' again. Note any abnormal movement or fixation of the cords.

Some patients are unable to cope with an indirect laryngoscopy because of an overactive gag reflex. In these cases it may be possible after spraying the oropharynx with lignocaine. After a few minutes the soft palate and uvula will be anaesthetized. If the patient is still unable to tolerate the procedure spray the nose with local anaesthetic and decongestant and use a flexible nasendoscope. This is usually well tolerated and allows a more thorough inspection and assessment of vocal cord movement. Be sure to tell the patient to avoid food and drink for the next hour because the gag reflex is impaired, and to avoid burning the throat and aspiration. Some patients still need to be assessed under a general anaesthetic. It is unlikely in an examination that the patient will have an overactive gag reflex as patients are specially selected.

Examination of the neck

Check the neck for any obvious skin lesion or ulceration. Be careful not to overlook a fading wound. Check that the patient does not have a stoma. Ask the patient to swallow and watch the larynx move. A thyroid goitre may also be seen moving with the larynx. An enlarged neck mass may be visible: note its position and inform the examiner that you have seen it. Ask the patient to count to 10 and assess the voice. Get the patient to breathe deeply in and out through the mouth and note any stridor.

The neck should be palpated from behind and in an orderly sequence so that no areas are missed. Be gentle. Ask the patient if there is any tenderness. Start at the mastoid bone and palpate down the line of the trapezius muscle and in the posterior triangle down to the clavicle. Feel for supraclavicular and infraclavicular nodes.

Then palpate down the line deep to the anterior border of the sternocleidomastoid muscle for deep cervical nodes. When your fingers reach the suprasternal notch, palpate up the anterior triangle, feeling the trachea, thyroid gland, laryngeal cartilages and hyoid bone. Loss of normal laryngeal crepitus (Trotters sign) may indicate a postcricoid neoplasm. Feel for submental lymph nodes, submandibular nodes, the parotid gland, preauricular nodes and finally occipital nodes. If a lump is felt note its site, size, shape, consistency and fixation to adjacent tissues or skin. If you think a lump is pulsatile or attached to the carotid, auscultate and listen for a bruit. If a lump is palpated in the anterior triangle see whether it moves on swallowing. If you think a lump is cystic see if it transilluminates.

Summary of examination of the throat
- Introduce yourself to the patient.
- Position the patient and expose the neck down to the clavicles.
- Assess speech.
- Oral examination (oral cavity and oropharynx).
- Nasopharynx.
- Indirect laryngoscopy.
- Examination of the neck.

Related topics of interest

Examination of the ear, p. 82; Examination of the nose, p. 84; Laryngeal carcinoma, p. 138; Nasopharyngeal tumours, p. 180; Oral cavity carcinoma, p. 197; Oropharyngeal carcinoma, p. 203.

EXTERNAL EAR CONDITIONS

Ear wax

This chapter confines itself to a discussion of ear wax, keratosis obturans, extostoses and osteomas. Foreign bodies in the ear canal, otitis externa and conjenital abnormalities are discussed elsewhere in separate topics (see Related topics of interest).

Epithelial migration

In all other parts of the body, the superficial keratinized squamous epithelium is constantly shed, usually as a result of friction from clothing or washing. This is not possible in the external ear canal and so it has developed the property of epithelial migration. Squamous epithelium on the tympanic membrane moves radially until it reaches the canal walls, when it moves laterally. When it reaches the hair-bearing cartilaginous portion of the canal the superficial layer starts to separate. It then mixes with the secretion of the ceruminous and pilosebaceous glands and any collected debris to form what we recognize as ear wax. The glands are found in the skin of the outer third of the external acoustic meatus and secrete a liquid material at the base of the hairs. After secretion, evaporation occurs to leave a sticky, waxy substance that is able to trap dirt, squames and microbes with relative ease.

Wax

Wax can be secreted in one of two forms. Wet wax is produced by most people of African origin and caucasians and is familiar as moist, sticky and honey-coloured. The dry type is more common in Mongoloid ethnic groups and tends to be greyer in colour, less sticky, granular and brittle. The gene for wet wax is dominant. Regardless of type, ear wax tends to become drier with age as a result of reduced glandular numbers and activity. Wax is then normally loosened by transmission of movement from the temporomandibular joint from chewing or talking, allowing its passage out of the external auditory meatus. This natural process can be upset by a number of factors and cause wax impaction. Impaction is commoner in males owing to the presence of thicker, coarser hairs in the lateral part of the external auditory meatus (EAM). Narrow canals, zealous use of cotton buds and even a hearing aid mould may impede the normal flow of wax to the periphery. In some people no obvious cause is found to account for the impaction and it has been suggested that desquamation of the superficial layer of the meatal epidermis is impaired.

Clinical features

Impaction of wax can cause a sensation of obstruction, deafness, otalgia, vertigo and coughing (via the auricular branch of the vagus – Arnolds nerve), although wax impaction is a relatively rare cause of hearing loss. Most of these symptoms are improved by removing the wax, which can usually be accomplished easily by syringing.

Management

Syringing involves the use of an old fashioned Higginson or a modern electric-pump syringe. These direct a jet of warm (body temperature) water along the roof or posterior canal wall so that it passes behind the wax and forces it outwards. The procedure is often best preceded by a week or two of ceruminolytic agent use (sodium bicarbonate drops are efficacious, safe and inexpensive). Although relatively safe, complications may occur and include coughing, pain, local trauma, otitis externa and rarely tympanic membrane perforation and otitis media. Contraindications to syringing include frequent previous episodes of otitis externa, a known or suspected perforation and a difficult ear, often caused by a narrow and/or tortuous external meatus. In these cases removal under direct vision with an operating microscope using microsuction or wax-hooks is a more appropriate and safer alternative.

Keratosis obturans

This uncommon condition occurs when there is a failure of the normal process of migration. Keratinocytes and keratin debris collect in the deep part of the external auditory meatus. As with collections of keratin anywhere, this sets up a low-grade inflammatory response. Osteoclast-stimulating mediators are produced, resulting in a resorption of bone and usually a widening of the bony canal.

Clinical features

Patients usually present with an acute exacerbation of the inflammatory process. Otalgia is usually the dominant feature, although there is inevitably a conductive hearing loss from the occluded canal. The otoscopic appearances are similar to an acute otitis externa around impacted wax. The keratin takes this appearance because the part in contact with the air oxidizes and changes colour.

Management

Removal of the keratin plug is essential to control the inflammatory process. This is often difficult as the patient is usually in considerable pain and a general anaesthetic is not infrequently required. Topical antibiotic/steroid combinations are advised to prevent a secondary otitis externa. In the long term these patients require periodic monitoring and aural toilet.

Exostoses and osteomas

Osteomas are uncommon benign tumours of bone usually arising from the tympanosquamous or tympanomastoid suture line. Exostoses, on the other hand, are common. They are hyperostoses of the tympanic bone of the external canal. They appear to be caused by a periosteal reaction to exposure to cold, usually from swimming. In both conditions, although the lumen of the canal may be reduced, they rarely result in symptoms. If problems do occur they are usually related to impairment of the normal process of epithelial migration. In these cases   surgical removal may be indicated. Osteomas can often be removed via the external canal,   while exostoses will more often require a formal postaural or endaural approach.

Further reading

Hanger HC, Mulley GP. Cerumen: its fascination and clinical importance: a review. *Journal of the Royal Society of Medicine*, 1992; **85**: 346–349.

Sheehy JL. Diffuse exostoses and osteomata of the external auditory canal: a report of 100 operations. *Otolaryngology – Head and Neck Surgery*, 1982; **90**: 337–342.

Related topics of interest

Examination of the ear, p. 82; Foreign bodies, p. 103; Otitis externa, p. 209.

FACIAL NERVE PALSY

Although the detailed anatomy of the facial nerve will not be discussed, it is important to appreciate that there are supranuclear or upper motor neurone (motor cortex to pontine facial nuclei) and infranuclear or lower motor neurone causes of a facial nerve palsy. The infranuclear portion can be divided into cerebellopontine angle, meatal, labyrinthine, tympanic, mastoid and extracranial portions.

Communication with the vestibulocochlear nerve occurs within the internal auditory meatus, with the otic ganglion and sympathetic afferents from geniculate ganglion branches and with the auricular branch of the vagus nerve from a branch of the mastoid segment of the facial nerve. Extracranially there are communications with the glossopharyngeal, vagus, greater auricular and the auriculotemporal nerves and multiple communications with branches of the trigeminal nerve. These interconnections explain the mastoid, ear, face and neck pain associated with herpes zoster and Bell's palsy, and the referred otalgia, face, occipital, throat and neck pain which may occur with malignant disease.

Injury may be classified into a neuropraxia, axonotmesis, neurotmesis, partial transection and complete transection. Evoked electromyography and maximal stimulation test response neurophysiological studies show that a neuropraxia injury gives normal results and an axonotmesis up to 10% of normal, but more severe injury gives no response. These studies can be used to provide a prognosis and to indicate if recovery is occurring.

Associated features

Altered facial nerve function occurs with a variety of conditions and in a variety of forms.

1. Synkinesis. The voluntary and reflex movement of groups of muscles that normally do not contract together. For example blinking, may be accompanied by movement of the corner of the mouth. This may occur after neurotmesis (or more severe injury) when the axons do not find their correct endoneural sheath.

2. Hemifacial spasm. This is an intermittent spasm of the orbicularis occuli muscle which may spread to include other or all muscles of facial expression. It is thought to be most commonly caused by compression of the nerve by an artery in the posterior fossa. If this is confirmed by an MRI scan and angiography the cause may be treated surgically. Cerebellopontine angle tumours may also cause this phenomenon.

3. Facial myokymia. In this condition there are multiple fine but asynchronous facial movements. It is associated with brain stem gliomas and multiple sclerosis.

4. Blepharospasm. This is unilateral or more commonly bilateral involuntary spasmodic eye closure. Injection of botulinum A toxin into the orbicularis oculi may provide temporary relief.

5. Crocodile tears. Lacrimation with eating can occur as a result of facial nerve injury in the region of the geniculate ganglion, where motor axons find the myelin sheath within the greater petrosal nerve.

Severity grading

The most commonly used system is that of House and Brackmann which grades from 1: normal function in all areas, to grade 6: total paralysis. Factors such as symmetry, resting tone and muscular movement at forehead, eye and mouth are used to score the dysfunction.

All ENT medical staff should grade all new facial palsy patients and follow-ups according to the House–Brackmann grading system (reproduced from House JW, Brackman DE. *Otolaryngology and Head and Neck Surgery* 1985; **93**: 146–147, with permission from Mosby Inc.).

Grade	Characteristics
I – Normal	Normal facial function in all areas

II – Mild dysfunction	Gross
	  Slight weakness noticeable on close inspection
	  May have slight synkinesis. At rest, normal symmetry and tone
	Motion
	  Forehead: moderate-to-good function
	  Eye: complete closure with effort
	  Mouth: slightly weak with maximum effort

III – Moderate dysfunction	Gross
	  Obvious, but not disfiguring difference between the two sides
	  Noticeable, but not severe synkinesis, contracture or hemi-facial spasm
	  At rest, normal symmetry and tone
	Motion
	  Forehead: slight-to-moderate movement
	  Eye: complete closure with effort
	  Mouth: slightly weak with maximum effort

IV – Moderately severe dysfunction	Gross
	  Obvious weakness and/or disfiguring asymmetry
	  At rest, normal symmetry and tone
	Motion
	  Forehead: none
	  Eye: incomplete closure
	  Mouth: asymmetric with maximum effort

V – Severe dysfunction	Gross
	  Only barely perceptible motion
	  At rest, asymmetry
	Motion
	  Forehead: none
	  Eye: incomplete closure
	  Mouth: slight movement

VI – Total paralysis	No movement at all

Causes

1. Bell's palsy (55%).   An acute lower motor neurone facial palsy of unknown aetiology and therefore a diagnosis of exclusion. It is probably a virally induced immune response that leads to inflammation, swelling and consequent impaired function of the facial nerve.

2. Ramsay Hunt syndrome (synonym: herpes zoster oticus) (7%).   Caused by herpes zoster virus.

3. Trauma (19%).   This may be external or iatrogenic. External trauma includes head injuries or penetrating trauma, usually in the parotid region.

4. Tumour (6%).   These may arise from the nerve (facial nerve Schwannoma), external compression of the nerve (vestibular nerve schwannoma), or invasion of the nerve (most commonly with parotid tumours).

5. Infection (4%).   A lower motor neurone facial palsy may occur with acute suppurative otitis media (in the 8% who have a dehiscent Fallopian canal), chronic suppurative otitis media either with or without cholesteatoma and malignant otitis externa.

6. Central causes.   For example secondary to multiple sclerosis, gliomas or cerebrovascular accidents.

7. Other causes.   For example sarcoid, drugs, myasthenia gravis and Guillain–Barré syndrome.

Clinical features

In Bell's palsy the facial nerve palsy is usually of rapid onset and associated with otalgia, altered facial sensation and taste. It recurs in 12%, more commonly on the contralateral side. Severe otalgia with vesicles involving the external ear associated with crusting, external ear canal oedema, a sensorineural hearing loss, tinnitus and vertigo are all common in Ramsay Hunt syndrome. The communications of the facial nerve may allow the face, neck tongue, palate and buccal mucosa to become involved. It rarely recurs, but only 60% recover to House and Brackmann grade 1 or 2. When trauma has caused the palsy, it is important to know the severity of a palsy as soon as possible after nerve injury as this will influence the management. Facial nerve palsies caused by tumours and infection are discussed elsewhere (see Related topics of interest).

Investigations

A high-resolution CT or MRI scan to include the petrous temporal bone will exclude cerebellopontine angle tumours as a source of the palsy, sometimes necessary in suspected Bell's palsy as this is a diagnosis of exclusion. It may localize injury in cases due to trauma or chronic suppurative otitis media. An evoked electromyogram (EEMG), in which a stimulating electrode is placed adjacent to the stylomastoid foramen and recording electrodes are placed either on the skin over the facial muscles or through the skin into the muscles, is helpful. If the EEMG response remains above 10% of normal during the first 10 days after injury there is an excellent chance of grade 1 or 2 recovery (85%). The prognosis overall for those below this level is only a 20% chance of achieving grade 1 or 2 recovery, and many surgeons will therefore advocate surgical decompression of the nerve in these circumstances.

Management

1. *General.* Reassurance and explanation are essential for all patients. Eye care is mandatory in order to prevent corneal ulceration and comprises artificial tears, eye closure with tape on to which is applied a light pressure dressing of cotton wool, ointment at night and eye protection when outdoors on windy or hot dry days with an eye pad. In patients with marked symptoms a lateral tarsorrhaphy or the insertion of a gold weight into the upper eyelid may be necessary as a permanent or temporary manoeuvre to ensure adequate eye closure.

2. *Specific.*

(a) *Bell's palsy.* Although no placebo-controlled double-blind trial has been reported, many practitioners advocate a short course of steroids provided there are no contraindications in the patient's medical history. Some groups also advocate the use of acyclovir as viral antigens have been found. Fisch advocates early decompression of the meatal portion of the facial nerve by a middle fossa approach, as this is the portion most often implicated as being affected in Bell's palsy.

(b) *Ramsay Hunt syndrome.* The commencement of acyclovir 800 mg five times daily for 7 days as early as possible during an attack may reduce the length of the infection and postherpetic neuralgia. Adequate analgesia is essential, and splinting the external ear canal with a pope wick expanded with antibiotic/steroid drops will reduce the otalgia.

(c) *Trauma.* If a complete lower motor neurone facial palsy is noted immediately after external trauma, this suggests that the nerve has been severed, and immediate exploration is indicated. It is preferable to anastomose the proximal to the distal stump after each has been prepared to present a clean surface. This must be performed without tension on the nerve, and should this not be possible after preparation of the stumps, perhaps because significant debridement was necessary or the injury involved a significant length of nerve, then a cable of sural or great auricular nerve is necessary. A partial palsy or a delayed onset of a palsy can be managed conservatively with sequential EEMG monitoring.

(d) *Tumour.* The facial nerve is usually sacrificed if it has been infiltrated by tumour which cannot therefore be teased off the nerve. A cable graft is indicated in these circumstances.

(e) *Infection.* The management in these circumstances is discussed elsewhere (see Related topics of interest). In summary, a palsy secondary to ASOM should be treated conservatively but that secondary to CSOM requires mastoid exploration to eradicate the underlying disease, although formal decompression of the nerve is probably unnecessary.

Follow-up and aftercare

If no recovery of function has occurred within a year of injury in those with a severe or complete palsy (grade 5 or 6), a permanent facial reanimation procedure, e.g. temporalis muscle sling or a gold weight for the upper eyelid, may be indicated.

Adequate counselling regarding eye care is essential. Maximum recovery may take 12 months so that no decision regarding permanent facial reanimation procedures should be undertaken until then.

Further reading

Bradford CR. Facial reanimation. *Current Opinion in Otolaryngology and Head and Neck Surgery*, 1994; **4**: 369–374.

El-Kashlan H and Kileny P. Outpatient facial nerve evoked electromyography testing. *Current Opinion in Otolaryngology and Head and Neck Surgery*, 1998; **6**: 334–337.

House JW, Brackman DE. Facial nerve grading system. *Otolaryngology and Head and Neck Surgery*, 1985; **93**: 146–147.

Related topics of interest

Acute suppurative otitis media, p. 5; Chronic suppurative otitis media, p. 38; Cosmetic surgery, p. 63.

FACIAL PAIN AND HEADACHE

A. Leach

The head and neck is an anatomically and neurologically complex region. It is unsurprising that pain arising from there is often misunderstood, misdiagnosed and mistreated. Up to 50% of cases of facial pain never receive a definitive diagnosis; tribute is paid to this fact by the plethora of treatment options.

If facial pain is to be successfully managed it is essential to spend sufficient time with the patient to elicit a full history. The reader is reminded of the definition of pain issued in 1986 by the International Association for the Study of Pain which reads as follows:

> Pain is an unpleasant sensory and emotional experience associated with actual or potential tissue damage or expressed in terms of such damage.

It is inevitable that the sufferer will have a significant emotional component to the pain, particularly if symptoms have been present for some time, and successful pain management will not be achieved without acknowledgement of this fact.

When taking a pain history, the patient will frequently find it difficult to convey the experience of pain to the listener. He should be encouraged to use descriptive terms, such as *burning, cramping, throbbing, stabbing* which are of more value in suggesting diagnosis than words that indicate intensity e.g. *sore, agonizing, excruciating.*

A number of pain assessment tools have been developed which may aid the clinician in accurately defining the pain. The McGill Pain Questionnaire attempts to define the qualitative aspects of pain, while the Visual Analogue Scale is the most widely-used pain intensity measure.

Classification of headache

Headache is a common presenting complaint. The International Headache Society has provided a detailed classification of headache. Some of the more common diagnoses and their management are discussed briefly.

- Migraine.
- Tension-type headache.
- Cluster headache and chronic paroxysmal hemicrania.
- Miscellaneous headaches unassociated with structural lesion.
- Headache or facial pain associated with disorder of cranium, neck, eyes, ears, nose, sinuses, teeth, mouth or other cranial or facial structures (referred pain).
- Cranial neuralgias, nerve trunk pain and deafferentation pain.
- Headache associated with:
  - head trauma
  - vascular disorders
  - nonvascular intracranial disorder
  - substances or their withdrawal
  - noncephalic infection
  - metabolic disorders
- Headache, non-classifiable.

The full classification has many subgroups within each diagnostic category (for example, there are seventeen subgroups within the 'migraine' section). It is beyond the scope of this chapter to list them all.

Migraine

The prevalence of migraine headache in the general population is said to be 10–15%. Onset of symptoms is usually between puberty and the fifth decade. It is more common in women and there is often a family history. Only about 10% of migraine headaches exhibit the classical signs of aura (most commonly a visual phenomenon, but may take the form of dysaesthesia in the ipsilateral limb or face and as a mood change) which precedes the headache by 10–60 minutes. The characteristic feature of migraine is its throbbing nature, which is usually unilateral in onset, but which may spread to involve the whole head and face and is accompanied by photo- and phonophobia and nausea. It lasts for 4–72 hours and the sufferer is free of pain between attacks. Precipitating factors include psychological stress, endocrine changes (such as menstruation) and dietary intake (especially tyramine-containing foods and irregular meals). The aetiology is not fully understood, although there is undoubtedly a vascular component. A rise in cerebral blood flow in the occipito-parietal cortex precedes the headache, and this is followed by a 25% reduction in flow spreading forwards from the occipital region. These changes seem to account for the symptoms of aura. The headache itself is probably due to the dilatation of cranial non-cerebral vessels. Experimental studies in animals suggest that the trigemino-vascular system is the final common pathway where the migraine headache is generated.

Treatment consists of symptomatic relief with analgesics and anti-emetics. An impending attack may be aborted with an ergotamine preparation taken orally or by inhaler. Also available is sumatriptan, a cranio-selective 5-HT1 agonist, which is effective at any stage of an attack when given by subcutaneous injection. Prophylaxis consists largely in avoiding precipitating factors. Drugs such as β-blockers, pizotifen, diltiazem, methysergide and cyproheptadine have all been used in an attempt to stabilize the cranial circulation.

Cluster headache

This is a rare but important cause of unilateral facial pain. It takes its title from the grouping together of attacks into clusters, consisting of 1–8 headaches per day for 3–12 weeks. Symptom-free periods of 3–18 months separate the clusters. Diagnosis is sometimes confused with trigeminal neuralgia. A careful history will reveal clear differences from TGN by duration of attacks, associated symptoms and temporal profile. Age of onset is between 20 and 40 years and there is a male–female ratio of 7:1. The pain is deep and throbbing and is extremely severe. It may appear at the same time each day during a cluster and may wake the subject from sleep. There are always associated autonomic phenomena such as nasal congestion, injected conjunctivae and facial sweating. Each attack lasts for 15 minutes to 3 hours.

Symptom relief during an attack may be achieved with oxygen, which causes transient cerebral vasoconstriction, ergotamine subcutaneously or by inhaler, or sphenopalatine ganglion block with intranasal local anaesthetic. For prophylaxis such drugs as prednisolone in a reducing dose, methysergide (long-term use may cause retroperitoneal fibrosis) and calcium channel blockers have all met with some success. Sumatriptan given by subcutaneous injection may relieve an attack.

Tension headache (also called myofascial headache)

Considering that muscle accounts for about 30% of body weight, it is overlooked surprisingly often as a source of chronic pain. Lack of a diagnosis rapidly results in frustration for the physician and loss of confidence in his or her abilities by the patient.

This is described as a deep, dull, aching, pressure-like pain which may be uni- or bilateral, and of gradual or sudden onset. There are no neurological abnormalities. Myofascial pain is usually associated with trigger points in the muscle and its surrounding fascia, which refer either locally or to a distant site which is usually unrelated dermatomally or myotomally. Trigger points are palpable as tender bands within the muscle which, when pressed, will either reproduce the patient's pain or refer it to a characteristic reference zone. Trigger points are thought to arise following muscle trauma, either as a single event or a repeated micro-trauma, such as poor posture or teeth grinding. Certain muscles appear to be particularly prone to developing trigger points, including sternomastoid, temporalis, pterygoids, trapeziums and neck strap muscles. Pain is often referred forward from the occipital region to the temple, forehead, orbit or ear.

Treatment consists essentially in restoring normal function to the affected muscles by gentle stretching and mobilization. To permit this it is helpful to reduce discomfort in the muscle body with cooling spray, ice, local anaesthetic injection or acupuncture needling of trigger points. The assistance of physiotherapists may be useful. If the pain has remained undiagnosed for some time it is common for a degree of pain behaviour to have developed. In this situation psychological therapy may be required, coupled with such techniques as deep relaxation and counselling to improve the patient's insight into the condition. Chronic tension headache does not respond well to analgesics and the most effective medication may be amitriptyline. Tension headaches and migraine may be related and may co-exist.

Temperomandibular joint (TMJ) dysfunction

When anatomical disturbance of the TMJ occurs, an associated myofascial syndrome commonly develops. TMJ problems manifest themselves as clicking or popping in the joint, pain on chewing or mouth opening and locking if the internal derangement is severe. Myofascial pain usually appears on the affected side, although it may in time become bilateral as a result of a general chronic tensing of head and neck muscles and assumption of a protective posture. A sensation of fullness or congestion in the ear may be mentioned. Diagnosis is confirmed by observing restricted mouth-opening (less than 40mm inter-incisal), eliciting TMJ tenderness and clicking, There will usually be trigger points in associated muscle groups, in particular the medial and lateral pterygoid muscles.

Treatment consists of physical therapy to the painful muscles and a dental splint which is usually worn at night to reposition the mandible and prevent bruxism (teeth grinding).

Trigeminal neuralgia (TGN)

The principal sensory nerve to the head is the trigeminal nerve. TGN, also called *tic douloureux*, is an agonizingly painful condition which usually affects 50–70-year-olds, although it has been described outside these age limits. It affects men and women equally. In the first half of the last (20th) century, before effective remedies were widely available, it was associated with a high incidence of suicide. Diagnosis must demonstrate three elements:

1. Pain occurs within one or more divisions of the trigeminal nerve.
2. Pain is described as a brief intense electric shock or knife-like sensation.
3. Pain is elicited by normally-innocuous stimulation of a trigger zone.

The mandibular (III) division is the most commonly affected, followed by the maxillary (II) and ophthalmic (I) divisions. The pain can induce spasms of the facial muscles on the affected side (hence *tic*). Bilateral symptoms are rare. It is believed to be caused by local demyelination of the trigeminal root entry zone, most usually due to compression by a small, tortuous artery or vein in the posterior cranial fossa. MRI of sufficiently high resolution may demonstrate such a vessel, and may also help to exclude other causes of these symptoms such as multiple sclerosis, acoustic neuroma, base of skull tumours and vascular anomalies such as aneurysms and vertebrobasilar atherosclerosis.

Treatment should start with an anticonvulsant. Carbamazepine (100–400 mg tds) is the most widely used drug, although other anticonvulsants such as clonazepam and phenytoin have been used. Gabapentin (100–300 mg tds) has had promising results in treating neuropathic pain and has been awarded a product licence for this indication. Side-effects may be problematic, especially in the elderly patient. Alternatively, destructive lesions to the Gasserian ganglion with alcohol or glycerol injection, or radio-frequencey diathermy are usually effective, although patients must be warned that symptom relief will be accompanied by sensory loss to the affected part of the face. Pain commonly returns 6 months to 5 years after this, necessitating a repeat.

If a vascular loop has been demonstrated by MRI, decompression of the nerve root via posterior fossa craniotomy has a high chance of prolonged symptom relief. However, surgery of this nature carries significant morbidity, especially in the elderly, and less invasive treatments are the rule. Although rarer, other cranial nerves may give rise to neuralgia whose manifestation is identical to TGN. Glossopharyngeal neuralgia (GPN) is characterized by stabs of pain in the ear, base of tongue, tonsillar fossa or beneath the angle of the mandible. Triggers include talking, swallowing and coughing. Adequate pain relief is important, as malnutrition due to inability to swallow is a distinct possibility. Neuralgia of the nervus intermedius is felt deeply in the ear, lasting for seconds or minutes, with a trigger zone in the posterior wall of the auditory canal. As with TGN, an aberrant vascular loop may be demonstrated near the nerve's origin. It has been suggested that GPN may be associated with an unusually long styloid process irritating the nerve.

Acute herpes zoster

Most individuals acquire varicella zoster virus during childhood infection with chicken pox. It appears that the virus may lie dormant in the dorsal root ganglia of peripheral nerves for many years until opportunistically reactivating, causing an antidromic infection along the nerve. Infection is commoner in the elderly and the immunocompromised. It presents with itching, pain, dysaesthesia and paraesthesia along the course of the affected nerve, followed a few days later by cutaneous vesicular eruptions. These form scabs within a week or so and heal within a month, though this may take longer in the immunocompromised patient. For reasons which are not understood, the ophthalmic division of the trigeminal nerve and the fourth to tenth thoracic nerves are more commonly affected than others.

Treatment of acute zoster consists of pain relief and in speeding resolution of skin lesions. Analgesics and acyclovir should be given systemically. Early treatment with tricyclic antidepressants has been recommended, both as an analgesic for the acute condition, and as an attempt to diminish the development of post-herpetic neuralgia (*vide infra*). Pain in ophthalmic zoster is relieved by stellate ganglion block with local anaesthetic, although such relief is limited to its duration of action. A number of small, uncontrolled studies have suggested that aggressive early therapy reduces the incidence of postherpetic neuralgia, although attempts to confirm this finding have been inconclusive. Constitutional upset frequently accompanies acute zoster and it may take weeks or even months for an elderly patient to recover fully.

Postherpetic neuralgia (PHN)

Diagnosis of PHN is rarely difficult, but treatment often defies the efforts of the most determined physician. A recent history of herpes zoster infection is followed by the development of pain in the affected area. The incidence is reported as being up to 50% following acute infection. It is more likely to develop in elderly patients, and two studies indicate that women are affected more than men in a ratio of 3:2. The pain experienced is usually burning, but occasionally throbbing or stabbing. There is commonly an accompanying sensory deficit and allodynia (pain caused by a normally innocuous stimulus) to light touch is often a feature. It is thought that this phenomenon is caused by alteration of the modulating effect of large-diameter sensory nerves (proprioception) at the dorsal root entry zone (i.e. the pain gate is held wide open) following viral damage during the acute infection. The ability of nerve fibres to repair themselves diminishes with age, which may account for the increased incidence of PHN with advancing years.

Treatment of burning pain and dysaesthesia is best achieved with tricyclic antidepressants such as amitriptyline in the lowest effective dose, since the incidence of dose-related side-effects is high in the elderly. The mechanism of action of these drugs is unknown, although they undoubtedly influence neurotransmitter systems high in the CNS. Anticonvulsants such as carbamazepine, gabapentin and valproate may help lancinating pain, and techniques such as transcutaneous electrical nerve stimulation (TENS) and acupuncture may also be of value. Also available is a topical preparation of capsaicin, extracted from chilli peppers, which acts by depleting substance P levels (an important neurotransmitter in pain fibres). It is most effective in treating burning pain.

Summary

> This is by no means a complete guide to diagnosis and treatment of facial pain. Careful consideration must be given to the history and symptomatology, and examination must always include full assessment of cranial nerve function.

Related topics of interest

Functional endoscopic sinus surgery, p. 108; Sinusitis, p. 285.

FOREIGN BODIES

Foreign bodies in the nose

Nasal foreign bodies are most commonly found in 2- to 3-year-old children. They may be inorganic or organic. Inorganic foreign bodies include buttons, beads, metal, plastic from toys, and stones. They are often asymptomatic and may be discovered only accidentally during an examination for an unrelated complaint. Organic foreign bodies include sponge, rubber, paper, wood, peas, and nuts. These are irritant and the nasal mucosa usually becomes involved in an inflammatory reaction causing a nasal discharge. A unilateral nasal discharge is nearly always due to a foreign body. This is initially mucoid, but will eventually become mucopurulent and finally odiferous mucopus, which may be blood stained. Inflammation and infection of the paranasal sinuses may complicate the problem. Occasionally deposits of calcium and magnesium carbonates and phosphates takes place around a foreign body to form a rhinolith, which will require removal under general anaesthetic.

Management

Confirmation of the presence of the foreign body is from the history and examination of the child. Examination of the anterior nares is often possible with a head mirror or electric head lamp, reflecting light on to the elevated tip of the nose. The child sits on either a parent's or nurse's knee. If nothing is visible then an auriscope may give a better view. It is possible in many children to remove the foreign body without the need for general anaesthesia. The child must be cooperative and the surgeon gently reassuring. Have good illumination and all the instruments possibly required to hand. The first effort will be the best and often the only attempt the child will allow. If this fails or if the foreign body is situated posteriorly in the nasal cavity then a general anaesthetic will be required.

Treatment

Removal is best accomplished with a wax hook or an old Eustachian tube catheter. It is passed point downwards above the foreign body, which is brought to the floor of the nose and raked anteriorly.

Cupped forceps are preferable for the removal of thin objects, such as buttons, or soft organic objects such as sponge.

In every case the nasal cavity must be examined afterwards as there may be a second foreign body more posteriorly. The child should be discharged with a supply of Naseptin nasal barrier cream and oral antibiotics if there is any obvious infection.

Foreign bodies in the ear

Foreign bodies are inserted into the ears more commonly by school children than by toddlers. The objects found can be organic (pieces of paper, rubber, pencil, seeds, peas and beans) or inorganic (beads, buttons, crayons and stones). Inorganic foreign bodies are often asymptomatic, but organic objects may give rise to otitis externa by local irritation of the epithelium of the meatal walls. One of the commonest causes of this is cotton wool, and it is not unusual to find this in adult patients who have been attempting to clean their ears.

Management

A foreign body in the external ear canal is usually easily seen on otoscopy. Removal may appear to be easy, but usually requires the skills and facilities of a specialist. Ill-directed attempts at their removal by the untrained may lead to complications. It is sometimes possible to remove the foreign body in the clinic, but a general anaesthetic may be required for children and sensitive adults.

Treatment

As a general rule, most foreign bodies can be removed by syringing. Objects of vegetable origin, such as peas, beans and nuts, are hygroscopic and should not be syringed. Large objects lying superficial to the external ear canal isthmus should not be syringed as there is a danger of wedging them in that area.

Suction or a fine hook may be used, with the object viewed with an operating microscope, to remove material of vegetable origin and large objects which lie superficial to the isthmus.

Forceps are useful for soft material such as paper, cotton wool or sponge. Forceps should never be used to remove smooth spherical objects such as beads, as they will tend to push them further down the ear canal.

Insects should be killed before syringing by instilling spirit drops into the ear canal. Maggots grip on the external ear-canal skin, so must be killed or anaesthetized with chloroform water prior to syringing.

It is rarely necessary to extract a foreign body through the posterior canal wall after a postaural incision. This is useful if permeatal extraction is not possible because of swelling of the canal walls from irritation, or if a large object has lodged at the isthmus. Once the object is out, the tympanic membrane should be examined to ensure it has not been damaged. If there is an otitis externa a swab should be taken, the ear should be cleaned, and antibiotic-steroid ear drops should be instilled.

Foreign bodies in the pharynx

Sharp and irregular foreign bodies may become impacted in the tonsils, base of tongue, vallecula or pyriform fossae. Small fish bones are the commonest and usually lodge in the tonsil.

Management

The patient, usually an adult, will be able to localize the side and site with reasonable accuracy. A thorough examination with light reflected from a head mirror, a tongue depressor and laryngeal mirror should reveal the offending bone. If the patient cannot tolerate indirect laryngoscopy and a foreign body is suspected in the vallecula or base of tongue, then examination with a nasendoscope is useful. In some patients there will be no abnormal findings and a lateral soft-tissue radiograph is indicated. If this too is normal they should be reassured and reviewed 2 days later. By this time the sensation will usually have passed, but if there are persistent symptoms the patient should be re-examined.

Treatment

After the foreign body has been visualized, the pharynx should be anaesthetized with lignocaine spray. It is then often possible to grasp the foreign body with forceps and remove it swiftly and painlessly.

Some fibreoptic nasendoscopes have a side arm which facilitate forceps and can be used to remove foreign bodies.

In a patient anaesthetized with lignocaine spray and positioned on a flat bed with the neck and shoulders supported on a pillow it is sometimes possible to pass the blade of a McGill laryngoscope to depress the tongue. This has its own light source and may help locate a foreign body in the pharynx. The surgeon's free hand can then be used to remove the object with forceps.

Patients who have been anaesthetized with lignocaine spray should be warned not to eat or drink for 2 hours as the pharynx will be relatively insensitive.

General anaesthesia is required to remove a foreign body from the pharynx if the patient is young or unable to tolerate the above manoeuvres.

Foreign bodies in the oesophagus

Impaction of a foreign body depends chiefly on the size and shape of the object. The presence of an abnormality in the patient's aerodigestive tract, for example a stricture, will make impaction more likely. A large bolus of food swallowed hurriedly may become impacted even in a normal oesophagus. Mentally handicapped and some psychiatric patients are at particular risk. The commonest objects are coins in children and fish or meat bones in adults. Impaction is commonest at the level of the cricopharyngeus muscle, but may also occur at the level where the oesophagus is crossed by the left main bronchus or at the cardia.

Clinical features

Adults are usually aware of having swallowed something and can localize fairly accurately the level at which it is impacted. Children and psychiatric patients may not be so reliable. Discomfort or pain in the oesophagus and difficulty in swallowing are the cardinal symptoms. Dysphagia may be total. The foreign body may cause coughing and excessive salivation. Clinical examination may be normal, but pooling in the pyriform fossae on indirect laryngoscopy is sometimes evident. There may be localized tenderness in the neck and crepitus owing to surgical emphysema if there has been an oesophageal perforation.

Investigations

Lateral and anteroposterior soft-tissue radiographs of the neck and chest radiographs are mandatory. Some foreign bodies are easily identified because they are radio-opaque. The inexperienced may confuse calcification in the laryngeal cartilages with an opaque foreign body. Widening of the postcricoid space or a persistent air bubble in the oesophagus may occur. If the foreign body has caused a tear, surgical emphysema will be shown radiologically. Barium swallow as an investigation is condemned because it makes subsequent oesophagoscopy and identification of a foreign body more difficult, though Omnopaque 500 contrast medium can be used because it is clear.

Treatment

If the obstruction is due to an impacted food bolus, the safest treatment is to admit the patient and give a dose of intravenous hyoscine butylbromide and diazepam. This will usually allow the oesophagus to relax and permit the passage of the bolus. Some surgeons have suggested that the ingestion of cola fizzy drinks will encourage this process. The patient should have a barium swallow 2 weeks later to exclude an oesophageal neoplasm. If there is sharp or bony object, the patient requires an oesophagoscopy as soon as possible. Using a rigid oesophagoscope the foreign body is identified and if possible drawn into the end of the scope using forceps. The scope and the foreign body should be withdrawn in unison under direct vision. The patient should remain in hospital for 24 hours postoperatively and receive nil by mouth for the first 4 hours and only water for the next 4 hours. If there is a mucosal injury the patient should have antibiotic cover. The neck should be examined to exclude surgical emphysema on the day of discharge. Perforation of the oesophagus should be treated with intravenous antibiotics and nasogastric feeding. Surgical repair should be considered depending on its site and extent.

Foreign bodies in the trachea and bronchi

Inhalation of a foreign object is most common in children under the age of 3 years. The event can easily escape a parent's notice. Any unexplained choking fit on the part of the child should be treated with suspicion, especially if any small object with which the child happened to be playing cannot be found. Adults usually give a clear history of foreign body inhalation. Most inhaled foreign bodies enter the right main bronchus, which is larger and more vertical than the left.

Clinical features

After the initial inhalation, which causes choking and coughing, and sometimes cyanosis, the foreign body may pass symptomless into the trachea. For this reason, if there is a good history suggestive of inhalation of an object, the child should have a bronchoscopy. There may, however, be a cough with inspiratory and expiratory stridor, or a wheeze. A foreign body which is causing a complete obstruction of a bronchus will produce a collapse of that lung segment, followed by consolidation. A foreign body may partly occlude the bronchus and act like a valve so that the partly obstructed lung becomes overinflated. Vegetable foreign bodies are particularly dangerous (nuts, pips, vegetables, fruits) as they will cause an intense inflammatory reaction of the bronchial mucosa leading to a pneumonitis.

Investigations

Lateral and anteroposterior chest radiographs are mandatory. Opaque objects are easily identified. Radiolucent objects are suspected when there is unexplained atelectasis, obstructive emphysema, mediastinal shift or consolidation of the lung.

Treatment

Bronchoscopy should be performed as soon as possible. A senior ENT surgeon and anaesthetist are required. A variety of bronchoscopes, suction tubes and forceps appropriate to the nature of the foreign body and size of the patient need to be readily available. Flexible fibreoptic bronchoscopes are used in some centres. Storz or similar instruments with Hopkins rod telescopes should be available with young children.

Removal via a thoracotomy is sometimes necessary if the foreign body cannot be retrieved by endoscopic methods.

Antibiotics and physiotherapy may be necessary if there is any sign of pneumonitis. A tracheostomy may be needed if there is oedema or obstruction of the larynx, either prior to or after bronchoscopy.

Further reading

Spector BC, Garret CG. Endoscopy and removal of foreign bodies. *Current Opinion in Otolaryngology and Head and Neck Surgery*, 1998; **6**: 416–420.

Related topics of interest

Paediatric airway problems, p. 232; Paediatric endoscopy, p. 237.

FUNCTIONAL ENDOSCOPIC SINUS SURGERY

Principle

Most infections of the sinuses are rhinogenic, i.e. disease spreads from the nose to the paranasal sinuses. The anterior ethmoid sinus air cells and clefts are regarded as pre-chambers of the dependant frontal and maxillary sinuses. Disease of these pre-chambers may interfere with ventilation and drainage of the dependant sinuses and cause acute or chronic mucosal disease. Similarly, disease of the posterior ethmoid sinuses may interfere with ventilation and drainage of the sphenoid sinus. Endo-scopic sinus surgery is minimally invasive surgery, which aims to provide ventilation and drainage of the ethmoid sinuses and the secondarily involved maxillary, frontal and sphenoid sinuses. The emphasis of surgery is to preserve, as far as possible, nor-mal anatomy and to preserve mucosa. Mucosal stripping leaves exposed sinus bone, which does not reline with ciliated respiratory epithelium, but usually a low colum-nella non-ciliated epithelium. Scarring and non-ciliation may lead to an irreversible impediment of ventilation and drainage, emphasising the importance of good sur-gical technique.

Pathophysiology

Mucus produced in the maxillary sinus is transported from the floor of the sinus along the sinus walls, to the natural ostium by the mucous ciliary transport. The frontal and maxillary sinuses communicate with the nose through a complex system of narrow clefts, which allow drainage and ventilation. These clefts are only a few millimetres wide and contain opposing mucosal surfaces lined with ciliated respira-tory epithelium. If extensive contact of opposing mucosal surfaces occurs, whatever the cause, the ciliary beat activity may be impeded so that spaces are blocked and do not drain. Common locations for contact areas in the sinuses include the frontal recess and ethmoidal infundibulum, the cleft between the uncinate process and the middle turbinate, between the ethmoid bulla and the middle turbinate, and in the lateral sinus, which lies above and behind the ethmoid bulla. Anatomical variance of the middle turbinate, uncinate process and the ethmoid bulla are common. The inci-dence of these variants is the same between a population with no history of sinus disease and a population with recurrent acute or chronic sinusitis. Therefore anatomical variations, while of academic interest, are not thought to predispose to sinusitis. Persistent mucosal disease of the ethmoidal infundibulum, frontal recess and posterior ethmoids may predispose patients to recurrent maxillary, frontal sinus and sphenoid sinus infection.

Indications for endoscopic sinus surgery

- Recurrent acute rhinosinusitis.
- Chronic rhinosinusitis.
- Polypoidal rhinosinopathy.

- Mucoceles.
- Sinus mycosis.
- Adjuvant surgery to allergy treatment.
- Antrochoanal polyps.
- Endoscopic bipolar diathermy for posterior epistaxis.

Extended applications
- Endoscopic spheno-palatine artery ligation for epistaxis;
- Endoscopic arrest of CSF rhinorrhoea;
- Endoscopic orbital decompression, most commonly for dysthyroid eye disease;
- Endoscopic drainage of an orbital abscess;
- Endoscopic dacryocystorhinostomy;
- Endoscopic optic nerve decompression;
- Endoscopic pituitary surgery.

Extensive experience and expertise is necessary in basic endoscopic sinus surgery before training in extended applications is undertaken. Certain patients may not benefit from endoscopic surgery. These include those with malignant sino-nasal tumours and those with inaccessible lateral frontal sinus disease, for example lateral frontal sinus mucoceles. Revision cases can be challenging, particularly if primary surgery performed by inexperienced surgeons has caused a lack of anatomical landmarks, significant scarring and narrowing of natural ostia due to mucosal stripping.

Investigations

A high definition CT scan of the paranasal sinuses on bone setting is required before undertaking endoscopic sinus surgery (except for the treatment of epistaxis). A common protocol would be a coronal CT scan with 5 mm cuts of 1 mm thickness, with two axial cuts to allow the orientation of the internal carotid artery and optic nerve in the region of the posterior ethmoid and sphenoid sinus to be identified. Variations from the standard protocol might be necessary from time to time, for example 1 or 2 mm coronal cuts of the frontal recess might be requested in difficult revision cases. In patients who have failed maximum medical therapy for recurrent acute or chronic rhinosinusitis or polypoidal rhinosinopathy, a CT scan should be requested to confirm that there is persistent disease amenable to endoscopic sinus surgery (the scan will provide details of sinus anatomy and disease extent). Patients should have agreed to surgery if the CT scan confirms this is necessary.

Surgical technique

Surgery limited to the anterior ethmoids may be performed under local anaesthetic with topical vasoconstriction and sedation, but more extensive surgery, for example frontal recess surgery and posterior ethmoid surgery requires a general anaesthetic. The aim of surgery is to re-establish ventilation and drainage of the affected paranasal sinus group. Surgery is performed in a stepwise manner from front to back (Messerklinger technique) or from the sphenoid forward (Wigand technique). Through-cutting instruments which cleanly cut through mucosa and bone of sinus air cells, and prevent avulsion and stripping of mucosa are a recent advance. The microdebrider cleanly cuts and aspirates tissue suctioned into the debrider opening.

In experienced hands the micro-debrider can be used for a complete spheno-ethmoidectomy. Although it is an extremely efficient way of clearing soft tissue disease, and in particular polypoidal rhinosinopathy, its detractors claim its usefulness for bone work is not proven as it may cause excessive scarring. It may, in the unwary, cause disastrous orbital injuries by rapidly sucking and debriding the orbital contents if the lamina papyracea is breached. The majority of experienced endoscopic surgeons in the UK have both through cutting instruments and the microdebrider to hand during surgery.

Complications

Complications of endoscopic sinus surgery may be life threatening or cause significant long term morbidity to patients. Complications may be reduced by a thorough understanding of sinus anatomy, extensive cadaver dissection and observation of experienced surgeons in the surgical technique. Attendance at a post graduate course would be of considerable benefit to those who are novices in endoscopic surgery. The inexperienced surgeon should be closely supervised by an experienced endoscopic sinus surgeon. Many complications occur due to not recognising sinus anatomy, or to working in a poor surgical field, due to intra-operative bleeding. Major complications are particularly likely to happen once the surgeon has gained some confidence and experience in the technique, but has not yet learned the finer points of anatomy, or when to stop during a procedure. If the surgeon is uncertain as to the anatomy, or cannot visualise landmarks due to bleeding, then he should ask for advice, or if this is not available then stop the operation. It is much better to complete the surgery with a second stage procedure than to cause a major complication at the initial procedure.

1. **Per-operative**
   - Anaesthetic reaction.
   - Bleeding.
   - Penetration of the lamina papyracea to cause periorbital bruising or an orbital injury such as a medial rectus or an optic nerve injury.
   - CSF leak due to penetration of the skull base.
   - Nasolacrimal duct injury.
   - Injury to structures impinging upon the lateral sphenoid sinus wall, namely the internal carotid artery and optic nerve.

2. **Immediate post-operative**
   - Intraorbital bleeding.
   - Epistaxis.

Blindness and diplopia from per-operative complications will only become apparent on patient waking.

3. **Early post-operative**
   - CSF leak (sometimes an unrecognised intra-operative complication).
   - Intracranial infection (meningitis, brain abscess).

4. Late complications

- Intranasal adhesions, particularly within the ethmoidal cavity, between the middle turbinate and septum, or between the lateral nasal wall and nasal septum.
- Sequelae of per-operative and early post-operative complications.
- Recurrent disease.

Management of major complications

1. CSF rhinorrhoea. A CSF leak is the commonest major complication of endoscopic sinus surgery. If the leak is identified at the time of surgery then the site of the leak should be confirmed and the leak arrested. There are many techniques described to arrest the CSF leak, but the commonest methods are using a middle turbinate flap, or a free turbinate graft to plug the defect, or to use temporalis fascia and muscle. Tisseel glue may be used to obtain a good seal with a piece of silastic used to separate the graft from intranasal packing, which is left *in situ* for several days. A lumber drain is usually unnecessary.

2. Intraorbital bleed. This is one of the most feared complications of endoscopic sinus surgery and occurs when the anterior ethmoid artery has been divided during surgery and retracts into the orbit while continuing to bleed. It is most likely to happen when the artery is divided when lying within a bony canal running from the orbit to the anterior cranial fossa, as in these circumstances there will be no soft tissue attachments preventing the artery from retracting into the orbit. An intra-orbital bleed caused by such an event will cause the eye to rapidly bulge and become tense, and rapid decompression of the orbit is ne-cessary to save the patient's vision.

It has been recommended that a lateral canthotomy be performed, perhaps with division of the orbital septum in the lower lid, to allow the orbital contents to flow laterally and anteriorly. However, most surgeons will not have seen nor performed this procedure before and with a patients vision in immediate danger it is arguably not the time to start. Most would advocate an external ethmoid approach to the anterior ethmoid artery which is diathermied or ligated. The lamina papyracea is removed and a formal orbital decompression performed with incision of the orbital septum as for dysthyroid eye disease. This will allow orbital fat and soft tissues to herniate into the ethmoids and will also provide drainage for any continued bleeding. An endoscopic medial approach is an alternative for the experienced. Since the surgeon has already performed an ethmoidectomy and the lamina papyracea is exposed, it can be removed endoscopically. Endoscopic orbital decompression has the dis-advantage of making identification of the bleeding anterior ethmoid vessel more difficult should a subsequent search be made for the vessel via an external approach.

Follow up and after care

Epithelialization of the ethmoid cavity is usually complete within 3 or 4 weeks of surgery. Some authorities still propose de-crusting of the ethmoid cavity every few days following surgery. Most surgeons now feel that this delays mucosal healing and removal of adherent crusts may predispose to greater scarring by causing delayed healing. Post operative nasal douching, morning and night, to remove nasal crusts and secretions is advised. This usually allows the ethmoid cavity to heal and to become crust-free at 2 weeks post surgery obviating the need to remove persisting crusts. Post operative steroids and antibiotics may be indicated depending on the surgeon's preference and the underlying disease process.

Future developments

The past three years has seen major advancements in the development of image guidance systems which provide three-dimensional images of the location of a probe within the sinuses. This system will be of especial use in patients with difficult anatomy and in revision cases. It can locate the frontal sinus ostium, the sphenoid sinus and the skull base. Its application is currently not justified for routine endoscopic work. This perception may change if a system is developed which can be set up rapidly in theatre or if medico-legal developments make it a requirement.

Further reading

Zweig JL, Schaitkin BM, Yang F, Barnes EL. Microdebrider technique: implications for endoscopic sinus surgery. *Am. J. Rhinol.* 2000; **1**: 27–33..

Neuman AM, Pasquale – Niebles K, Bhuta T, Sillers MJ. Image-guided transnasal endoscopic surgery of the paranasal sinuses and anterior skull base. *Am. J. Rhinol.* 1999; **6**: 449–455.

Related topics of interest

Allergic rhinitis, p. 11; Nasal polyps, p. 174; Sinusitis, p. 285.

GLOBUS PHARYNGEUS

Globus pharyngeus (globus syndrome, globus hystericus) is the sensation of a lump, discomfort or foreign body in the throat for which there is no obvious cause.

Pathophysiology

A number of organic aetiological theories have been proposed; the two most strongly supported are the suggestion that it represents a manifestation of reflux oesophagitis or is a disorder of pharyngeal and oesophageal motility. Disorders of motor function have certainly been demonstrated in globus patients, including elevation of cricopharyngeal sphincter pressure, mid-oesophageal dysmotility and poor lower oesophageal sphincter relaxation, but there is still debate as to whether these are primary or secondary phenomena. Pharyngeal pH measurements tend to be normal in such patients. What is undisputed is that globus patients have much higher levels of psychological distress (than the general population) in the form of anxiety, somatic concern, neuroticism and even depression. Many people suffer from globus sensation for whatever underlying reason at some time in their life. It is the patient's psychological profile that dictates whether it becomes a problem. In this group of patients a vicious cycle is created where somatic concern and anxiety only serve to further aggravate the symptom. This cycle of events is very similar to that seen in tinnitus and thus may represent another disorder of perception.

Clinical features

Patients are more often women, usually in their fifth decade. The complaint is typically of a lump in the throat, usually at the region of the sternal notch, although it may be felt higher and to be unilateral. Although patients may complain of some subjective difficulty in swallowing, true difficulties are never a feature; for many the symptom actually improves during feeding. The sensation is often intermittent and variable in severity. Many patients seem anxious and introspective. Physical examination is normal, although one must be alert for any physical cause for the symptom such as a foreign body or an inflammatory cause. Occasionally tenosynovitis of the digastric tendon as it runs through its sling on the hyoid may be the cause. This can be very rewarding to treat with a local anaesthetic/steroid injection. In particular, a neoplastic lesion should be excluded, which is what many of these patients are most concerned about.

Investigations

Most clinicians would perform a chest radiograph and a barium swallow in spite of a typical history and a normal clinical examination and the likelihood that these will be normal. The radiologist should be encouraged to pay particular attention to the hypopharynx during the examination. In those patients with persistent or suspicious symptoms, endoscopy is indicated. Ambulatory pH measurement and manometry are sometimes used although they rarely add much to the clinical picture.

Management

There is no specific treatment for globus pharyngeus. Strong and appropriate reassurance at all stages is invaluable. Reflux oesophagitis should be treated with antacids, H2 antagonists (e.g. ranitidine) or a proton pump inhibitor (e.g. lansoprazole or omeprazole). Relaxation therapy can be suggested for those who are tense and over-anxious. Antidepressants may be required for those patients who are clinically depressed. Smoking should be discouraged.

Follow-up and aftercare

Most patients are happy once reassured that they do not have cancer or other serious pathology, and follow-up is not usually required.

Further reading

Wilson JA. Globus sensation. *Clinical Otolaryngology*, 1992; **17**: 105–106.

Related topics of interest

Hypopharyngeal carcinoma, p. 124; Pharyngeal pouch, p. 246.

HALITOSIS

Aetiology and pathophysiology

Halitosis is a problem that not uncommonly presents to the ENT surgeon and may be subjective or objective. The causes can be divided into three broad categories: local, general and drugs. Local and general causes overlap when general or systemic conditions give rise to a dry mouth.

1. Local causes.   Saliva plays a crucial role in the oral cavity and is involved in taste, lubrication, water balance and oral hygiene. Saliva acts as a mechanical cleansing agent, its contained buffers combat acid/alkali excesses and the secreted immunoglobulins have an important anti-infective function. Any significant reduction in salivary flow allows an increase in the local bacterial flora. These micro-organisms break down proteins with the production of odiferous volatile gases and consequent halitosis (as well as leading to an increase in dental caries and peri-odontal disease, in themselves a cause of halitosis). A decrease in saliva production can occur temporarily, as during sleep and with anxiety, or more permanently as a result of previous radiotherapy, cardiac and renal failure and some autoimmune conditions (Sjögren's syndrome). Any local inflammatory lesion is likely to become secondarily infected and lead to halitosis. Examples include any oral ulcerative lesion (from aphthous to neoplastic), tonsillitis, pharyngitis and nasal and sinus infections.

2. General causes.   Certain foods, alcohol and cigarettes all give rise to a charac-teristic unpleasant smell on the breath. A reduction in food intake during any sys-temic illness will lead to ketosis and typical ketotic breath. Diabetes can lead to a sweet acetone smell, uraemia a smell of ammonia, liver failure a smell of decaying blood and chest infections a peculiarly foul anaerobic smell. The latter is particularly common in bronchiectasis. Reflux of partially digested stomach contents into the oesophagus as a result of hiatus hernia is another cause. There are some patients who complain bitterly of halitosis for which there is no objective support. This may rep-resent a monosymptomatic hypochondriacal condition, and these patients may be severely depressed.

3. Drugs.   Drugs can cause halitosis by several mechanisms: they may cause a dry mouth (anticholinergics), they may alter the normal oral and pharyngeal flora (antibiotics) or their metabolites may be excreted by the lungs (chloral hydrate, iodine-based medications).

Clinical features

Halitosis is usually due to local causes. It is commonest in those with poor dental hygiene and peridontal disease. There is a natural decline in salivary flow and increase in dental disease with age. A full history should be taken to establish any possible systemic or drug causes. Clinical examination should establish objective evidence of halitosis. A useful manoeuvre is to ask the patient to breathe through the mouth and the nose separately; if the smell is still present when breathing through the nose, an extraoral cause should be suspected.

Investigations

Investigations should be directed at the suspected cause and might include a chest radiograph and blood tests to exclude systemic disease.

Management

Management should obviously be directed at the underlying cause and will often fall outside the remit of the ENT surgeon. Those with systemic causes and severe chest disease will require referral to an appropriate physician. Patients with a psychological problem may require referral to a psychiatrist. Periodontal disease will require the services of a dental practitioner. Most oral inflammatory conditions will resolve spontaneously, but any that persist demand biopsy and subsequent definitive treatment. Pharyngitis, tonsillitis and sinonasal disease can all be treated appropriately by the ENT surgeon.

General advice on adequate dental care, good fluid intake should be given. In some patients with objective halitosis and little pathology, a lengthy (2 to 3 months) trial of low dose antibiotics to alter the local bacterial flora can be helpful.

Follow-up and aftercare

This will be dictated by the underlying cause.

Further reading

Symposium on dry mouth and halitosis. *The Practitioner*, 1990; **234:** 603–619.

Related topics of interest

Sinusitis, p. 285; Intrinsic rhinitis, p. 131; Tonsil diseases, p. 330.

HEARING AIDS

A hearing aid is any device that amplifies sound or assists the hearing-impaired individual, but in the present context will be taken to mean an electro-acoustic device used to amplify sounds. Cochlear implants can be included in this definition, but they are described in a separate topic.

Design

It is important to be familiar with the basic design of the hearing aid as many patients attending the ENT department are prescribed them. There is a good chance you will be handed one and asked to describe it in an examination.

The basic components of any hearing aid are a receiver (microphone and/or induction coil), an amplifier/processor, a sound transmitter (earphone, bone conductor) and a power source (primary cell). There are two types of signal processing systems – analogue and more recently digital.

1. Analogue systems. In analogue systems, an acoustic signal is converted to its electrical analogue at the microphone stage of the hearing aid circuit. That is, an acoustic signal is constantly varying in sound pressure. When converted to an electrical analogue, the varying sound pressure is changed to a varying voltage. The amplitude of these voltages can be controlled so as to emphasize selected frequency regions, as well as carrying out other processing tasks.

In order to avoid the problem of excessive amplification of loud sounds which may cause discomfort to the user, analogue amplifiers can use one of two methods of reducing sudden peaks of sound.

(a) *Peak clipping.* In essence this system basically chops the tops off the peaks of sound. It has the advantage of being simple and instant but does result in some distortion.

(b) *Automatic gain control.* This system involves some complicated circuitry that picks up the signal and compresses it so that the maximum sound peak is never above a set maximum value. It is a little more complicated but produces less distortion.

The external controls are usually a selector switch and a volume control. The selector switch has three markings; O is for off, T is for a television or telephone induction coil and M is for the microphone. Internal controls on the amplifier/processor are often available to alter the frequency response and spread of volume control available to the user. Some analogue aids can now be digitally programmed to alter their processing performance.

2. Digital signal processing. Digital is best defined as sound that is represented mathematically. When digital signal processing (DSP) is used, the acoustic signal is converted to its electrical analogue at the microphone stage of the hearing aid system. After this conversion, a frequency filter is introduced to reduce possible distortion of the input signal, which is then sampled a defined number of times per second (normally, 10 000 times per second or greater). The analogue signal is then converted to its digital equivalent at the analogue to digital stage (A/D). Each of the samples receives a digital code. Binary numbers (0 and 1) are used to represent the digital value of each sample. Following the digitization of the signal, the digital representations are processed by a central processing unit (CPU) or microprocessor. The digital values can be multiplied, divided, added, subtracted and grouped in defined ways. In the microprocessor are various algorithms. For example, one algorithm may control the frequency response of the instrument, another may control loudness growth, a third may function to enhance the speech signal in a background of noise, etc. After the microprocessor has performed its tasks, the digitized signal must be converted back to its analogue equivalent. This is accomplished at the digital to analogue conversion stage (D/A). It is then again frequency filtered and amplified in the conventional manner and submitted to the 'loud-speaker' of the hearing aid.

The obvious advantage of digital signal processing is that there are unlimited ways in which the signal can be manipulated. The numbers of parameters that can be utilized are significantly greater than those found in conventional analogue systems. As such, the ability to manipulate the signal to the acoustic needs of the patient is greatly enhanced, and this without excessive battery current demands.

Types of aid

As things currently stand most NHS aids are analogue in design. However the government have recently announced a 'Beacon Site project' to look at the logistics and feasibility of providing digital hearing aids through the NHS. Most digital aids are the same basic design as NHS aids, but as the DSP 'chip' is so much smaller than the corresponding analogue circuit they tend to be smaller and are often 'in the ear' (ITE) or even 'in the canal' (ITC) aids.

1. ***Postaural aids.*** In most common usage are the standard behind-the-ear (BEHA) aids, available on the NHS. The body of the aid sits behind the wearer's ear and is normally connected by a hollow plastic tube to an ear mould, which allows sound passage to the ear. There are three main groups of BE aids, the 10, 30 and 50 series, with the power of the aids increasing correspondingly. Within each series are a number of models with differing patterns of frequency response. All contain an induction coil which can be used with telephones, televisions and in theatres and cinemas, fitted with induction loops, to bypass much of the unwanted background noise.

2. ***ITE or ITC aids.*** These commonly available commercial aids sit in the concha or canal. Their external shell is usually of acrylic and conforms to the shape of the wearer's ear. They are less obtrusive than the standard BE aids but are expensive and occasionally prone to feedback problems due to the proximity of microphone and 'speaker'.

3. ***Body-worn (BW) aids.*** These rather cumbersome, ugly aids are usually worn with a strap around the neck and the body of the aid on the patient's chest. By virtue of their size they can be made very powerful, and the distance between microphone and earphone means that, even with high amplification, feedback is rarely a problem. They are, however, prone to picking up the sounds of rustling clothes. There are two series available on the NHS: BW 60 and BW 80.

4. Bone conduction aids. These are very similar to the standard body-worn aid but feed their output to a bone conductor rather than an earphone. They are indicated because of meatal discharge or stenosis, or subjective preference for bone conduction reception.

5. Osseointegrated hearing aids. Conventional bone conduction aids have drawbacks, such as bulkiness and discomfort. In addition, the skull cannot be vibrated directly, but only through the energy-absorbing skin and soft tissues. Bone-anchored hearing aids largely overcome these problems. There are two devices in clinical use, both relying on the transmission of mechanical vibrations to the bone of the skull.

(a) In the bone-anchored hearing aid (BAHA) a percutaneous titanium abutment is fixed to a titanium screw implanted in the mastoid. A vibrator is then mounted directly on to the abutment, which is fed either from a microphone and circuit in a small box with the vibrator or from a body-worn hearing aid (for higher output power).

(b) The Xomed audiant bone conductor consists of an encased rare earth magnet implanted completely under the skin and fixed into bone with a titanium screw. Externally, another magnet serves to hold its surrounding induction coil in place over the implanted magnet. By passing electric currents (derived from what is essentially a hearing aid) through the induction coil, an electromagnetic field is set up that causes the implanted magnet, and hence the skull, to vibrate.

6. Implantable middle ear aids. The Symphonix sound bridge works on a similar principle to the Xomed audiant except that the external magnet vibrates a coil that is attached to the patient's incus, thus directly vibrating the ossicles.

7. Spectacle aids. These involve modification of standard spectacle frames to incorporate a hearing aid. They can then be used in a number of ways: as a standard hearing aid, as a bone conductor or for contralateral routing of signal (CROS). In this last variation, sound is picked up from one side of the head and fed to the contralateral side, which is often the good side.

Choice of aid

Many factors will influence the choice of hearing aid. The actual degree and nature of the hearing loss will dictate the amplification characteristics. The cause of the deafness will influence the type of aid chosen, as will vanity and available finance. It is important to establish the patient's requirements and to remember that an aid will not cure the underlying disease.

1. Type. A spectacle-type aid is useful for those people who regularly wear glasses as they are relatively inconspicuous. They are often chosen when there is one very deaf ear and a requirement for contralateral signal routing. A bone conduction aid is ideal in those cases where a hearing loss exists in association with active outer- or middle-ear inflammatory pathology. A body-worn aid is useful for anyone with a profound hearing loss. For most NHS patients an ear-level aid will be found to be suitable.

2. Amplification characteristics. The pattern of frequency response chosen depends very much on the shape of the audiogram. As for amplification, a hearing aid must function in a relatively narrow dynamic range, providing adequate amplification to overcome the hearing loss, but not over-amplifying sound and causing recruitment and consequent discomfort and intolerance. In an effort to overcome this problem, a number of formulae have been developed to calculate the appropriate amplification for the patient's hearing loss (half-gain rule, Berger's procedure, POGO 2, NAL-R, etc.). All formulae give differing importance to differing frequencies, with maximum importance for hearing loss at the main speech frequencies of 1000 and 2000 Hz. Many patients with deafness have a high frequency loss with comparative sparing of the lower frequencies. Most hearing aids can be adjusted to alter their frequency response, for instance high tone boost and base tone cut. More flexibility exists with digital signal processing.

3. Ear moulds. A number of modifications can be made to the ear mould. These may be made for both auditory and medical reasons. Venting the mould will reduce the low-frequency response. In patients prone to otitis externa, it is useful to ventilate or even skeletonize the mould to provide aeration. Unfortunately, feedback becomes more likely with a high-power aid if the mould is vented.

4. General. Although it is preferable to provide binaural aids in cases of bilateral hearing loss, this is rarely possible in the NHS on the grounds of cost, although the National Institute for Clinical Excellence (NICE) have recently endorsed this approach. Which ear to fit the aid in will then depend on a number of factors, including patient preference, available dynamic range and discrimination scores in each ear. The presence of any active inflammatory process in either ear, as well as other medical factors such as manual dexterity relating to arthritis, strokes, amputations, etc. also have a bearing.

Follow-up and aftercare

After the initial fitting, a period of support and rehabilitation is essential to allow the patient to gain confidence, iron out early teething troubles and achieve useful function with the hearing aid. In fact some would argue that this process is more important than the aid itself.

Further reading

Ballantyne D. *Handbook of audiological techniques.* London: Butterworth-Heinemann, 1990.
The Hearing Aid revolution. *ENT News,* Jan/Feb 2000, Volume 8(6).
National Institute for Clinical Excellence. *Technology appraisal guidance No. 8. Guidance on hearing aid technology,* July 2000.

Related topics of interest

HIV INFECTION

Aetiology

Acquired immunodeficiency syndrome (AIDS) is caused by two of five human retroviruses: human immunodeficiency viruses (HIV) 1 and 2. (The other three are T-cell leukaemia viruses and are associated with lymphomas and leukaemias.)

Pathology

HIV-1 is prevalent worldwide, while HIV-2 is found mainly in west Africa. HIV infects cells bearing the CD4 antigen, which acts as a virus receptor. Such cells are monocytes, macrophages and T-helper cells. The HIV-1 glycoprotein, gp120, binds to CD4 and allows the virus to enter the cell. Viral replication may occur in cells in which HIV-1 DNA has been integrated (productive infection), although in some cells containing integrated HIV-1 DNA, the virus does not replicate except when the cell is activated by antigenic stimulation (latent infection), for example by Epstein-Barr virus or cytomegalovirus infection. Ultimately, a functional impairment and depletion of T-helper cells occurs, but to a degree that is disproportionate to the number of cells infected. The mechanism of this has yet to be elucidated, but may relate to damage to lymph node architecture. The ultimate consequence is a compromise of the host immune system. Immunosuppression places the victim at risk of developing opportunistic infections and unusual malignancies, particularly B-cell lymphoma and Kaposi's sarcoma.

Clinical features

AIDS is defined as the development of a complication of immunosuppression such as malignancy or opportunistic infection in an HIV-positive individual. The CD4+ T-cell count will be less than 200/mm^3. Although the time to development of AIDS is variable, the majority of infected individuals in developed countries will develop AIDS about 10–11 years after infection with HIV, in the absence of treatment. So far only about 2% of infected individuals have avoided progression to AIDS. It is invariably fatal, with nearly two-thirds of reported sufferers in the USA already dead. There are various methods of transmission, but all demand close contact with infected body fluids, particularly blood. High-risk groups include intravenous drug users, homosexual males, heterosexual contact with an infected partner and children of infected mothers. Although transfusion of blood products, particularly in haemophiliacs, resulted in a significant number of cases, the screening of all blood products for HIV-1 and HIV-2 antibody has greatly reduced but not irradicated the risk because it may take up to 4 months for seroconversion (the interval between infection and the appearance of antibody).

AIDS-related complex (ARC) comprises persistent fever lasting longer than 3 months, weight loss, leucopenia, anaemia and diarrhoea. The CD4+ T-cell count is less than 400/mm^3. Typical patients are in one of the high-risk groups and, excluding children, are usually between the ages of 20 and 40.

ENT disorders and HIV infection

Between 40 and 70% of patients will have head and neck manifestations. AIDS patients are prone to a variety of conditions:

1. Otological. Otitis media and externa (particularly fungal) are more common. Kaposi's sarcoma of the pinna or external auditory meatus may occur.

2. Rhinological. Chronic rhinosinusitis may occur because of the debilitated state of the patient. Acute sinus infections may occur and unusual organisms such as yeasts and fungi are not uncommon. Kaposi's sarcoma and lymphomas may be found in the nasopharynx.

3. Oropharyngeal. The oral cavity is one of the most commonly affected sites. Kaposi's sarcoma is not uncommon. Severe candidiasis is frequent and may spread to involve the pharynx and larynx. Herpes simplex ulceration is also common and tends to be widespread and severe. Xerostomia is a frequent complaint and epiglottitis is reported to occur more often.

4. Neck. Neck abscess may occur and tend to be deep. They often culture unusual organisms, e.g. atypical mycobacteria. Salivary glands may enlarge.

Generalized cervical lymphadenopathy is a frequent finding in all AIDS patients.

Investigations

The diagnosis of HIV infection depends on detecting the virus or the host response to it in the blood. Usually this is done by identifying a specific antibody, using first an enzyme-linked immunosorbent assay (ELISA) as a screen, followed by western blot confirmation. Plasma HIV RNA assays give useful information when measured sequentially about both disease progression and response to anti-viral treatment. Monitoring of the CD4+ T-cell count is helpful as a surrogate measure of immune function. Opportunistic infections are diagnosed by appropriate sampling and microbiological culturing. Neoplastic lesions are confirmed histologically on biopsy. Other investigations (e.g. radiology) are dictated by the clinical conditions.

Management

The management of HIV infection as it presents to the ENT surgeon and the management of the patient so as to avoid the risks of infection pose separate problems. The occurrence of unusual organisms requires a high index of suspicion to make the diagnosis followed by appropriate therapy. Radiotherapy and chemotherapy may be used for Kaposi's sarcoma and lymphomas.

Risk of infection

The risk of infection to a health care worker from an HIV-positive patient is extremely low and invariably relates to blood exposure. To reduce this risk, two sets of common sense recommendations have developed.

- Universal precautions should be adopted for all patients and involve the use of gowns and gloves to avoid blood contamination. All non-intact skin surfaces should be covered and sharps should be handled with appropriate caution.

- Theatre precautions apply to any invasive procedure on a proven or suspected HIV-positive patient. A high level of discipline is required in these cases. The most senior or experienced surgeon/clinician should operate and theatre/ancillary staff should be kept to a minimum. All staff should be fully gowned and double gloved and boots and eye protection should be worn. Drapes should be disposable and double bagged at the end of the procedure. The patient need not be last on the list, but the theatre should be thoroughly cleaned with hypochlorite solution prior to the next case. There is no evidence of infection risk from the anaesthetic system, but sensible hygienic measures should be employed.

Should inoculation occur, and for other HIV infected individuals, combination therapy may be used. Appropriate serological monitoring is then required over a period of several months. Current effective anti-viral agents include Protease Inhibitors (PI), Non-Nucleoside (NNRTI) and Nucleoside Analogue (NARTI) Reverse Transcriptase Inhibitors. Generally 'triple' therapy is recommended to avoid drug resistance in a very similar fashion to treatment of tuberculosis.

The General Medical Council recommends that a HIV-positive clinician should not perform invasive procedures.

Follow-up and aftercare

In general terms these patients are best cared for in a centre with a team with a particular interest in AIDS.

Further reading

Gold JWM. HIV-1 infection: diagnosis and management. *Medical Clinics of North America*, 1992; **76**: 1–18.

Joint Working Party of the Hospital Infection Society and Surgical Infection Study Group. Risk to surgeons and patients from HIV and hepatitis: guidelines on precautions and management of exposure to blood or body fluids. *British Medical Journal*, 1992; **305**: 1337–1343.

Lucente FE. Otolaryngologic aspects of the acquired immunodeficiency syndrome. *Medical Clinics of North America*, 1991; **75**: 1389–1399.

Related topics of interest

Cervical lymphadenopathy, p. 29; Salivary gland diseases, p. 271; Sinusitus, p. 285; Halitosis, p. 115; Otitis externa, p. 209.

HYPOPHARYNGEAL CARCINOMA

The hypopharynx extends from the lower limit of the oropharynx at the level of the hyoid bone down to the lower level of the cricoid cartilage at the opening of the oesophagus. For the purposes of tumour classification the UICC recognizes three anatomical sites:

1. *Postcricoid* (The pharyngo-oesophageal junction). Extends from the level of the arytenoid cartilages and connecting folds to the inferior margin of the cricoid cartilage, thus forming the anterior wall of the hypopharynx.
2. *Piriform fossa*. This extends from the pharyngoepiglottic fold to the opening of the oesophagus. It is bounded medially by the aryepiglottic folds and laterally by the inner surface of the thyroid cartilage.
3. *Posterior pharyngeal wall*. Extends from the level of the floor of the vallecula to the level of the inferior border of the cricoid cartilage.

Pathology

More than 90% of tumours of the hypopharynx are squamous cell carcinoma. Other epithelial and mesodermal tumours of benign and malignant behaviour do occur, but they are rare.

Carcinoma of the hypopharynx in itself is an uncommon disease with a prevalence of less than 1 per 100 000 population. It is a disease of the elderly and the incidence is higher in men than in women. In the postcricoid site the reverse is true. Although tobacco smoking and alcohol have been implicated as aetiological agents, the association is not as clear as with other upper aerodigestive tract tumours. Approximately 2% of patients with the Paterson-Kelly-Brown syndrome (iron deficiency anaemia, glossitis, angular stomatitis, pharyngeal web, koilonychia and splenomegaly) will develop postcricoid carcinoma. A few patients who had irradiation for thyrotoxicosis many years ago are now presenting with pharyngeal carcinoma after a latent period of 25–30 years.

Hypopharyngeal tumours are sometimes so advanced when first seen that it is difficult to determine the site of origin, but the piriform fossa (60%) is the most common site, with postcricoid carcinoma (30%) and posterior pharyngeal wall tumours (10%) occurring less often. Tumours of the posterior pharyngeal wall and the upper piriform fossa tend to be exophytic, whereas an ulcerated lesion is typical of the other parts of the hypopharynx. Tumours of the lateral wall of the piriform fossa may invade the thyrohyoid membrane and present as a palpable neck mass which may represent direct extension of the tumour rather than an enlarged lymph node. Medial wall tumours invade the aryepiglottic fold and into the paraglottic space, causing fixation of the vocal cord and consequent hoarseness. Dissemination of hypopharyngeal tumours in the submucosal lymphatics leads to a high incidence of 'skip lesions'. More than 10% of patients have a second tumour in the oesophagus. Hypopharyngeal tumours also have a propensity to metastasize to cervical lymph nodes. The piriform fossa has the richest lymphatic drainage, and more than two-thirds of these patients will have lymph node metastases at presentation, with half of these being bilateral. Postcricoid tumours have a tendency to spread to paratracheal nodes.

Clinical features

Early symptoms include the sensation of a lump or discomfort in the throat. Later the patient will usually present with dysphagia, at first for solids then for fluids. Hoarseness may occur as a result of invasion of the larynx or vocal cord paralysis. The patient with advanced disease may have anorexia and weight loss. There may be a history of food sticking and repeated aspirations which will cause pneumonia. Indirect laryngoscopy may reveal an obvious tumour or oedema of the arytenoids with pooling of saliva in the piriform fossa. There may be vocal cord fixation. The neck must be examined for lymph node metastases. Laryngeal crepitus is lost in postcricoid tumours and occasionally a direct extension of the tumour through the thyrohyoid membrane is palpable.

Investigations

1. Laboratory tests. A full blood count to exclude anaemia and biochemical tests are required as electrolyte disturbances are not infrequent.

2. Radiography. A soft-tissue neck radiograph is of limited value, but it may show a shadow posterior to the trachea. This can be regarded as abnormal if it is wider than the thickness of a vertebral body. Every patient who presents with swallowing difficulty or the sensation of a lump in the throat should have a barium swallow, which will usually demonstrate the presence and extent of any hypopharyngeal tumour or oesophageal lesion. MRI is preferable to CT scanning in delineating the extent and spread of tumour. A chest radiograph is mandatory to exclude metastases and to demonstrate any consolidation due to aspiration.

3. Endoscopy. Direct laryngoscopy and oesophagoscopy should be performed in every patient who has an abnormal barium swallow or persistent symptoms despite a normal barium swallow. This allows staging of the tumour and a representative biopsy to be taken. Bronchoscopy should be performed to look for any spread to the trachea. The extent of the lesion, particularly its upper and lower limits, need to be assessed. Digital examination of the tumour is appropriate if there is superior spread, and all patients should have their necks palpated again while they are under the general anaesthetic. Management of the patient will depend on, among other factors, the site and extent of the disease.

TNM Stage

T1 Tumour limited to one subsite of hypopharynx and 2 cm or less in greatest dimension

T2 Tumour invades more than one subsite of hypopharynx or an adjacent site, or measures 2–4 cm in greatest dimension.

T3 Tumour measures more than 4 cm in greatest dimension, or with fixation of the hemilarynx.

T4 Tumour invades adjacent structures e.g. thyroid/cricoid cartilage, neck soft tissues, prevertebral fascia, and/or oesophagus.

Management

Hypopharyngeal carcinoma generally has a poor prognosis even with extensive surgery, and 60% of patients are dead within a year of diagnosis. Because of the low survival and high recurrence rate the choice of treatment is particularly important. The optimal treatment modality should provide the best chance of cure, the lowest mortality and morbidity, the shortest hospital stay and the highest chance of good upper aerodigestive tract function (speech and swallowing).

All patients should have some treatment to their neck. In patients with an N0 neck the overall risk of occult nodal metastases may be as high as 40–60%. Bilateral nodal involvement is common. Therefore treatment of both sides of the neck and the retropharyngeal lymph nodes with either surgery or radiotherapy must be considered electively. Metastases are most common in levels II, III and IV. A lateral selective neck dissection is therefore appropriate if surgery is the preferred modality.

Treatment may consist of radiotherapy, surgical resection, combined therapy or palliative therapy.

1. Radiotherapy. Early hypopharyngeal cancer may be treated with radiotherapy, with the option of salvage surgery if there is a recurrence. Radiotherapy may be reserved for the patient without enlarged lymph nodes, but it has been proposed that in selected cases radiotherapy can be given to the primary tumour and a radical neck dissection carried out for nodal metastases.

2. Surgery. Surgical resection is preferred for large tumours or in the presence of bulky cervical metastases. A lateral pharyngotomy can be performed for posterior wall tumours and the defect repaired with a radial forearm free flap. Extensive and circumferential lesions will require total pharyngolaryngectomy and then reconstruction of the residual defect. A variety of techniques to reconstruct have been used including skin grafts, cervical and deltopectoral skin flaps, myocutaneous pectoralis major and latissimus dorsi flaps and visceral interposition of stomach, jejunum or colon. The main complications are failure of the graft or flap, postoperative fistulae and stenosis, which are all more likely if there has been previous radiotherapy. There is also a significant mortality rate of 1% for skin flaps and revascularized loops and up to 10% for gastric transposition. The choice of reconstruction depends largely on the experience of the unit.

3. Combined therapy. Postoperative radiotherapy is carried out within 6 weeks of surgical resection as a combined treatment, with the aims of destroying metastases and maximizing the recurrence-free life interval. It is indicated if: surgical resection margins are close to or involved in tumour, in most large tumours requiring surgery, when there is vascular or perineural invasion, more than 2 lymph nodes are involved, or if there is extra-capsular rupture.

4. Palliation. This therapy is for those patients with advanced end-stage disease, severe intercurrent illness, poor general condition, distant metastases, or those who refuse treatment. Palliative radiotherapy can be offered to produce tumour shrinkage and symptom relief in some cases.

Follow-up and aftercare

On the 10th postoperative day, if there is no evidence of graft failure or leak, the patient can be tested with a methylene blue or gastrograffin swallow. If there is no evidence of extravasation, the patient can be commenced on fluids and then soft diet. Most patients will require thyroid, calcium and calciferol replacement for life. Speech rehabilitation is difficult in these patients, although there are some encouraging reports with low-pressure speech valves (e.g. Provox or Blom-Singer), the voice is not as good as after a total laryngectomy. Patients should be regularly reviewed in the clinic and their nutritional status and swallowing ability should be monitored along with a careful examination for primary and secondary recurrence.

Further reading

Jones AS, Roland NJ, Husband D and Gati I. Free revascularised jejunal loop repair following total pharyngectomy for carcinoma of the hypopharynx, a report of 90 cases. *British Journal of Surgery*, 1996; **83**: 1279–1283.

Schetter GL. Cancer of the hypopharynx and cervical oesophagus. *Current Opinion in Otolaryngology and Head and Neck Surgery*, 1998; **6**: 97–101.

Wilson J (ed). *Effective Head and Neck Cancer Management. Second Consensus.* British Association of Otolaryngologists, Head and Neck Surgeons, 2000.

Related topics of interest

Globus pharyngeus, p. 113; Laryngeal carcinoma, p. 138; Oral cavity carcinoma, p. 197; Oropharyngeal carcinoma, p. 203.

IMPEDANCE AUDIOMETRY

Physics and physiology

The middle-ear and mastoid air cells communicate with the nasopharynx via the Eustachian tube. As a closed system, air is being continually absorbed by the lining mucosa but is periodically replaced when the Eustachian tube opens, during the act of swallowing. Sound transmission from the external to the inner ear is optimal when the compliance of the middle-ear system is maximal, i.e. when the pressure in the middle ear is equal to the pressure in the external auditory meatus. Compliance (or admittance) is the measure of this system to allow the passage of sound energy through it, and is inversely related to impedance, which is the resistance to the passage of sound energy. The mass, stiffness and frictional resistance of the medium through which the sound wave travels contribute to the impedance, which at low frequency is stiffness dominated. Strictly speaking, compliance is the reciprocal of stiffness so that impedance measurements at low frequency are usually referred to as the compliance.

Basic principles

Impedance audiometry consists of three tests: tympanometry, acoustic reflex testing and static compliance. All three tests work on the same basic principle. The test probe consists of a sound producer, a sound receiver and a device for altering the air pressure within the EAM. The probe has a soft plastic or rubber tip to allow an air-tight seal in the EAM. A test tone is made (220 Hz, 65 dB) into the EAM, of which some will be absorbed (admitted) by the middle-ear system (drum and ossicles) and some reflected. The reflected sound energy is measured by the probe microphone. The compliance, that is the amount of sound absorbed by the middle-ear system, can be determined either by measuring the reflected sound level in the ear canal or more commonly by measuring the amount of energy required to keep the sound level constant at varying ear canal pressures. The compliance will be maximal when the ear canal pressure is equal to middle-ear pressure, that is when there is no pressure differential across the tympanic membrane. A tracing of the compliance as ear canal pressure alters allows this and other parameters to be determined.

Clinical uses

1. Tympanometry. This test is the most commonly used aspect of impedance audiometry and is particularly useful in evaluating children with otitis media with effusion. Here compliance is measured continuously while the pressure in the EAM is automatically varied from +200 to –400 mm H_2O. This gives a graphical result which can be classified into one of three groups:

(a) *Type A*. Maximal compliance occurs when the pressure in the EAM is between +50 and –100 mm H_2O. A normal maximal compliance value is between 2 and 4 ml. A low value for maximal compliance indicates stiffness of the middle-ear system as in tympanosclerosis or otosclerosis. A high or unrecordable peak of compliance indicates excess mobility of the middle-ear system as in ossicular discontinuity or atelectasis.

(b) *Type B.* A low-value flat or horizontal compliance trace occurs, implying persistently low compliance. This is usually taken to indicate fluid in the middle-ear cavity, and in young children (< 7 years) with glue ear can be correlated with audiometric hearing loss. A type B tympanogram will also occur in the presence of a perforation in the tympanic membrane but the ear canal volume will be large (> 6 ml) because it is measuring that of the middle-ear cleft too. It can occasionally be useful in confirming this diagnosis or to test the patency of a ventilation tube.

(c) *Type C.* This group give a peak compliance when the pressure in the EAM is < −100 mm H_2O. This indicates a significant low pressure in the middle-ear system and is a sign of eustachian tube dysfunction. The C curve can be subdivided into C1, when the peak is between −100 and −199 mm H_2O, and C2, when the peak occurs at less than −200 mm H_2O.

2. *Acoustic reflex measurement.* Acoustic reflexes are measured at the ear canal pressure producing maximum compliance, which corresponds to middle-ear pressure. Ipsilateral reflexes are recorded using the tympanometry probe; contralateral reflexes use a monaural headset to deliver sound to the non-probe ear. It is usual to test at 0.5 kHz and then at either 1 or 2 kHz. A sound intensity of 70–90 dB above the pure tone threshold at that frequency is required to elicit a reflex in a normal-hearing subject, although in one who has a recruiting sensorineural hearing loss a reflex may be present only 10 dB above threshold. The compliance, which is constant for the ear canal pressure selected, is recorded as a horizontal line and shows a dip on contraction of stapedius muscle, representing a reduction in compliance. The stapedial reflex is a complex crossed reflex and demands an intact afferent arm, brain stem and VIIth cranial nerve. As such, the acoustic reflex can provide diagnostic information with regard to the site of a neurological lesion based on the pattern of response to ipsi- and contralateral testing.

It is important to remember that a conductive hearing loss of only 5 dB may result in an absent ipsilateral and contralateral (for reasons that have not been satisfactorily explained) reflex, although it is not until there is a 15 dB air–bone gap that the reflex is absent in 50% of cases.

Adaption (stapedial reflex decay) is determined by producing a persistent tone in the test ear and measuring the reflex in the contralateral ear. Normal adaption occurs only after 10 seconds, decay being no more than 50%.

Summary of the value of measuring the acoustic reflex:
(a) Assesses the integrity of the facial nerve up to the branch to stapedius tendon.
(b) Assesses recruitment and stapedial reflex decay, the latter in particular being an accurate pointer in distinguishing a cochlear (recruiting) from a retrocochlear (abnormal decay) lesion.
(c) Assess the presence of a conductive hearing loss.
(d) Assess brainstem function.

3. Static compliance.   The least used of the three tests. The compliance is measured with an air pressure of +200 mm H_2O in the EAM, and this figure is subtracted from the maximal compliance, regardless of the pressure in the EAM at which this occurs. The normal range for this is from 0.3–1.6 ml. A figure greater than 2.0 ml implies the presence of a tympanic membrane perforation.

Conclusion

Impedance audiometry is rapid and easy to use. It provides an objective measure of middle-ear function, can help to distinguish cochlear from retrocochlear hearing loss, as well as localizing brainstem and facial nerve lesions. It is, however, essential that the results are interpreted in the context of other clinical findings.

Further reading

Ballantyne D. *Handbook of Audiological Techniques*. London: Butterworth-Heinemann, 1990.
Jerger J, Hayes D. Clinical use of acoustic impedance testing in audiological diagnosis. In: Beagley HA (ed.) *Audiology and Audiological Medicine*, Oxford: Oxford University Press, 1981.

Related topics of interest

Acoustic neuroma, p. 1; Clinical assessment of hearing, p. 45; Facial nerve palsy, p. 92; Otitis media with effusion, p. 213; Pure tone audiogram, p. 254; Speech audiometry, p. 301.

INTRINSIC RHINITIS

Intrinsic rhinitis (IR) is an inflammatory condition of the nasal mucosa which is probably better described by the title non-infective, non-allergic rhinitis. As such it represents, to some extent, a diagnosis of exclusion.

Pathology

IR has been divided into two types, eosinophilic and non-eosinophilic, on the basis of the numbers of eosinophils found in the nasal secretions. However, recent research evidence has cast doubt on this distinction. It is likely that the condition represents more than one pathological process. Upsets to the autonomic nervous system have been postulated, but it would appear that immunological abnormalities are common. Of particular recent interest has been the separate findings of anti-IgE antibodies and elevated nasal IgE levels. A number of patients demonstrate an intrinsic mucosal disorder of prostaglandin metabolism. In this type there is an association with aspirin hypersensitivity, asthma and nasal polyposis.

Regardless of the underlying aetiology most patients demonstrate glandular hyperplasia and submucosal vascular dilation. The nasal mucosa becomes hyperaemic and hypertrophic, particularly on the turbinates. Eosinophil-laden polyps are more common in IR than in allergic rhinitis.

Predisposing factors

- Familial tendency.
- Preceding infection (nasal mucosal hyper-reactivity following viral or bacterial rhinitis).
- Psychological and emotional factors.
- Endocrine (puberty, menstruation and pregnancy).
- Drugs (hypotensive agents, e.g. beta blockers and methyl dopa, aspirin, oral contraceptives).
- Pollution (atmospheric pollution, fumes, dust, industrial detergents and cigarette smoke).
- Atmospheric conditions (changes in humidity and temperature).
- Alcohol.
- Smoking.

Clinical features

IR accounts for 40–70% of all cases of perennial rhinitis and becomes more common with increasing age. All patients exhibit nasal obstruction and rhinorrhoea or post-nasal discharge, but itching and sneezing are less common than in allergic rhinitis. Patients vary in their degree of nasal obstruction and discharge. There may be associated nasal polyps with anosmia. Co-existent sinus pathology is frequently found (up to 50%) which may be primary, causing a secondary rhinitis, or secondary due to the inevitable compromise of sinus aeration and drainage. Examination generally reveals a rather red and angry mucosa, often with copious secretions and hypertrophy of both middle and inferior turbinates, causing a consequent reduction in the airway size.

Investigations

IR is a diagnosis of exclusion, and the aim of investigations is to identify other causes of rhinitis. IgE estimation by PRIST and RAST and skin testing can be used to indicate allergy. Radiological examination of the nose and sinuses with CT scanning may help diagnose structural abnormalities and any coexistent sinus infection.

Management

1. Medical. Antibiotics may be used to treat any co-existent infective component and a short course of oral steroids is often helpful to get an initial response. However the mainstays of maintenance treatment are as follows:

(a) Intranasal steroids. Many cases respond well to topical intranasal steroid preparations although in some the response is disappointing.

(b) Antihistamines are useful in some cases. Older preparations such as chlorpheniramine have anticholinergic effects and are to be preferred but sedative side-effects may be troublesome. Topical preparations can sometimes have an impressive local effect.

(c) Topical ipratropium bromide is useful for its anticholinergic effect in reducing rhinorrhoea.

(d) Systemic sympathomimetics can be helpful (e.g. pseudoephedrine), though they may produce unpleasant side-effects such as dry mouth, constipation and excitability. They should not be used long term or in children.

(e) Local nasal decongestants. Self-medication with topical vasoconstrictors (e.g. xylometazoline, ephedrine) is common and initially successful in bringing relief to the patient with enlarged turbinates by reducing blood flow in them. Unfortunately, when the effects wear off, there is a reflex vasodilatation causing increased blood flow and turbinate engorgement (rebound phenomenon). Prolonged use leads to an aggravation of symptoms, which eventually become unresponsive to the decongestant, and rhinitis medicamentosa may supervene. The treatment is to stop the decongestant and prescribe topical nasal steroids.

(f) Interleukin antagonists. Although not yet established in the management of this condition, it is likely that developments in this area will ultimately prove helpful. Some clinicians are already using them on a limited basis and with some success.

2. Surgical. Surgical treatment is useful for the control of symptoms, particularly nasal obstruction, when medical treatment is ineffective.

(a) *Treatment of concomitant problems.* Associated nasal polyps are treated with excision or topical intra-nasal steroids as appropriate. Correction of septal deflections and spurs should be considered to relieve an obstructed airway.

(b) *Turbinate surgery.* Most procedures are aimed at reducing the bulk of the inferior turbinate to improve the airway. Submucosal diathermy, linear diathermy, laser cautery, cryosurgery and multiple out-fractures are all successful in the short term, but obstruction recurs after 1–2 years. Inferior turbinectomy is associated with slightly higher morbidity from postoperative haemorrhage but is more successful for long-term symptom control. The theoretical risk of atrophic rhinitis has not materialized in UK practice.

(c) *Vidian neurectomy*. This operation divides the parasympathetic nerve supply to the nose as the nerve of the pterygoid canal (Vidian nerve) enters the pterygopalatine fossa. Initial enthusiasm for Vidian neurectomy for the relief of rhinorrhoea without nasal obstruction waned when it became apparent that over 50% of patients relapsed within 1 year.

(d) *Functional Endoscopic Sinus Surgery* (FESS). There is no doubt that any associated sinus disease can be addressed with FESS. Some clinicians will also trim the middle turbinates in this procedure to achieve significant improvements in the nasal airway.

Further reading

Jones AS, Lancer JM. Vasomotor rhinitis (editorial). *British Medical Journal*, 1987; **294**: 1505–1506.
Carney AS and Jones NS. Idiopathic rhinitis: idiopathic or not? *Clinical Otolaryngology*, 1996; **21**: 198–202.
Banfield GK and McCombe AW. Partial resection of the middle turbinate at functional endoscopic sinus surgery. *Journal of the Royal Army Medical Corps*, 1999; **145**: 18–19.

Related topics of interest

Allergic rhinitis, p. 11; Examination of the nose, p. 84; Nasal polyps; p. 174; Functional endoscopic sinus surgery, p. 108.

LABYRINTHITIS

Labyrinthitis is an inflammation of the labyrinth and may be classified into serous labyrinthitis, suppurative labyrinthitis, perilabyrinthitis and paralabyrinthitis. Three important definitions are provided to aid their understanding.

Labyrinthine fistula

A labyrinthine fistula is a bony erosion of the labyrinthine capsule to expose, but not breach, the endosteum of the labyrinth. A breach will usually result in a dead ear. A fistula most commonly occurs in the dome of the lateral semicircular canal.

Tullio phenomenon

The Tullio phenomenon is defined as vertigo in the presence of loud sounds. The phenomenon occurs when sound energy is transmitted from a mobile stapes footplate to the labyrinth which is distensible only when there is a fistula. Historically the phenomenon occurred if a fenestration procedure was performed in the presence of a mobile footplate, this scenario arising in the 1950s in patients with severe adhesive otitis. The phenomenon may also arise in those with endolymphatic hydrops when it is thought to be secondary to sound energy transmission from the footplate to the distended saccule which may be touching the undersurface of the footplate in advanced cases.

The fistula sign

In the presence of a labyrinthine fistula, raising the ear canal pressure of the affected side may cause conjugate deviation of the eyes away from the affected ear. The mechanism is pressure transmission to the labyrinth causing endolymph movement and stimulation of the labyrinthine sense organs. This occurs either directly if there is labyrinth endosteum exposed to the ear canal after mastoid surgery or indirectly if endosteum is covered by disease that can transmit the pressure wave such as cholesteatoma. On occasion it may occur by a similar mechanism to the Tullio phenomenon. Releasing the pressure allows the deviated eyes to return to the midline.

Perilabyrinthitis

Perilabyrinthitis is a *syndrome* caused by a labyrinthine fistula *after mastoid surgery* in the presence of retained labyrinthine function. The fistula may have been present, but silent, before surgery. For example when secondary to cholesteatoma, the mass of the cholesteatoma sac prevents distension of the labyrinthine endosteum. Alternatively the fistula may be iatrogenic. The hallmarks of perilabyrinthitis are the *Tullio phenomenon* and a *positive fistula sign*. Vertigo may also arise in perilabyrinthitis on windy days when the relatively cooler wind produces a thermal gradient across the labyrinth and a difference in the specific gravity of endolymph at each end of the semicircular canal to cause circulation of the endolymph within the canal.

Treatment consists of occluding the meatus with cotton wool when outdoors or grafting the fistula with temporalis fascia, sealing the graft with fibrin glue and a temporalis muscle flap.

Paralabyrinthitis

This is vertigo occurring in the presence of CSOM when inflammation close to the endosteum of the labyrinth causes an irritative nystagmus, that is a nystagmus towards the affected ear.

Serous and suppurative labyrinthitis

Serous labyrinthitis is a retrospective diagnosis and depends on there being some recovery of cochlea and vestibular function after an attack of postulated bacterial labyrinthitis. The symptoms and signs are identical to suppurative labyrinthitis except in the latter the loss of inner ear function is irreversible.

Clinical features

Labyrinthitis is most commonly virally induced but may be secondary to CSOM, or may also be a complication of ASOM via the round window. Typically, there is an acute onset of violent, overwhelming vertigo that is so severe it inhibits the perception of tinnitus and hearing loss. There may be a short period of irritative jerk nystagmus towards the affected ear, but soon a paralytic jerk nystagmus to the healthy ear ensues. Tiny movements of the head exacerbate the vertigo so that the patient prefers to lie completely still on his side and in the presence of a paralytic nystagmus the affected ear will be uppermost. In this position the patient will tend to voluntarily look in the direction of the affected side (especially when they have visitors), reducing the drive from the unaffected ear so that the corrective nystagmus and therefore the vertigo will be less severe. This can be understood when we explain the normal labyrinth causes conjugate deviation of the eyes to the opposite side so that if one labyrinth is paralysed the opposite labyrinth will become dominant and deviate the eyes to the side of the affected ear, the nystagmus occurring as a corrective measure. Initially there is third degree nystagmus, that is nystagmus in any direction of lateral gaze. (As compensation gradually occurs second degree nystagmus develops (nystagmus when gazing straight ahead or looking in the direction of the nystagmus) and then first degree nystagmus (nystagmus only when looking in the direction of the nystagmus). Finally there is absence of nystagmus on optic fixation. In parallel with these changes is an improvement in mobility and symptoms.

Investigations of labyrinthitis

The diagnosis is made on the clinical features occurring in the presence of a precipitating factor. The ears should always be examined under the microscope and if any debris is found it should be removed. A labyrinthine fistula may be visible. If there are no features to suggest a meningitis the important diagnosis not to miss is a cerebellar abscess. Here the symptoms and signs are different, but may be difficult to recognize in a patient continuously vomiting. An enhanced CT or MRI scan will be necessary in these circumstances. Sequential pure tone audiometry and electronystagmography (ENG) will allow the monitoring of recovery although hearing loss and vestibular failure is permanent with purulent labyrinthitis.

Management of labyrinthitis

Treatment of both the precipitating factor and the labyrinthitis is necessary.

- An ear culture swab if there is evidence of middle ear infection and appropriate antibiotics, broad spectrum until results of the swab are available.
- Bed rest, avoiding head movements.
- Vestibular sedatives.
- Intravenous fluids if vomiting.
- If the precipitating factor was CSOM, exploration of the mastoid after recovery from the acute symptoms, should be considered. A labyrinthine fistula may have arisen from chronic osteitis or cholesteatoma. The chronic disease should be eradicated and if a fistula is identified the treatment is described above.

Follow up and aftercare

- After recovery from the acute infection, Cooksey-Cawthorne exercises may accelerate central compensation.
- Counselling is a necessary but often overlooked part of the management. Even with complete central compensation patients with unilateral labyrinthine failure will still be unsteady in the dark, if they develop a severe illness (allows inhibition of central compensation) or if they should develop a neuropathy affecting the peripheral proprioceptors.

Future advances

Growth factors and antioxidant cocktails may provide protection to the labyrinth from progressive damage and may allow regeneration of vestibular receptors. Growth factors of particular interest are brain-derived neurotrophic factor (BDNF) and glial cell line-derived neurotrophic factor (GDNF). The BDNF gene, using a herpes simplex virus (HSV) vector has been injected into the cochlea of mice whose hair cells had been killed with neomycin which allowed a near total rescue of cells within 4 weeks. Cochlea hair cells are more susceptible to injury than vestibular receptors which suggests the latter receptors should respond well to such attempted rescue and further work is on going. Osmotic pump infusion and viral vector delivery of GDNF into perilymph has attenuated kanamycin and ethacrynic acid sensory cell loss. Furthermore changes in BDNF expression following trauma are correlated with the degree of regeneration. Antioxidants will reduce sensory hair cell loss due to cisplatin and the protective function of antioxidants to gentamicin ototoxicity and to acoustic trauma has also been demonstrated. Neurotrophic factors and antioxidants may therefore have a significant future role to play in the protection and recovery of inner ear receptors from injury of any aetiology.

Further reading

Shepard NT, Telian SA, Smith-Wheelock M, Raj A. Vestibular and balance rehabilitation therapy. *Annals of Otology, Rhinology and Laryngology*, 1993; **102**: 198–205.

Staecker H, Dazert S, Malgrange B, *et al*. Transforming growth factor alpha treatment alters intracellular calcium levels in hair cells and protects them from ototoxic damage in vitro. *Int J Dev Neurosci*, 1997; **15**: 553–562.

Related topics of interest

LARYNGEAL CARCINOMA

Pathology

Squamous cell carcinoma of the larynx is the commonest head and neck cancer in the Western world and represents approximately 1% of all malignancies in men. In some areas of India and Malaysia it is the most common cancer and is probably related to variations in smoking habit. It is about five times commoner in males than in females. The incidence increases with age, but the peak age of presentation is in the seventh decade. The cause of cancer of the larynx is not known, but persons who smoke tobacco and drink alcohol are predisposed to the disease. It is very rare in non-smokers. Alcohol on its own is probably not a cause of laryngeal cancer but it is highly synergistic with smoking. Verrucous carcinoma is a distinct variant of well-differentiated squamous cell carcinoma. Adenocarcinoma, adenoid cystic carcinoma, fibrosarcoma, chondrosarcoma and lymphomas are all rare.

For classification purposes, the larynx is divided into three regions which each include a number of sites:

1. Supraglottis. This comprises the larynx superior to the apex of the ventricle. It includes the ventricle, vestibular folds, arytenoids, aryepiglottic folds and the epiglottis (laryngeal surface, tip and lingual surface).

2. Glottis. This comprises the vocal cords and the anterior and posterior commissures. It extends from the apex of the laryngeal ventricle to 1 cm below. Some authorities hold that the superior and inferior borders of the glottis correspond to the superior and inferior arcuate lines, respectively.

3. Subglottis. This extends from the inferior border of the glottis to the lower border of the cricoid cartilage.

Clinical features

The clinical features of malignant disease are dictated by the primary tumour, secondary deposits and the general effects of cancer. The symptoms and signs of a laryngeal tumour depend on the way in which it is related to the upper aerodigestive tract. Hoarseness is the commonest and often the only presenting symptom. Dyspnoea and stridor are late symptoms and almost invariably indicate an advanced tumour. Pain is an uncommon symptom but is most typical in supraglottic tumours. Patients with a cancer in this site may complain of a unilateral sore throat. There may be referred otalgia. Dysphagia indicates invasion of the pharynx. Swelling of the neck may be due to direct penetration of the tumour outside the larynx or to lymph node metastases. Cough and irritation of the throat are occasional symptoms. The general symptoms of anorexia, cachexia and fetor imply advanced disease.

There should be a general examination to identify distant metastases and an assessment of the overall physical status of the patient. Indirect laryngoscopy should allow an inspection of the primary tumour site and size. Vocal cord mobility should also be assessed. There are three areas which are difficult to examine by this technique: the subglottis, the laryngeal surface of the epiglottis and the laryngeal ventricle. All patients should, therefore, also undergo fibreoptic laryngoscopy. The neck should be carefully palpated for the presence of enlarged lymph nodes. Examination must include an assessment of the number, mobility and level of the nodes. Laryngeal tumours usually metastasize to the upper deep cervical lymph nodes, but supraglottic tumours may cause bilateral nodes, and some subglottic tumours may spread to the upper mediastinal nodes.

Investigations

A chest radiograph, full blood count and serum analysis are baseline investigations prior to a general anaesthetic. The serum analysis may show deranged liver function raising suspicion of liver metastases, or hypoproteinaemia, which may indicate malnourishment and a possibility of poor wound healing. The chest radiograph should be carefully examined to exclude metastases or to assess intercurrent lung disease. MRI or CT scans of the larynx and neck provide further information about the primary tumour. Imaging may also uncover the presence of impalpable or occult nodes. A CT scan of the chest may be indicated if suspected lung metastases need further delineation. An ultrasound scan of the liver is required if hepatic metastases are suspected and in some units this is routine prior to major surgery. An isotope bone scan is indicated only if symptoms suggest bony metastases or there is a raised serum calcium or alkaline phosphatase. Distant metastases are unusual in laryngeal carcinoma at presentation (1–5%).

Direct laryngoscopy under general anaesthesia is mandatory. In addition, the patient should have a full panendoscopy including bronchoscopy. The incidence of a synchronous second primary tumour in the head, neck or lung is in the region of 1–5%. All the larynx sites should be inspected systematically. The tumour's position and extension should be recorded by means of a diagram in the case notes. Biopsy material should include an adequate amount of representative tissue to obtain a definitive diagnosis of malignancy, identification of the tumour type and tumour differentiation. While the patient's neck muscles are relaxed under general anaesthetic the neck should be palpated for nodes which may not have been noted previously. Cord mobility should be assessed as the patient wakes if not done already. The information from the investigations of the patient allow the surgeon to 'stage' the tumour according to the TNM classification and manage it accordingly.

Staging

Laryngeal tumours are diverse in their behaviour and prognosis and thus there have been many endeavors to classify them. Clinical staging attempts to group together features which may share a level of prognosis or a certain treatment. In cancer of the larynx, clinical staging is the only generally reliable criterion of any prognostic significance, and even with this standard there is considerable variability. An accurate anatomical description of tumour extent (with a case file diagram or photograph) is therefore essential in treatment selection.

Supraglottis.

T1   Tumour limited to one subsite of the supraglottis.

T2   Invasion of more than one subsite of the supraglottis or glottis or adjacent region outside the supraglottis (e.g. mucosa of tongue base).

T3   Confined to larynx with a fixed vocal cord or invades the postcricoid area, pre-epiglottic tissues, base of tongue.

T4   Extends beyond the larynx.

Glottis.

T1(a)   Tumour limited to one vocal cord.

T1(b)   Involves both vocal cords.

T2   Tumour extends to supraglottis and/or subglottis, or impaired cord mobility.

T3   Confined to the larynx with a fixed vocal cord.

T4   Extends beyond the larynx.

Subglottis.

T1   Tumour limited to subglottis.

T2   Extends to vocal cords with normal or impaired mobility.

T3   Vocal cord fixed.

T4   Extends beyond the larynx

The presence of palpable lymph nodes is the most important factor in determining prognosis, but assessment of lymphadenopathy is subjective. About one-third of patients with no palpable lymph nodes have histologically invaded nodes, and a similar number of palpable nodes are not invaded by tumour. The supraglottis has a rich lymphatic drainage, and a high proportion of these tumours spread to cervical lymph nodes. The subglottis drains to paratracheal and mediastinal nodes in addition to the cervical lymph node. The glottis has virtually no lymphatic drainage, so metastases usually only occur when the tumour has spread to involve the supraglottis and subglottis in the so-called transglottic tumour. Some authorities maintain that transglottic tumours arise from the laryngeal ventricle.

Management

Each patient will fall into one of the following treatment categories depending on their age, general condition, and stage of the tumour: curative treatment or palliative treatment.

1. Curative treatment may involve radiotherapy, surgery or a combination of these two modalities. As a general rule, small tumours are treated by radical radiotherapy in the first instance, with surgery reserved for recurrence. Preservation laryngeal surgery is also an option with small tumours. Larger tumours tend to be treated with primary surgery, usually with postoperative radiotherapy. Patients who present with stridor should have endoscopic debulking carried out when possible. Tracheostomy, although not desirable, may be necessary. Management of the neck will depend on nodal status (see Cervical Lymphadenopathy and Neck Dissection chapters). Supraglottic tumours have a high incidence of overt and occult nodal metastases and the N0 neck needs elective treatment in these cases. Bilateral dissection of levels II–IV with inclusion of level I if tongue base involvement and level VI if subglottic spread. N1 disease in cancers from all sites of the larynx can be treated by modified radical neck dissection and N2/N3 by radical neck dissection with a modified dissection on the contralateral side if required.

2. *Palliative treatment* includes pain relief, tracheostomy, insertion of a percutaneous gastrostomy, palliative radiotherapy, chemotherapy and occasionally surgery. Early involvement of the palliative care team.

Glottic tumours.

T1   In the UK, radiotherapy has been the conventional treatment of choice for T1 glottic tumours, giving cure rates in excess of 90%. Alternatively, small tumours confined to one vocal cord can be treated by endoscopic laser resection or open cordectomy.

T2   They can be similarly managed by radiotherapy or by partial laryngectomy. Radiotherapy may be better for extensive superficial tumours because of the better functional results obtained.

T3   Many T3 glottic tumours are treated in the first instance by radiotherapy, but vertical partial laryngectomy is sometimes an alternative. Larger tumours causing stridor will need a total laryngectomy, sometimes as an emergency procedure. Radiotherapy has the advantage of leaving the patient with his larynx, but there is often persistent oedema, sometimes with aspiration and poor function of the larynx. The results of salvage surgery for recurrences after radiotherapy are poor. Furthermore, approximately 50% of T3 laryngeal carcinomas are understaged and are in fact T4 tumours due to extension through the cricothyroid membrane or from unsuspected cartilage invasion. Primary surgery with post-operative radiotherapy is therefore recommended for high volume lesions.

T4   Tumours will be treated by total laryngectomy and a radical neck dissection if there are any nodal metastases with post-operative radiotherapy.

Supraglottic tumours.

T1–T2   Usually treated by radiotherapy or conservation surgery. Endoscopic resection may have a role in selected T1 cases, but its use is controversial.

T3–T4   Larger tumours will require treatment by either a supraglottic laryngectomy or total laryngectomy, combined with a neck dissection.

Subglottic tumours.

Pure subglottic cancer is very unusual. The subglottis becomes involved in extensive glottic and transglottic carcinoma. Small tumours may be treated by radiotherapy, but these tumours often present late and the patient needs a total laryngectomy. It is important that the upper mediastinum is included in the radical treatment regimen.

Follow-up and aftercare

Patients who have had potentially curative treatment should be carefully examined for signs of primary recurrence, neck node spread and distant metastases, and have their weight recorded in the outpatient clinic on a regular basis. This should be monthly for the first 6 months, then every 2 months for 6 months, every 3 months for 12 months, then 6 monthly for the next 3 years. Some units continue to monitor patients as the incidence of second primary tumours is in the region of 10–20%. Patients who have had a laryngectomy will require speech therapy. All patients should have had modern method of voice restoration following laryngectomy including valved speech. They will also require monitoring of their thyroid function and calcium levels if there has been a thyroid gland excision.

Further reading

DeSanto LW. Cancer of the larynx. *Current Opinion in Otolaryngology and Head and Neck Surgery*, 1993; **1**: 133–136.

Stell PM. Review. Prognostic factors in laryngeal carcinoma. *Clinical Otolaryngology*, 1988; **13**: 399–409.

Wilson J (ed). *Effective Head and Neck Cancer Management. Second Consensus Document.* British Association of Otolaryngologists, Head and Neck Surgeons, 2000.

Related topics of interest

Cervical lymphadenopathy, p. 29; Laryngectomy, p. 143; Neck dissection, p. 185; Radiotherapy, p. 264; Tracheostomy, p. 336.

LARYNGECTOMY

The choice between surgery and radiotherapy as treatment for carcinoma of the larynx should be made according to the likely effective control of the cancer, the general health of the patient and the relative consequences of the treatment. With both a laryngectomy and radiotherapy there is invariably some or total loss of normal voice and compromise of airway protection and function. Radiotherapy has the advantage of vastly reduced morbidity compared with surgery. Although patients may undergo speech rehabilitation and may swallow well after removal of the larynx, the main handicap associated with this procedure, according to quality of life studies, appears to be the need for a permanent stoma. Conservative approaches which attempt to preserve as much of the larynx and its function as possible, are popular in the USA and Continental Europe. The goals of conservative laryngeal surgery are to control cancer and obtain a functional outcome of speech and swallowing without the need for a permanent tracheostomy. It is apparent that the modern surgeon should not manage laryngeal cancer on the basis of one surgical option (total laryngectomy). The repertoire must include conservation techniques including laser surgery, partial laryngectomy and surgical voice restoration.

In general in the UK, radiotherapy is reserved for smaller tumours (T1 and T2), whereas surgery is considered more effective for larger tumours (T3 and T4) and when there are secondary deposits of carcinoma in the lymph nodes of the neck. The other less common malignant neoplasms of the larynx (adenocarcinoma, verrucous carcinoma, fibrosarcoma, chondrosarcoma, etc.) are invariably treated by laryngectomy.

Types of laryngectomy

1. Vertical partial resection.
(a) Cordectomy.
(b) Hemilaryngectomy (frontal, lateral and fronto-lateral).

2. Horizontal partial resection.
(a) Epiglottectomy.
(b) Supraglottic laryngectomy.

3. Near-total laryngectomy.
(a) Supracricoid partial laryngectomy.
(b) Vertical subtotal laryngectomy.

4. Total laryngectomy.

Investigations

A panendoscopy should always be performed by the surgeon prior to operation. This will allow a representative biopsy to be obtained, the tumour to be staged and the appropriate operation planned.

The patient should be investigated to allow surgery to proceed and to exclude distant metastases. A CT or MRI scan of the larynx should be obtained. A chest radiograph and liver ultrasound scan are essential (in addition many authorities would advocate a chest CT scan). Serum urea and electrolytes, liver function tests and a full blood count will be required. The patient should be cross-matched for 2 units if a total laryngectomy is proposed. Written confirmation of the histological diagnosis must be in the case notes or the surgeon should have personally spoken to a senior pathologist to confirm the diagnosis of cancer when a frozen section result is presented.

Patient preparation

The patient should have a clear explanation of the diagnosis and what it means. The operation should be described and the patient should have knowledge of the wounds, drains, nasogastric tube and sutures, etc. It should be remembered that this situation will be distressing for the patient, who should have a relative or close friend present. The patient should be warned before any treatment that there is no guarantee of cure. Specifically for a laryngectomy the patient must be warned that the voice box will be lost and a new technique to speak will need to be learned, a permanent end tracheostome will be necessary, and thyroid and parathyroid supplements may be needed for life following the operation. The explanation and warnings should be logged in the case notes. The speech therapist should see the patient preoperatively. Consent for total laryngectomy should always be obtained before embarking on any partial resection.

Cordectomy

This is indicated for a T1–T2 cancer of the glottis which does not reach the anterior commissure or the arytenoid cartilage. It can be performed by an endoscopic or open approach. Excision can be performed using the KTP or CO_2 laser. It is performed much less frequently in the UK owing to the equally effective results achieved by radiation. However, new perspectives will continue to challenge old ones and the current trend is for endocopic laser resection to be offered to patients more often. Cordectomy also remains a suitable operation for the removal of benign laryngeal tumours.

Hemilaryngectomy

This technique can be used to remove tumours confined to the vocal cord, with an adequate margin of healthy tissue. It involves removal of half of the thyroid cartilage, with the false and true vocal cords, part of the supraglottis and the upper half of the cricoid cartilage. The resulting gap is closed by the strap muscles, fashioned so as to form a new fixed vocal cord. This procedure therefore has the advantage of allowing some protection for the airway and a reasonable voice for the patient. However, if on histological examination there has been incomplete resection of the lesion, either postoperative radiotherapy or total laryngectomy should be performed.

Supraglottic laryngectomy

This is indicated for cancer of the supraglottis (epiglottis and laryngeal vestibule). The technique involves removing the entire supraglottis from the vallecula to the ventricle, and joining the lower half of the larynx to the base of the tongue. Cricopharyngeal myotomy is considered an essential manoeuvre to make swallowing easier. The operation is not suitable if the tumour extends to the base of tongue or vocal cords, if the patient is over the age of 65 years or if there is intercurrent lung disease. It should be preceded by direct laryngoscopy to assess the extent of disease and likelihood of successful resection. If the operation is to be carried out for post-radiotherapy recurrence, it is important that the extent of the original lesion is known.

Supracricoid partial laryngectomy

In the spectrum of procedures available for the surgical management of laryngeal carcinoma, the supracricoid partial laryngectomy (SCPL) falls between the vertical partial laryngectomy and the supraglottic laryngectomy at one extreme and total laryngectomy at the other. There are actually two groups of SCPLs. The first is used for selected glottic carcinomas in which both true and false cords, the whole thyroid cartilage, and a maximum of one arytenoid cartilage are resected. Closure is between the cricoid, the hyoid and the remaining epiglottis and tongue base, hence the name crico-hyoid-epiglottopexy. The procedure that is used for selected supraglottic and transglottic carcinomas results in a more extensive resection, with removal of the entire epiglottis and pre-epiglottic space. In this case closure is performed by pexy between the cricoid and the hyoid and tongue base; therefore, the procedure is called cricohyoidopexy. The aim of these two procedures is excision of tumour and to allow speech and swallowing without a permanent tracheostomy.

Total laryngectomy

Total laryngectomy is indicated for the curative treatment of laryngeal carcinoma when the tumour is considered to be unsuitable for either radiotherapy or a partial resection. It is also indicated as salvage surgery in failed radiotherapy, as a palliative measure in some advanced cases of carcinoma and as a last resort in those who have no voice and chronic aspiration due to palsy of the IXth, Xth and XIth cranial nerves. The technique involves removing the hyoid bone, thyroid and cricoid cartilages and several rings of the proximal trachea and an ipsilateral thyroid lobectomy or total thyroidectomy. The main disadvantages of this procedure are that the patient's normal voice is lost and a permanent end tracheostome is required. All patients having a total laryngectomy should have a speech valve inserted at the time of the operation.

Emergency laryngectomy

An emergency laryngectomy is a laryngectomy performed on a patient with airway compromise due to carcinoma, within 24 hours of presentation, without a prior tracheostomy.

The procedure should be avoided by proper planning and if possible by establishing an airway when such patients present. The laser can be used to debulk the tumour and improve the airway, after laryngoscopy and biopsy. This has the advantage of avoiding any surgical disturbance of the regional anatomy, yet secures the airway while the biopsy results are awaited, the patient counselled and further treatment planned.

The rationale for emergency laryngectomy is based on the dismal prognosis for any patient who develops a tumour recurrence in their tracheostome: so-called stomal recurrence. Performing a tracheostomy for the relief of airway obstruction due to carcinoma prior to any definitive treatment is associated with a high rate of stomal recurrence. This could be due to tumour seeding at the time of tracheostomy, to inadequate resection or to a second primary. A number of solutions have been offered to this problem. Some groups have argued that if definitive treatment is undertaken within 48 hours of the tracheostomy the rate of stomal recurrence is not increased.

Follow-up and aftercare

Voice rehabilitation and periodic surveillance for recurrence or second tumour are the main features of follow-up. Thyroid function and calcium levels should be checked appropriately.

Further reading

Gibson A, McCombe AW. The psychological consequences of laryngectomy. *Journal of Laryngology and Otology*, 1999; **113**: 349–352.

Jones AS, Cook JA, Phillips D, Soler Lluch E. Treatment of T3 carcinoma of the larynx by surgery or radiotherapy. *Clinical Otolaryngology*, 1992; **17**: 433–436.

Robin PE, Olofsson J. Tumours of the larynx. In: Scott-Brown's Otolaryngology, Vol. 5, 6th edn. London: Butterworths, 1997; Chaper 11.

Wilson J (ed). *Effective Head and Neck Cancer Management. Second Consensus.* British Association of Otolaryngologists, Head and Neck Surgeons, 2000.

Related topics of interest

Laryngeal carcinoma, p. 138; Lasers in ENT, p. 147; Stridor and stertor, p. 311; Tracheostomy, p. 336.

LASERS IN ENT

Laser is an acronym for light amplification by the stimulated emission of radiation.

Historical

The theoretical foundations for lasers were postulated by Einstein in 1917. In essence, he proposed that electromagnetic radiation (including light) could be produced by an electron of an atom jumping from a high-energy atomic shell to a lower energy shell, thereby releasing a photon of energy. The wavelength of the photon would depend on the energy difference between the two energy shells and so would be identical for all atoms of a specific element or molecule. Should this photon strike an atom or molecule identical to that which released the photon and which is in a high-energy state, another photon will be released, travelling in the same direction as that which stimulated the emission, the electron which released the photon dropping to a lower energy level. The electron must first be stimulated into the higher energy shell by an external energy source, usually electrical. In 1955 microwaves were produced in this fashion and in 1960 the first laser was built by Dr T. Maiman using synthetic ruby crystals.

Technical background

All currently available medical laser devices work in a similar fashion. An optical resonating chamber has a fully reflective mirror at one end and a partially reflective, partially transmitting mirror at the other. Through this chamber is pumped the laser medium, which is stimulated by an electrical current. This results in emitted photons, which bounce around the inside of the chamber; only those parallel to the long axis of the resonating chamber are able to escape through the partially transmitting mirror as laser light. This light is monochromatic (same colour), collimated (parallel and unidirectional) and coherent (intense and in phase) and therefore represents an extremely powerful, high-energy beam. It may then be passed through a lens system for focusing. As this whole process results in the production of heat, the optical chamber is surrounded by a water-jacket cooling system.

Tissue effects

The wavelength of light produced, and so its tissue effects, depend on the laser medium used. All the effects of lasers are due to the local absorption of energy and the subsequent production of heat in the tissues. This laser burn is extremely accurate, and will cause tissue damage which varies with its penetration. Total energy delivery to the tissues is dependent on the power density of the beam and the duration of exposure. It can be controlled by three methods. The total power of the beam (watts) is set at the laser control panel. The area of the spot is altered by adjusting the focus of the beam. Exposure time (seconds) can also be set at the control panel in pulsed mode or left as continuous mode. Pulsing reduces the exposure time, with a concomitant increase in the power delivered in that time. Techniques exist for further shortening of the pulse (ultrapulse and Q-switching). These are important for the confinement of the thermal energy.

Types

1. The carbon dioxide laser produces light in the far-infrared range (wavelength 10 600 nm). Consequently it is invisible to the human eye and the system is usually provided with a low-power helium–neon laser carried coaxially to act as a sighting beam. The energy of the CO_2 laser is strongly absorbed by any water-containing tissues, regardless of pigmentation, and its effects are extremely localized (0.3 mm penetration). It kills cells by boiling the water content of cells (80% water), which causes a sudden increase in volume and vaporization. The advantage of this is that it can accurately destroy small volumes of tissue with minimal surrounding tissue injury, but its disadvantage is that its poor penetration will certainly not coagulate blood vessels more than 0.5 mm in diameter.

2. The Nd-YAG laser has a crystal of neodymium doped-yttrium aluminium garnet stimulated by a krypton arc lamp, produces light of wavelength 1064 in the near-infrared range, and so is also invisible. The Nd-YAG laser is prone to light scattering and so tissue effects may be evident 2–4 mm from the target site. It is therefore less precise than the other lasers but will coagulate vessels 1.5–2 mm in diameter. It can be used in contact mode with a sculptured quartz or sapphire tip. Its effect then is that of a hot knife cleaving tissue bloodlessly without deeper effects. The Nd-YAG is mostly used in fibreoptic bronchoscopy and oesophagoscopy, although the KTP laser, by being more precise, may gradually take over this work.

3. The KTP laser is a modification of the Nd-YAG laser, in which a crystal of potassium titanyl phosphate is stimulated by a krypton arc lamp, to produce a beam of 532 nm visible green light. When excising lesions in tissue with larger vessels, such as the tongue, a bloodless field will only be gained with a more penetrative laser, the KTP being ideal.

4. The erbium YAG (Er:YAG) laser. For skin surgery in order to achieve correct energy densities, the CO_2 laser needs to be pulsed (e.g. ultrapulse system) or flash scanned (e.g. silktouch system). The Er:YAG has a water absorption coefficient 10 times that of these systems. Thus it vapourizes narrower, thinner segments of tissue and has more control of the zone of thermal necrosis. It main use has been in laser skin resurfacing.

5. The argon laser produces visible blue/green light with light at a number of wavelengths, but mostly 488–514 nm. Energy from the argon laser is particularly well absorbed by pigmented tissues, notably haemoglobin, which is advantageous in areas where small haemorrhages will prove disastrous, such as the retina of the eye. Tissue penetration is about 1 mm and so it will accurately and reliably coagulate vessels of this diameter.

6. The holmium:YAG (Ho:YAG) laser. With a wavelength of 2100 nm, this can vapourize bone with little collateral damage. This property has made the Ho:YAG laser a candidate for use in sinus surgery which necessitates the removal of bone.

7. Diode lasers. These are becoming increasingly available. To date they are being manufactured to offer wavelengths in the region of 630–1000 nm, but those with shorter wavelengths tend to be much less powerful. They may be used with optical fibres and have properties similar to those of the Nd-YAG laser with respect to coagulating tissue in non-contact mode and as a 'hot knife' in contact mode.

Safety

Medical lasers are class 4 and their use requires extreme caution. A number of protective measures are required and include:

1. **Environment.** The operating theatre should be designated a laser area and appropriate warning signs displayed. It should be equipped with remote door-locks to prevent non-essential personnel straying into theatre during laser use.

2. **Personnel.** Access should be limited to essential personnel only and there should be nominated laser users who are fully conversant with the operation and risks of the laser. All theatre personnel are required to wear eye protection.

3. **Anaesthetic.** There is a potential explosion risk with volatile anaesthetic agents and oxygen. To protect the endotracheal tube, metal tubes, coated tubes and even jet venturi are used.

4. **Patient.** All exposed parts of the patient adjacent to the operating area are covered with damp swabs to prevent any burns.

Clinical uses

A greater range of conditions are now being treated with a variety of lasers. Sometimes the laser is not proven to be of greater efficacy than conventional techniques. It is important to remember that just because a procedure *can* be done with a laser, it does not mean that it *should* be done with a laser.

1. **Ear.** The KTP laser has been used (as a weightless knife) for work around the ossicles, minimizing cochlea trauma. It has been suggested that a defocused beam be used to reduce the incidence of residual cholesteatoma in mastoid surgery. The argon laser can be used in stapedectomy to divide the crura and fashion a stapedotomy. It has also been used to spot weld tympanoplasty grafts in place. Current research is evaluating the use of lasers for atrophic tympanic membranes and outpatient myringotomies.

2. **Nose.** The CO_2 laser has been used to perform linear cautery to the inferior turbinates and turbinectomy, in the symptomatic treatment of rhinitis, as well as removing a variety of localized benign intranasal mucosal lesions. However, the KTP laser will be less likely to cause troublesome bleeding in these instances and will vaporize tissue more efficiently. This laser has been used, with some success, to perform endoscopic dacrocystorhinostomy under local anaesthetic. The Ho:YAG has been advocated for use in sinus surgery as it is powerful enough to ablate bone. However, tissue splatters and coats the endoscope lens and charring of the tissues obscures the operative field. These disadvantages have reduced the popularity of the use of lasers in this instance. This may change with the evolution of image-guided surgery. The CO_2, argon and Ho:YAG laser have all been described as being of benefit in the management of hereditary telangiectasia. The benefit is, however, relatively short lived.

3. Throat.   The CO_2 laser has found most application in ENT in the treatment of laryngeal conditions. Treatment with this laser results in minimal injury to surrounding tissue and minimal postoperative oedema, so there is less chance of postoperative airway compromise. Scar tissue formation is also minimized and so the CO_2 laser is the method of choice in the excision of benign lesions from the vocal cord. These include papillomata, which may be vaporized at a high power setting, polyps, nodules and the division of webs. It can be used to perform an arytenoidectomy and cordectomy in airway compromise due to vocal cord palsy. Recent studies have shown that cordectomy for T1 vocal cord squamous cell carcinoma provides a similar prognosis to radiotherapy regarding tumour recurrence. It provides at least as good voice preservation after healing. Carefully controlled trials are needed to confirm these preliminary findings. Obstructing laryngeal and tracheobronchial tumours may be debulked with this or the KTP laser, and on occasion small tumours have been completely excised. Although the CO_2 laser may be used for excising lesions of the tongue and oral cavity, the KTP laser is the method of choice as bleeding is minimal because of its better penetration.

4. Facial skin.   Rhinophyma has been treated with the CO_2 laser and is cited as causing less intra and post-operative bleeding when compared to scalpel or electrocautery. Cutaneous telangiectasia and port wine stains or flat macular lesions can be reduced by a flashlamp pulsed dye laser and need several treatments. Thick cutaneous haemangiomas do not do well with laser treatment. Ultrapulsed CO_2 and Er:YAG lasers are used for resurfacing facial scars and wrinkles.

5. Photodynamic therapy.   This technique has found its greatest use in the treatment of skin cancers. A photosensitive haematoporphyrin derivative which shows preferential uptake by the tumour is administered to the patient. A gold vapour laser emitting a red light is used to activate the photosensitizer, which is stimulated to release singlet oxygen atoms. These are extremely cytotoxic and result in tumour necrosis. This technique has not found a significant application in ENT although its potential for treating laryngeal cancers and papillomatosis has been investigated.

Further reading

Carruth J, Jones N, Robinson JM, Dilkes MG, Steiner W, Prescott C. A review of lasers in otolaryngology. *ENT News*, 1999; **8**(4): 10–24.

Related topics of interest

LITERATURE EVALUATION

G. Browning

Reading the literature is something that most medical post-graduates spend a considerable amount of time doing, unfortunately most of it being poorly directed. This is mainly because a journal is readily to hand, perhaps because it is free, we subscribe to it or it is in the library and we feel it has to be read to keep 'up-to-date'.

Whilst this objective is highly desirable, the problem is that the majority of what is written, repeats what is already known. Or, if it attempts to add to knowledge, the research is so poorly designed or executed that the findings are likely to be so grossly biased as to make them invalid.

Peer review

This is the process of reviewers critically evaluating an article that is submitted to a journal for consideration for publication. The reviewers advise the editor on the scientific merit and suitability of the paper for publication. Unfortunately, many reviewers, often chosen for their prominence in a specialty, are unable nor have the time to do this properly. *Table 1* is a list of journals most frequently read by otolaryngologists, which are informally ranked by the quality of their peer review process. Using this should make one focus attention on articles from some journals more than others, though it does not remove the need to be critical of articles, even in the highest ranked journals.

Table 1. Journals relevant to otolaryngology ranked by the quality of their peer-reviewer process

Rating	Journal
XXXX	*British Medical Journal*
	Lancet
	JAMA
	New England Medical Journal
XX	*Ear and Hearing*
	British Journal of Audiology
X	*Clinical Otolaryngology*
	Journal of Laryngology and Otology
	American Journal of Otology
	Archives of Otolaryngology
	Laryngoscope
None	*Continuing Medical Education*
	ENT News

This topic takes a systematic approach to evaluating an article, most of which will not be read further than the title or the abstract. It does not cover editorials, which are non-reviewed personal opinions, nor reviews, most of which are biased selections of the literature rather than 'structured reviews' for which there is a formal process (e.g. Cochrane). In addition, it does not apply to meta-analyses, which are a compilation of papers on the same topic in an attempt to improve the power of the analysis. The more knowledge a reader has on scientific methods and the topic being written about, the easier the process becomes. Reading articles in the top (*Table 1*) journals, even though not the readers' specialty, can increase the former. Reading a good text book should provide knowledge of what is already known, rather than the literature itself where the introduction in papers are often biased reviews of the existing literature.

Abstract

This will be scanned to ascertain, alongside the title of the article, the question being addressed. This task will be made easier if the abstract is 'structured' in its format (*Table 2*) and an objective clearly stated.

Table 2. Example of a structured abstract

Intratympanic gentamicin titration therapy for intractable Meniere's Disease.
Objective: To assess the efficacy and morbidity of intratympanic gentamicin titration therapy on patients with intractable unilateral Meniere's disease.
Study design: Retrospective chart review and patient interviews.
Setting: Tertiary referral ambulatory dizziness clinic.
Intervention: Eighty-three patients received weekly intratympanic gentamicin injections in their diseased ear. Treatments were terminated after four injections or sooner if patients met clinical or audiologic criteria.
Main outcome measures: Vertigo frequency, hearing status, personal disability ratings, tinnitus level, and caloric responses before and after gentamicin therapy were measured.
Results: Eighty-four per cent of patients showed complete, and an additional 6% showed substantial, vertigo control. At 24 months, 17% of patients demonstrated a clinically significant (10-dB) reduction in hearing, but 26% showed a significant hearing improvement. No patients had an 'extreme' drop in hearing (>30 dB).
Conclusions: Intratympanic gentamicin titration therapy provides excellent vertigo control with a low incidence of hearing loss.

The reviewers should then ask themselves whether it is a question that would enhance their knowledge or be of practical value to them. In the example in *Table 2*, most would answer 'Yes'. The next question is 'What is already known about the topic?' In this case, we know that there are multiple papers on the topic, to which this one does not appear to add anything. In this case, read no further. On the other hand, if the question posed had been 'To assess the efficacy . . . in comparison to the natural history' or '. . . in comparison to sac surgery' the reader would move on to their next question.

Study designs

What is the ideal study design to answer the question posed? For studies that assess the efficacy of management, there is a well-established hierarchy of levels of evidence

Table 3. Levels of evidence in studies of management

Grade	Level	Source
A	Ia	Evidence obtained from meta-analysis of randomized controlled trials
	Ib	Evidence obtained from at least one randomized controlled trial
B	IIa	Evidence obtained from at least one well-designed controlled study without randomization
	IIb	Evidence obtained from at least one other type of well-designed quasi-experimental study
	III	Evidence obtained from well-designed non-experimental descriptive studies, such as comparative studies, correlation studies and case studies
C	IV	Evidence obtained from the expert committee reports or opinions and/or clinical experiences of respected authorities

Table 4. Levels of evidence in studies which assess methods of diagnosis of a disease or condition

Step 1	State the gold (reference) standard and, if this is not histology, present the evidence, if any, that relates the gold standard to histology
Step 2	List the tests/investigations that can be used to arrive at the gold standard. Thereafter, having reviewed the literature, identify the papers at the highest level of evidence for studies of diagnostic methods
Level 1	An independent, masked comparison with reference standard among an appropriate population of consecutive patients
Level 2	An independent, masked comparison with reference standard among non-consecutive patients or confined to a narrow population of study patients
Level 3	An independent, masked comparison with an appropriate population of patients, but reference standard not applied to all study patients
Level 4	Reference standard not applied independently or masked
Level 5	Expert opinion with no explicit critical appraisal, based on physiology, bench research, or first principles

Data which should be presented: Clear definition of characterization of subjects being studied. For dichotomous outcomes (e.g. disease/no disease on X ray), state sensitivity/specificity/predictive value of diagnostic algorithms versus accepted gold standard. For continuous outcomes (e.g. results of a laboratory investigation such as audiology), 'Receiver-operating characteristics' (ROC) curve showing test performance over a range of cut-off values.

(*Table 3*). The abstract *Table 2* suggests a paper at level III, which is the level of evidence for all current papers on this particular topic. What is being looked for is the highest level available. Papers on diagnostic tests and on aetiology/epidemiology have different criterion (*Tables 4* and *5*).

Table 5. Levels of evidence in studies which investigated the aetiology or epidemiology of a condition

Level 1	Evidence from at least one randomized controlled trial of risk factors (this is the ideal study design, but virtually always impracticable to carry out because of the timescale involved)
Level 2	Evidence from at least one well-designed prospective controlled study without randomization
Level 3	Evidence from at least one well-designed retrospective controlled study over the same time frame
Level 4	Evidence from at least one well-designed study with historical controls
Level 5	Evidence from non-controlled studies

Data which should be presented: (i) clear definition of category of subjects being reported; (ii) clear definition of category of controls being reported; (iii) univariate analysis of risk factors with P-values; (iv) multivariates analysis of risk factor with P-values; (v) odds ratios of significant risk factors with 95% confidence intervals; (vi) proportion of population to whom risk factors apply with probability of disease occurrence.

Bias

Very few papers are unbiased to some extent, most often unintentional rather than in an attempt to mislead. The most difficult examples of bias to detect are where there is a lack of information. To help detect these a list of things to look for are given. Having identified potential bias, a decision has to be made as to whether it is so gross that the results of the paper are invalid or whether they should be taken with a degree of caution.

1.   *Population sample bias.* How similar is the population being studied to the patients the reader deals with? Patients treated in tertiary centres are at the extreme range of the spectrum.

2.   *Exclusion bias.* In retrospective studies, patients can be excluded in a biased manner if they do not fit. This also can occur in prospective studies, because they need treatment. Look for a description of those excluded.

3.   *Response bias.* This most often occurs with postal questionnaires where less than 85% of individuals respond. One of the reasons why people do not respond could be that they are dissatisfied or at the extreme end of the range of subjects studied (e.g. unhappy about the results of treatment). What the reader ought to do is to pose the question 'What if the non-responders had all replied in a particular way, would the range of outcomes be?' Using the following example: '89% of otolaryngologists always discuss facial nerve damage with a patient prior to mastoid surgery' based on a 45% response rate. A sample of 100 ENT surgeons produces the following table:

	n	Yes discuss	No discuss
Responders	45	40 (89%)	5 (11%)
Non-responders	55	0	55 (100%)
Total	100	40 (40%)	60 (60%)

The paper should have read 'between 40 and 89% of otolaryngologists always discuss facial nerve damage with a patient ...'.

4. Control bias. Controls should be identical to the study population in everything but the condition being studied. Think of what factors affect the outcomes and see if they have been controlled for. These factors are called 'effect modifiers'. If controls are not identical, consider what magnitude the 'effect modifier' might have on the results.

5. Non-blinding bias. Blinding is necessary whenever the outcomes can be biased by knowledge of what happened to the patient. This particularly applies to subjective rather than objective outcomes, e.g. to quality of life questions rather than death or an audiogram. Blinding of the individual recording the outcome is usually possible but not of the patient if surgery is being compared with a no surgery aim. The placebo effect of surgery is large, hence objective outcomes are important when this is being assessed.

6. Randomization bias. In randomized controlled trials, those allocating treatment should not in any way be able to decide on what the patient gets, nor to decide that once allocated the treatment is inappropriate and exclude the patient. Randomisation by an independent party is the ideal method.

7. Bias in choice of outcome. Designing questionnaires to assess subjective outcomes is a complicated science and is frequently done incorrectly if at all. Do not be misled by statements such as 'a validated questionnaire was used'. The means of assessment to ascribe validity are complicated, but the easiest question to ask is whether a specific questionnaire is appropriate to use in the population being studied. 'Generic' questionnaires *cannot* be used in all conditions. Thus a generic Quality of Life Questionnaire for cancer patients is quite inappropriate to use for hearing-aid patients.

Before reading a paper, the reader should think of the outcomes that they would consider important and then to look to see if the ones chosen satisfy that requirement. This will help exclude papers that describe unimportant outcomes. Thus in papers on chronic rhinosinusitus, whether the bacteria are eradicated or the X ray has improved are irrelevant outcomes. It is the patient's symptoms that matter. These should be assessed in detail by questions, proven to be relevant in this disease and not covered by a 'Are you better?' type question.

8. Bias in timing of outcome. Here the reader must ask whether the timing of the outcome is an applicable one. The take-rate of myringoplasty 1 week after surgery is irrelevant, it must be at least 6–12 months later.

9. Analysis bias. In randomized controlled trials the results should be quoted on an 'intention to treat' basis rather than what the patient actually received. Switching between randomization arms is most likely to apply to those allocated to medical management and surgical management. The temptation here is to compare those actually treated surgically with those treated medically. Whilst this is of interest, it is not the main question being addressed, that is 'What is the outcome of management strategy A versus strategy B, knowing that some will change arms during the study?' (which reflects real life).

Following is an example of a trial of surgery versus medical management for coronary heart disease with death as the main outcome.

Example of how analysis on an intention to treat basis produces different results from on an 'abstracted' basis in a randomized controlled trial.

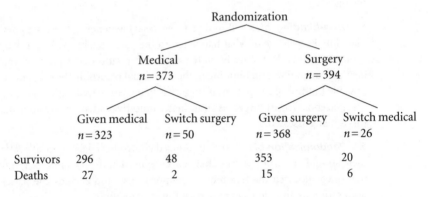

% Death rates

Method of analysis	Medical	Surgery	Difference (95% CI)
Intention to treat	7.8 (29 of 373)	5.3 (21 of 394)	2.4 (−1.0, 6.1)
As treated	9.5 (33 of 349)	4.1 (17 of 418)	5.4 (1.9, 9.3)

Of the 373 patients randomized to medical management, 50 subsequently switched to surgery. Of the 394 patients randomized to surgical management, 26 did not undergo surgery for various practical reasons. The data shows the number of patients that died, from which the percentage mortality on an 'intention to treat' basis and an 'as treated' basis can be calculated. If the 95% confidence interval (CI) of the differences between surgical and medical management are looked at, and taking the statistical rule that if they straddle zero (0) the result is not significant; when analysed on an 'as treated' basis, there are significantly fewer deaths in the surgical arm, but not when analysed on an 'intention to treat' basis. The latter is the result to take because in real life patients initially allocated to surgery or medical management will switch, and the question being addressed is what should the initial management strategy be. In this particular study it does not matter, the results are the same.

10. Statistical bias. The majority of statistical errors are relatively easy to spot. Different statistical methods are required for 'parametric' (i.e. numerical results with an equal spacing such as height) and 'non-parametric' results which may be numerical but not of an equal spacing (e.g. 0 = no change, 1 = better, 2 = a lot better). The former can be reported as means, with standard deviations and confidence intervals whilst the latter cannot.

Type II errors are where no statistical significance was found in a study, but this could be due to insufficient numbers of subjects being studied to show this, i.e. there is a lack of power. Thus, when a statistically insignificant or negative result is being reported, look at the number of patients studied. Tables are available which can be consulted to see whether this is the case, but in many instances too few a number of subjects is obvious.

P-values should be interpreted with caution. A P-value of 0.05 means that there is a 5% chance that the association is not statistically significant. Take 20 different outcomes and with a P-value of 0.05 one outcome will be significant as a matter of chance.

11. Interpretation bias. Many papers on aetiological factors fall into the trap of inappropriately linking cause and effect, particularly if it fits in with preconceived ideas. As an example, let us assume that there is a strong link between lower socio-economic group and otitis media with effusion (OME). Papers that looked at maternal smoking as a single factor would have a positive relationship because smoking is common in the lower socio-economic groups. Such papers could say that this is evidence for mothers to stop smoking to prevent their children getting OME. On the other hand, if a study were to look for it, there would also be a positive association of having OME with non-ownership of a car, but nobody would suggest giving cars to those that don't have them to prevent children getting OME.

Such misinterpretations would be less likely if a multifactorial analysis were performed on a full range of factors. Such biases are usually unintentional, based on a lack of understanding of scientific methodology. Others can be intentional.

Following is an example of the results of a study where death rates between two management arms are being compared:

- Reduces rate of deaths by 20%.
- Produces an absolute reduction in deaths of 3%.
- Increases survival from 84% to 87%.
- 31 people needed to be treated to avoid one death.

Four different methods of describing the difference are shown, based on the data in the third line. Each one is valid but gives a different impression of the difference between the two management strategies.

Finally, having read this topic, your critical skills should be honed and regularly used. To do this with colleagues in a group or at a course immensely increases their educational value.

Further reading

Dixon RA, Munro JF, *et al.* The evidence based medicine workbook. Critical appraisal for clinical problem solving. Butterworth Heinemann, 1997.

Sackett DL, *et al.* Clinical epidemiology. A basic science for clinical medicine. Little Brown and Company, 2nd edition, 1991.

Sackett DL, *et al.* Evidence-based medicine. How to practice and teach EBM. Churchill Livingston, 1997.

Greenhalgh T. How to read a paper. The basics of evidence based medicine. British Medical Journal   Publishing Group, 1997.

MASTOIDECTOMY

T.H.J. Lesser

Mastoidectomy is an operation undertaken on the mastoid air cells to remove disease. The disease is usually infective but may occasionally be neoplastic. It may also be performed as part of a procedure for access to deeper structures, for example endolymphatic sac surgery or insertion of a cochlear implant.

Incisions

Either an endaural or postaural incision is used. Both are equally popular in the UK. A properly performed endaural incision will allow good access to the attic, tegmen and sigmoid sinus even in well-aerated mastoids. It provides better access to the sinus tympani and is ideally suited for a small cavity mastoidectomy. It will not allow sufficient posterior access for a subtotal petrosectomy; this degree of bone removal is routinely performed by some if there is mastoid disease to allow the postauricular soft tissues to fall into the smooth defect, obviating the need for an obliteration procedure. Neither will the endaural incision allow an adequate angle of approach to the middle ear in those who perform a posterior tympanotomy (required for combined approach tympanoplasty and to access the round window in cochlear implants).

Cortical mastoidectomy

This is also known as the Schwartze operation and is used for the treatment of the acute non-cholesteatomatous mastoiditis when medical treatment has failed or complications have set in. If cholesteatoma is found, the posterior canal wall may be removed and the procedure converted to a modified radical mastoidectomy. A cortical mastoidectomy can also be used as treatment for chronic suppurative otitis media when there is no cholesteatoma, to clear granulation tissue from the mastoid air cells and the antrum. A myringoplasty is performed at the same time, if indicated. Occasionally a cortical mastoidectomy is performed for severe glue ear.

Procedure

A postaural incision is made at least 1 cm behind the skin fold down to the periosteum, which is elevated to expose the whole of the mastoid, including the tip. A high-speed drill is used to remove the outer cortex of the mastoid bone and then all air cells, leaving cortical bone over the sigmoid sinus and middle fossa dura. The pos-terior canal wall is left intact and the middle-ear contents are not disturbed.

Modified radical mastoidectomy

The routine procedure for cholesteatoma is a modified radical mastoidectomy. This is an operation to remove all middle-ear and mastoid disease, exteriorizing both into a common cavity. Disease-free remnants of the tympanic membrane and ossicular chain are preserved. If all the tympanic membrane, the malleus and incus are removed, the procedure is termed a 'radical mastoidectomy'.

Procedure

In a modified radical mastoidectomy the disease is either approached from behind or followed back from the attic. When approached from behind, a cortical mastoidectomy is performed and the bridge of the posterior canal wall drilled away to continue removal of the disease from the antrum, attic and middle ear (atticoantrostomy). When followed backwards, the attic is removed first, the middle ear explored and then the antrum opened and the bone removed only as far back as the disease. This has the advantage that the cavity is only as big as the extent of disease. Some cases require an atticotomy only. There are a large number of modifications in the way this operation is performed, for instance some surgeons try to remove the canal wall in one piece and then replace it at the end of the procedure.

There are even more variations in the way the reconstruction is done to minimize the chances of chronic or repeated discharge and maximize the hearing. The basic reconstruction involves including the Eustachian tube opening in a reconstructed middle ear using a fascial graft. The graft, usually temporalis fascia, is placed under the drum remnant and often over the whole of the mastoid cavity. This appears to encourage squamous epithelium to cover the cavity and it may allow air from the Eustachian tube to fill deep to it and effectively reform a soft posterior canal wall and a near-normal ear canal. The cavity can also be obliterated with bone dust, muscle flaps, artificial substances, e.g. hydroxyapatite, or free muscle. The bony work on the cavity itself is of greater importance than the obliteration substance. All air cells should be removed, the cavity edges must be well saucerized, the mastoid tip removed as far medially as the digastric ridge, the facial ridge lowered to the level of the inferior canal wall and a wide meatoplasty fashioned. These procedures will improve the chance of a dry ear and are especially useful in revision surgery. When all the cells of the mastoid are removed, in particular those in Trautman's triangle, the perifacial, the retrosigmoid, the zygomatic root, and all perilabyrinthine cells, the operation is called a subtotal petrosectomy. This may be combined with Eustachian tube obliteration, closure of the external auditory meatus and filling the cavity with free abdominal fat graft in particularly difficult ears.

Hearing reconstruction

The reconstruction of hearing is dealt with elsewhere, but has to be considered at the same time as the primary surgery even if the tympanoplasty is done as a second stage. Most British surgeons prefer to accept a type III tympanoplasty with the new eardrum in direct contact with the head of the stapes if it is present. This gives a 5–25 dB conductive loss but profers long-term stability. This type III can be encouraged if the posterior annulus is medialized when lowering the facial ridge so that the head of the stapes is relatively more prominent. It is also useful if an edge of bone is formed for the new tympanic membrane to take off from. If the stapes superstructure is not present, the hearing reconstruction is best left to a second stage. Many patients opt for no further surgery or a hearing aid if given the choice. If a second stage is performed, a deep middle ear is helpful and this should be encouraged at the first stage by leaving a lateral annulus. At the second stage a piece of bone or an artificial total ossicular chain prosthesis is placed between drum and footplate.

Combined approach tympanoplasty

This operation removes disease from the mastoid and middle ear. A cortical mastoidectomy is extended to remove bone posteriorly over the lateral sinus to allow an adequate angle to visualize the middle-ear contents via a posterior tympanotomy in which the posterior part of the middle ear is entered lateral to the mastoid segment of the facial nerve in the angle between it and the chorda tympani. This allows access to disease via the ear canal as well as via the mastoid. The combined approach tympanoplasty is the main canal wall up procedure. It has a high rate of recurrent cholesteatoma, but if performed skillfully it is suitable for patients who are available for long-term follow-up and second- and third-look surgery.

Complications of mastoidectomy

Injury to the anatomical structures of the temporal bone is the main danger for the patient. The facial nerve is always at risk and damage to it is the most obvious disaster that can occur. The dura and lateral sinus are also at risk, as is the otic capsule. Great care is necessary when removing disease from the lateral semicircular canal as a fistula can be opened and the resulting loss of perilymph may lead to a dead ear. Indeed it may be better to leave disease in situ on such occasions. The middle-ear part of a mastoidectomy needs equal care to avoid damage to undiseased ossicles.

Prior to mastoid surgery each patient should be warned about the risk to the VIIth cranial nerve, the risk of deterioration in hearing, the possibility of a dead ear and a chance of postoperative vertigo. It is important to document this discussion in the case notes.

Further reading

Ear. In: Ballantyne JC and Morrison A (eds). *Rob and Smith's Operative Surgery*. London: Butterworths, 1986.

Related topics of interest

Cholesteatoma, p. 35; Chronic suppurative otitis media, p. 38; Tympanoplasty, p. 341.

MEDICOLEGAL ISSUES IN ENT SURGERY

M.F. Ramadan and N.J. Roland

> *'The regimen I adopt shall be for the benefit of the patients according to my ability and judgement, and not for their hurt or for any wrong.'*
>
> Hippocratic Oath

The aims of the medical practitioner may be laudable, but all too often when problems occur they become accountable. Rarely a day passes now without the media focusing on some issue of disputed medical practice, medical ethics or medical litigation. One day the doctor is hailed as the saviour. The next he is condemned as authoritarian or uncaring. Public opinion will affect our patients perceptions. It is appalling to contemplate the treatment of patients on the basis of what will be the least likely to land the practitioner in court. However, whilst the practice of defensive medicine should be condemned, it is naïve for any medical practitioner not to have a thorough knowledge of the law and how it is applied. It is surprising how often this is overlooked in postgraduate courses and texts. This chapter summarizes the key medicolegal issues and in particular their application to the practice of otolaryngology and head and neck surgery. The main areas covered are:

- confidentiality;
- consent;
- malpractice
  - negligence
  - litigation in ENT surgery
- complaints against doctors.

Confidentiality

In 1947, the Declaration of Geneva strongly reinforced the Hippocratic Oath on this issue. It states 'I will respect the secrets which are confided in me, even after the patient has died'. However, there are many complex pressures brought to bear on practitioners to leading them to consider breaching confidentiality. The vast majority of cases of breach of confidentiality occur inadvertently, for example overhearing a conversation in a lift or at a reception desk. All healthcare workers should therefore remain constantly vigilant. In contrast to Continental Europe, confidentiality is not currently enshrined in statutory law in the UK. A patient may enforce confidentiality through a court injunction and an action for damages in a civil court may follow any breach. All staff employed by the NHS may be subject to disciplinary proceedings following a breach of confidentiality, which may result in dismissal. In general practice and private practice the doctor is responsible not only for themselves, but also any staff in their employment. It usually falls to the GMC to enforce patient confidentiality on ethical rather than legal grounds. A breach can lead to a charge of serious professional misconduct and erasure from the Register.

Consent

The competent adult patient has a fundamental right to give, or withhold, consent to examination, investigation or treatment. This right is founded on the moral principle of respect for autonomy.

1. **Types of consent.** Consent may be *implied* or *expressed* in the oral or written form. Consent is implied, for example, when a patient undresses voluntarily for examination. Express consent is in an oral or written form. Oral consent is valid but should be recorded in the case notes. For major procedures, written consent is usually obtained. This provides evidence that consent has been obtained and this should be kept safe in the patient's record.

2. **Obtaining consent.** A surgeon has a duty to explain to the patient in layman's terms the nature, purpose and material risk of the proposed procedure and, if necessary, to supplement verbal explanation using drawings or diagrams to ensure that the patient has sufficient knowledge to make an informed decision.

Consent is obtained before the procedure and before sedation. It may be taken in the out-patients to allow the patient to consider the matter further, or take advice, but this needs to be checked again on admission in case there has been a change in the patient's condition. The person who obtains the consent should, whenever possible, be the one who will do the procedure and, if not, should be appropriately qualified and familiar with all the details and risks of the procedure. The patient must have sufficient time to think of the procedure and should not be taken under any form of duress.

3. **Material risk.** Material risk is that to which a reasonable person in the patient's position would be likely to attach significance. Doctors should answer any question as truthfully and as fully as possible. The legal position on whether, or not, a doctor is negligent in failing to mention a risk to a surgical patient was determined in the UK in the case of Sidaway. Under the terms of the Bolam test, a practitioner can expect to avoid liability if the court finds a reasonable body of opinion which would support the practitioner's decision. In the Sidaway case, the court retained the right to overrule medical opinion if disclosure was obviously necessary for an informed choice by the patient. In some cases a practitioner may reasonably omit to mention a material risk if, after proper consideration of the patients condition, he believes that a warning would be harmful to the patients health (therapeutic privilege).

4. **The consent form.** If alteration to the consent is needed, the patient should be consulted and a new form should be signed. Abbreviation on the consent form should be avoided. Consent should be counter-signed and dated by the same person who gave the explanation.

Negligence

Negligence is established if the duty of care of a doctor towards his patient has been breached (that is when a person has not taken reasonable care to avoid acts or omissions which can cause injury and which can reasonably be foreseen). However, negligence that did not cause damage is not sufficient to bring a medical negligence claim.

The standard of care provided is not an absolute, but a doctor is expected to display the skill and care of a reasonably competent colleague. Naturally, standards will change with the passage of time (more progress and knowledge). Duty of care can be discharged if the patient is referred to or advice taken from a senior colleague.

Different doctors genuinely vary in their management of an illness. Therefore, it is acceptable to provide different treatment from a colleague as long as it is accepted by a reasonable body of medical opinion skilled in that specialty, not necessarily the majority.

In the Bolam case (Bolam vs. Frien HMC, 1957), ECT treatment was given to a patient without a muscle relaxant. The patient suffered injuries and fractures but because some doctors do avoid muscle relaxants because of their side effects, the judge directed the jury that a doctor is not guilty of negligence if he has acted in accordance with a practice accepted as proper by a responsible body of medical men skilled in that particular art.

The Bolam test now applies extensively in all areas of medicine, including diagnosis, treatment and information disclosed to patients to obtain a true consent.

Complaints against doctors

Complaints against doctors are rising and the main cause for this is lack of or inadequate communication with the patients. Doctors need to communicate better, to listen to the patient and to speak to the patient in a language which can be understood, avoiding medical jargon.

Patients do not like to be rushed out of the clinic. Patients like to know that he or she is the most important person in your life during the consultation and always want to feel that their personal agenda has been expressed fully during the consultation. Patients do not like, and indeed often do not understand, medical terms and one needs to speak to the patient clearly when diagnosis and treatment are explained and risks and realistic expectation of treatment are quoted. For example, the patient must know what facial paralysis means and looks like and one must quantify for the patient the percentage of risk and success, if possible.

A clear and honest explanation to the patient often avoids or aborts an imminent complaint. For most patients, all that is required is an explanation of what happened and why things went wrong. This, again, highlights how important it is that obtaining consent for surgery requires a great deal of clarity.

Failure of communication among the hospital staff can also be a source of complaint, such as when one hands over care of patients when going on holiday. The art of good communication also covers the areas of patients calls to you or your secretary. Patients' letters, patients' suggestions for further investigation or different treatment by correspondence should be respected. One should always believe the patient. Your communication with the patient should also be expressed clearly in the records.

Many complaints arise as a result of poor communication (informed consent, unrealistic expectations, lack of clarity. For example, the case of the patient who was told that there is a 2% risk to the hearing. This was perceived by him as insignificant, but when he had a 'dead' ear after the operation, lack of communication was evident, because the patient had thought that it was 2% loss of his ability to hear clearly not

2% risk of absolute deafness). The majority of patients seem to react reasonably to warnings of facial paralysis, but when they actually understand what it looks like, reaction is different.

It will do no harm to improve the line of communication by checking with the patient in plain words whether he or she has understood all that has been said, whether he or she would like to ask further questions and to ask the patient to get in touch if there is a problem with follow-up arrangements.

What to do when things go wrong

- Explain clearly and honestly what happened, for often that is all the patient or their relatives need.
- Write clearly in the case notes what happened and what has been said.
- Avoid being defensive.
- If appropriate, contact the Legal Adviser or Medical Defence Union immediately.
- Do not file your copy to the Legal Adviser in the case notes.
- Never tamper with the patients records.
- Always date clearly any addition to the notes.
- Educate yourself further in the subject.

Unclear medical notes will not help the case against you. Complete and contemporaneous medical records are essential. They provide invaluable evidence of treatment given in the event of a claim. Medical records which are tampered with or missing may turn a defensible case into an indefensible one.

Finally, because of the pride and faith doctors have in their own profession, it is naturally very upsetting when a complaint is made against a doctor who treated their patient with the best intent. But remember not to let self-doubt creep in, continue to keep a good relationship with the patient, give a follow-up appointment, keep good records, keep your Legal Advisor informed and keep faith, for things have the habit of not turning out to be as bad as they first appear.

Areas of litigation in ENT

Medical Defence Union figures show that the most common reason for the notification of an ENT claim relates to some form of sensory loss following surgery, i.e. diminished hearing, sight, smell or taste. The most common reason for a completed ENT claim involves some sort of dental damage during an ENT procedure.

1. Outpatients Procedures. In a busy out-patient department, informed consent can be forgotten and this causes complaint. Patients unsatisfied for being hurried out of the consulting room may feel the cause for a complaint. Figures from general practice show that almost 20% of all claims arise from ear syringing (a procedure often delegated to a practice nurse). The common reasons for this are poor technique, faulty equipment, excess pressure and failure to examine the ear.

Potential harmful effects of prescribed medication should be clearly explained and documented. For example there has recently been successful litigation in this area by patients receiving ototoxic ear drops. Useful advice on this is given by the BAO-HNS. Patients receiving systemic ototoxic medication ought to be assessed audiometrically and the risks explained to the patient, not only of the medication but of the options without the medication. Similarly, the pros and potential problems of oral/topical steroids should always be explained.

Failure or delayed diagnosis is particularly risky in certain areas, such as malignancy. It can be difficult in others, such as untypical presentation of acoustic neuroma. Litigation for delay or failure to diagnose is on the increase.

2. *In-patient procedures* Good communication in layman's terms continues to play a major role so that the patient forms realistic expectations. It is not sufficient to warn the patient who is to undergo mastoid surgery of facial palsy. It is necessary that the patient understands what facial palsy is. A written account of what is said, investigations and pre-operative photography should be documented.

Areas where special precautions should be taken are diathermy and laser (burn) and damage to the teeth during endoscopy. Make sure that all swabs are correct after surgery and that bandages are not too tight. Each patient is a different individual. His or her circumstances, age, occupation and type of disease have to be taken into account when taking consent.

Conclusion

Although there are exhaustive lists of moral, ethical, legal and political issues that affect the way in which we work, one should remember that courtesy, competence and communication are the cornerstone of good medical practice (the three Cs).

Further reading

Handbook of Medicolegal Practice, Butterworth, 1991.
Journal of MDU, Vol. 13, No. 1 February 1997.
MDU Consent to Treatment, MDU Ltd., 1996 revised November 1997.
General Medical Council, Seeking Patients Consent – the Ethical Consideration, GMC Publications.
Bolam -v- Frien, Hospital Management Committee, 1957.

MENIÈRE'S DISEASE

Menière's disease has been recognized since the first description by Prosper Menière, in 1861, of a condition characterized of episodic vertigo, tinnitus and deafness.

Pathophysiology

Despite mountains of research, the aetiology of this condition still remains unknown. Current theories of aetiology include labyrinthine ischaemia and an autoimmune response following a viral infection. Regardless of the primary cause, there follows expansion of the endolymphatic compartment, endolymphatic hydrops, which is thought to give rise to the classical symptoms. The increased endolymphatic pressure leads to an alteration in basilar membrane mobility, resulting in hearing loss and tinnitus. The same pressure increase leads to distortion of the ampullae of the semicircular canals with subsequent vestibular dysfunction. In severe cases rupture of Reissner's membrane may occur, leading to the delicate neural tissues being exposed to potassium-rich and neurotoxic perilymph with further provocation of symptoms.

Clinical features

Menière's disease accounts for between 10–20% of cases of true vertigo in a typical outpatient population. Patients are typically in their fifth decade at presentation with no gender bias. Episodic vertigo and hearing loss are the main complaints, although tinnitus and a sense of fullness in the affected ear are not infrequent. Attacks vary in frequency but typically last between 1 and 24 hours and are often associated with systemic upset in the form of nausea and vomiting. Movement may exacerbate the vertigo so the patient will lie as still as possible during an attack. Nystagmus is present but its direction is not indicative of the side of origin of the symptoms. In the early stages of the disease the hearing may return to normal after the attacks, but if the condition progresses and attacks recur deafness becomes established and more severe.

Patients are usually seen in the clinic between attacks, and consequently physical examination is normal. The condition is punctuated by frequent remissions and relapses over a time period of many years. There is no doubt that a large psychological component exists. In the long term (10 years) over 75% of patients' vertiginous symptoms will improve regardless of treatment type, although hearing in the affected ear invariably tends to deteriorate. Bilateral disease is thought to occur in about one-third of cases.

Investigations

An audiogram is essential and may show evidence of a sensorineural hearing loss. Classically this loss is described as low frequency, but in fact is flat in two-thirds of cases. A fluctuating sensorineural loss shown on consecutive audiograms over a period of time, with an appropriate history, is good evidence for the diagnosis.

Electrocochleography may show an enhanced negative summating potential indicative of altered cochlear function, and caloric tests may demonstrate impaired vestibular function. The glycerol dehydration test works on the principle that dehydrating the cochlea and thus reducing the endolymphatic hydrops will produce an improvement in the audiogram and the ECochG; it can be used as a preoperative assessment of the potential response to conservative surgery, but is unpleasant for the patient as it causes nausea and headache. The triad of symptoms of episodic vertigo, tinnitus and deafness is sometimes described as Menière's syndrome. There are causes of this other than Menière's disease. In those patients with an asymmetrical hearing loss, it is essential to exclude a cerebellopontine angle tumour (e.g. acoustic neuroma). Other causes of intermittent vertigo should also be excluded.

Management

It is important to bear in mind that Menière's disease is a condition that responds well to a supportive and sympathetic therapeutic approach, regardless of which treatment modality is ultimately used (i.e. strong placebo effect). Treatment can be either medical or surgical and can be regarded as a therapeutic ladder, climbing from the simple to the complicated.

1. Medical. Medical treatment starts with the manipulation of diet in an effort to reduce salt and fluid intake, and strong psychological reassurance. Betahistine 16 mg t.i.d., a labyrinthine vasodilator, has been shown to give significantly greater symptom control than placebo. Vestibular sedatives, such as prochlorperazine and cinnarizine, are without doubt useful in short-term symptom control and are best prescribed to be taken at the onset of any attack. Diuretics, thiazides in particular, are frequently prescribed but there is no good study to demonstrate any greater efficacy than placebo in this condition. Medical treatment should provide adequate symptom control in about 80% of patients.

2. Surgical. The simplest surgical procedure is the insertion of a grommet in the affected ear. This procedure is without any logical or scientific support and probably works by placebo effect alone. The mainstay of surgery for this condition has been decompression of the endolymphatic sac with the aim of treating the underlying pathophysiological abnormality without destroying the function of the ear, particularly hearing. This is accomplished via a cortical mastoidectomy approach to the sac as it lies in the posterior cranial fossa. Decompression is achieved by exposing and opening the sac with or without the use of a shunt to provide prolonged drainage. Although 90% of patients report initial satisfactory symptom control, by 5 years this figure is down to 60%. The greatest controversy surrounding endolymphatic sac surgery concerns the Danish sham study in 1981, in which sac surgery was prospectively and randomly compared with simple cortical mastoidectomy. The study was blind and demonstrated no significant differences between the two surgical options.

More radical surgery for this condition involves vestibular nerve section, which abolishes signals from the troublesome labyrinth while still preserving hearing. Control rates of 90%, maintained for up to 10 years, have been reported, although the morbidity is higher as a neurosurgical approach is required.

The vestibular labyrinth may be selectively destroyed by the use of ultrasound, but this technique does also risk cochlear damage. It can also be achieved by the local application of gentamicin at the round window, or by insufflation of gentamicin using an indwelling middle ear catheter. Finally, in those ears with poor hearing a surgical labyrinthectomy may be the procedure of choice.

Follow-up and aftercare

By the very nature of the condition, these patients are often 'long-term' attenders at an ENT department. However, with appropriate support and encouragement, they need not be 'frequent' attenders.

Further reading

Ludman H. Menière's disease. *British Medical Journal*, 1990; **301**: 1232–1233.

Ruckenstein MJ, Rutka JA, Hawke M. The treatment of Menière's disease: Torok revisited. *Laryngoscope*, 1991; **101**: 211–218.

Commins DJ and Nedzelski JM. Topical drugs in the treatment of Menière's disease. *Current Opinion in Otolaryngology and Head and Neck Surgery*, 1996; **4**: 319–324.

Related topics of interest

Caloric tests, p. 27; Vertigo, p. 346; Evoked response audiometry, p. 78; Vestibular function tests, p. 350.

NASAL GRANULOMATA

A granulomatous reaction is a specific type of chronic inflammation characterized by the local accumulation of macrophages and their morphologically and functionally diverse derivatives. These comprise the epithelioid cell and multinucleate giant cell. Usually surrounding and interacting with these is a zone of lymphocytes.

Most nasal granulomata are formed as a result of specific chronic infections. The most important of these are tuberculosis, syphilis, leprosy and fungal infections. Non-specific granulomata occur when no infectious agent can be defined and comprises sarcoidosis and Wegener's granulomatosis (WG). The formerly and inappropriately named lethal midline granuloma is now recognized to be a high grade T-cell lymphoma.

Wegener's granulomatosis

Wegener in 1939 described a granulomatous disease of unknown aetiology comprising destructive lesions of the upper and lower respiratory tracts and glomerulonephritis. Histological examination showed granuloma formation and necrotizing vasculitis. It is now accepted that only a single system may be affected by the disease or there may be multi system involvement, affecting not only the three classical systems but also virtually every organ in the body including the ear. These are considered to be variations of WG, but no consensus view exists on the nomenclature in these situations.

Pathogenesis

Current knowledge suggests that an infection, usually viral, in susceptible individuals triggers an immunological response to produce the features of WG.

Clinical features

In the nose and when active WG classically causes a sanguinous discharge, crust formation and friable ulcerated mucosa. Chest features comprise haemoptysis and dyspnoea. Oliguria and micro or macroscopic haematuria suggests renal involvement. The patient feels weak and lethargic and experiences marked weight loss. Untreated there is a 93% two-year mortality. WG may effect the external and middle ear causing a serosanguinous discharge and a conductive hearing loss. Vestibulocochlear symptoms, a facial palsy and a secondary infection may occur. On examination the appearances are similar to a carcinoma and the diagnosis can only be made by a representative biopsy. Friable, ulcerative lesions in the mouth, oropharynx, and larynx have also been described.

Investigations

A chest radiograph may show single or multiple opacities up to 5 cm in diameter compatible with areas of infarction with or without cavitation. Alveolar infiltrates, pleural opacities or atelectasis may be present. Urinalysis may show red cells, protein and casts. Creatinine clearance declines. Renal biopsy, if indicated, shows focal necrotizing glomerulonephritis and vasculitis. A recent meta-analysis of patients with active WG calculated a sensitivity of 91% and a specificity of 99% for cytoplasmic anti-neutrophil cytoplasmic antibody (c-ANCA). Between 20 and 40% have raised titres against p (perinuclear)-ANCA. Both antibodies are detected by indirect immunofluorescence. Both antibodies are directed against proteinase 3 and therefore low titre samples can be checked by an antigen-specific enzyme-linked immunosorbent assay. These titres parallel changes in disease activity. The classical three system involvement and a representative biopsy of an active area is both necessary and sufficient to make the diagnosis. Random biopsies of normal looking upper respiratory mucosa in subjects suspected of having the disease provide a zero WG diagnostic yield and therefore the biopsy of an active area is stressed.

Treatment

Long-term, low-dose antibiotic therapy aimed at preventing an infectious trigger or immunosuppressive therapy aimed at dampening the immunological response is the current strategy. Low-dose co-trimoxazole has been shown to prevent relapse in many patients. Septrin has been shown to increase host cytotoxicity and enhance intracellular killing. Cell mediated immunity against viruses involves the intracellular killing of free virus particles and the killing of virus infected cells by macrophages. Co-trimoxazole's mechanism of action may be to enhance virus killing sufficiently to prevent immune complex formation which causes inflammation and granuloma formation when deposited in the micro circulation (see Related topic). Cyclophosphamide and prednisolone are the current immunosuppressive drugs of choice, the doses of which are adjusted to reduce side effects to a minimum while maintaining remission. In patients with resistant or fulminant disease plasma exchange, high-dose intravenous steroids or extracorporeal immunoabsorption with protein. Disease activity can be monitored by the ESR and serum C-reactive protein level.

High grade T-cell lymphoma

This was often confused with WG, but with the advent of modern immunocytochemical techniques, a representative biopsy will allow an accurate diagnosis.

Clinical features

The nasal features are similar to WG but there is little systemic disturbance and in particular no bronchial or renal disease. There is progressive destruction of the mid-facial structures. Untreated the patient succumbs from secondary infection or cachexia.

Investigations

A representative biopsy will show huge numbers of small cells with a high incidence of mitoses. There may be zones of acute inflammatory cells if a secondary infection supervenes. Necrotizing vasculitis and granuloma formation are absent. As the small cells may represent a poorly differentiated squamous cell carcinoma, malignant melanoma, neuroblastoma or rhabdomyosarcoma immunocytochemical analysis is necessary to confirm the diagnosis. Staging should be undertaken by a medical oncologist to determine optimum treatment.

Treatment

1. Antibiotics to control secondary infection.
2. Surgical debridement of necrotic tissue.
3. A curative dose of radiotherapy, usually 60–66 Gy in 30 fractions if stage I (localized) disease, followed by further debridement if indicated.
4. Reconstructive surgery to the nose and mid facial regions as required.

Syphilis and tuberculosis

Only tertiary syphilis produces a granulomatous reaction, the pathological lesion being the gumma. This can invade mucous membrane, cartilage or bone, the bony septum being the site most commonly involved. The usual presentation is nasal swelling, putrid discharge, bleeding and crusting. A red nodular swelling which can be diffuse or localized may be visible. The treponema pallidum haemagglutination test (TPHA) and fluorescent treponemal antibody test (FTA) for syphilis are positive and a biopsy of the lesion shows perivascular cuffing of arterioles by chronic inflammatory cells and endarteritis. There may be a septal perforation, erosion of the nasal bridge with a saddle deformity, stenosis of the nares or atrophic rhinitis. Tuberculosis and sarcoid affect mainly the cartilaginous septum. In tuberculosis there may be apple jelly nodules around the vestibular skin and signs of pulmonary involvement. Biopsy shows caseating granulomata and acid fast bacilli may show on a Ziehl-Neelsen stain or following culture. Biopsy of a sarcoid lesion shows non-caseating granulomata, angiotensin converting enzyme levels are raised, the Kveim test is positive and there may be evidence of multi-system involvement.

Scleroma and rhinosporidiosis

Scleroma is a disease affecting any area of the upper and lower aerodigestive tract and caused by a gram-negative diplococcus *Klebsiella rhinoscleromatis*. It is endemic in India, the Middle East and parts of Africa but unusual in Western countries when it usually arises within the immigrant population. Nasal symptoms are the most common and usually comprise nasal obstruction and foul smelling mucopurulent rhinorrhoea. Signs of a severe bacterial rhinosinusitis with mucosal injection and oedema, and mucopurulent discharge may be present on endoscopic examination. There may be submucosal swelling in the vestibular area. Atrophic rhinitis like crusting and septal perforation may occur in the cicatricial phase. The diagnosis is made by culture of the diplococcus. Mikulicz cells (macrophage with clear cytoplasm containing the encapsulated organism) and Russell bodies (bright-red degenerated plasma cells) are classically seen on histology. Ciprofloxacin or co-trimoxazole are the antibiotics of choice and need to be continued for at least a month as the organism is difficult to kill because of its mucopolysaccharide coat.

Rhinosporidiosis is a chronic disease which can affect any skin lined or mucosal surface of the body and occasionally the viscera. It is caused by *Rhinosporidium seeberi* and it is thought to be a fungus rather than a protozoan. It is transmitted by swimming in infected water. It is most commonly found in India and Sri Lanka. The nose is the mostly commonly infected site and the disease is typically insidious in onset and runs a slow course. In the early stages a thick, sticky nasal discharge may be seen and there is usually a history of recurrent epistaxis. Thereafter pedunculated or sessile, soft, injected polyps form typically around the nasal vestibule. The organism has not been cultivated *in vitro* or transmitted to animals in the laboratory. Chemotherapy is universally unsuccessful and the only treatment is surgery to excise the lesions.

Further reading

Van der Woude FJ, Van Es LA, Daha MR. The role of the c-ANCA antigen in the pathogenesis of Wegener's granulomatosis. A hypothesis based on both humoral and cellular mechanisms. *Netherlands Journal of Medicine*, 1990; **36**: 169–171.

Rao JK, Weinberger M, Oddone EZ, Allen NB *et al.* The role of antineutrophil cytoplasmic antibody (c-ANCA) testing in the diagnosis of Wegener's granulomatosis. *Annals of Internal Medicine*, 1995; **123**: 925–932.

Marfatia HK, Kirtan MV. Management of rhinosporidiosis – newer concept. *Indian Journal of Otolaryngology Head and Neck Surgery*, 1997; **49**: 73–74.

Related topic of interest

Sinonasal tumours, p. 280; Sinusitis, p. 285.

NASAL POLYPS

Aetiology

In certain predisposed individuals, any inflammatory nasal condition can lead to marked swelling of the sinus and nasal mucosa. This seems particularly to affect the mucosa in the region of the middle turbinate and middle meatus. When this swelling becomes sufficiently pronounced, polyp formation may result. The initiator of this inflammatory response may be chronic infection, allergy or intrinsic rhinitis, but in some cases the cause is unknown. Recent work suggests that patients who develop nasal polyps have a subtle immunological disorder of the upper (and often lower) airway; co-existent asthma is common.

Pathology

Pathologically, polyps demonstrate marked oedema of the connective tissue stroma, which also contains a variety of inflammatory mediators such as histamine, prostaglandins and leukotrienes. There is a marked eosinophilic and histiocytic infiltrate and the epithelium displays goblet cell hyperplasia and in some areas a squamous cell metaplasia. A polyp forms when the oedematous stroma ruptures and herniates through the basement membrane. Nasal polyps are rare in childhood, and if they occur one should suspect cystic fibrosis or immune deficiency. Recurrence is common after surgical removal, although it may often be delayed for many years. It is more likely and tends to occur sooner in those patients with coexistent asthma and aspirin hypersensitivity.

Clinical features

Nasal polyps may be asymptomatic, but even when small most patients complain of a feeling of congestion or obstruction high in the nose and a hyponasal quality to their speech. As the polyps enlarge there is associated worsening of nasal obstruction and usually a profuse watery nasal discharge causing rhinorrhoea or a postnasal space drip. At the same time patients frequently complain of loss of taste and smell. Headaches, pressure sensation in the face and sinusitis may occur. In severe cases the polyps may be visible at the external nares and widening of the intercanthal distance may occur. The polyps are insensitive. A history of epistaxis or contact bleeding should raise suspicion of the possibility of a neoplastic polyp. Clinical examination of the nose is not complete without an endoscopic examination (rigid or flexible), as without it small polyps in the middle meatus may be missed.

Investigations

There are few essential investigations. It is worth performing skin tests or a PRIST and RAST to identify an allergic cause. Sinus radiographs may be helpful in demonstrating maxillary sinus involvement but are rarely used. In recurrent cases and those to be treated by FESS, coronal CT scanning of the sinuses is essential and provides far more anatomical and diagnostic information. Following surgical removal the polyps should always be sent for histological analysis, especially unilateral polyps or unusual-looking polyps.

Management

1. Medical. In patients with small polyps and following surgical removal it is worth trying medical therapy. This consists of intranasal steroids, as either drops or spray, with the addition of oral antihistamines if there is an allergic element. Short courses of low-dose oral steroids may be extremely useful in those patients with particularly aggressive polyposis.

2. Surgical. If sufficiently troublesome surgical clearance can provide marked symptomatic improvement. Good symptom control can be obtained with a 'simple' intranasal polypectomy under either local or general anaesthetic. It is likely that a more thorough clearance can lead to better longer-term disease control and so an ethmoidectomy may also be performed. The majority of surgeons would now probably undertake this procedure endoscopically. With appropriate preparation of the operative field and the excellent vision afforded by the endoscope, an exceptionally thorough clearance can be undertaken. This is now often augmented with the aid of powered suction and microdebriders. Computer-aided navigation systems for ethmoid sinus surgery are available and may increase safety in difficult regions, such as the frontal recess.

Follow-up and aftercare

In simple cases no long-term follow-up is required after the first post-operative check; the patient can be asked to return should future problems arise. Intranasal steroids have been shown to reduce recurrence in the first year and may make a difference to the recurrence rate given long term. In severe cases oral steroids may be needed following surgery. Periodic surveillance and follow-up are usually required.

Antrochoanal polyp

The antrochoanal polyp is uncommon. It is typically unilateral and commences as oedematous lining from the maxillary sinus. This lining prolapses through the ostium into the nasal cavity and enlarges towards the posterior choana and nasopharynx.

The patient, commonly a young adult, complains of unilateral nasal obstruction, which is worse on expiration owing to the ball valve-like effect of the polyp in the posterior choana. If sufficiently large, it may produce bilateral obstruction and cause otological symptoms as a result of blockage of the Eustachian tube orifice. Anterior rhinoscopy may look normal as only the thin stalk may present in the nose. The enlarged posterior end may be seen on posterior rhinoscopy. All suspected cases should therefore have proper endoscopic examination.

A CT scan is the best investigation, but a plain sinus radiograph of the maxillary sinus may show complete opacification of the affected antrum.

Treatment is by complete nasal avulsion with removal of the antral portion. This can usually be achieved endoscopically. An intranasal antrostomy is the usual approach. Failure to remove the antral lining may result in a recurrence. With recurrence a Caldwell–Luc procedure may be required to clear the sinus.

Further reading

Rowe-Jones JM, and Mackay IS. Management of nasal polyps. *Current Opinion in Otolarygology and Head and Neck Surgery.* 1998; **6**: 41–46.

Related topics of interest

Allergic rhinitis, p. 11; Functional endoscopic sinus surgery, p. 108; Intrinsic rhinitis, p. 131; Sinusitis, p. 285.

NASAL TRAUMA

The commonest causes of nasal trauma are assault, road traffic accident and sports injuries. Nasal trauma does not imply only nasal fracture. Injury to the nose may result in a combination of soft-tissue injury, fracture of the nasal bones, fracture or dislocation of the septum, septal haematoma, CSF leak and facial bone fracture.

Classification of fracture of the nasal bones

An isolated nasal fracture is usually caused by low-velocity trauma. If the nose is fractured by high-velocity trauma then facial fractures are often an accompaniment. Nasal fractures are classified on a 1–3 scale depending on their severity and extent.

A *class 1* fracture is usually due to a frontal or fronto-lateral blow and results in a vertical fracture of the septum (Chevallet fracture) with a depressed or displaced distal portion of the nasal bone.

A *class 2* fracture is nearly always due to lateral trauma and results in a horizontal (Jarjavay fracture) or C-shaped fracture of the septum involving the perpendicular plate of the ethmoid and the septal cartilage in combination with a fracture of the frontal process of the maxillae.

A *class 3* fracture indicates that the velocity of the trauma has been even greater and results in a nasal fracture which extends to include the ethmoid labyrinth. The perpendicular plate of the ethmoid rotates backwards and the septum collapses into the face, turning up the tip of the nose and revealing the nostrils. There is a marked depression of the nasal bones, which are pushed under the frontal bones, and there is an apparent widening of the space between the eyes (telecanthus).

Clinical features

Trauma to the nose may be part of a more extensive injury to the facial skeleton and base of skull. It should be remembered that the most important consideration in maxillofacial injuries is the maintenance of an airway. A history of trauma to the midface accompanied by epistaxis, a noticeable deformity and nasal airway obstruction are the usual complaints. Nasofrontoethmoid fractures may produce symptoms of diplopia and epiphora. It is important to carefully record the time and nature of the trauma, previous episodes of trauma and whether the nasal deformity is new or old. Remember to enquire about any trauma to the head and neck and any other injuries.

Tenderness, haematoma and swelling may make the assessment difficult. It is appropriate in uncomplicated cases to reassess the patient 5–7 days after the injury. The nasal swelling is often accompanied by periorbital and subconjunctival ecchymosis. Check the nasal airways and examine the septum; note any deformity and exclude a septal haematoma. Ocular movements should be tested and Vth nerve function (infraorbital sensation) and dental occlusion should be checked. All injuries should be carefully documented in the case notes supplemented with drawings and occasionally photographs. The elucidation and documentation of these clinical symptoms and signs should be standard medical practice. They are also important for medicolegal purposes.

Investigations

In the majority of simple uncomplicated fractures no investigations are required, but in more serious injuries radiographs are an important investigation. They should include views of the skull, face and nasal bones depending on the extent and severity of the injury. They may be important for medicolegal purposes. A CT scan on bone setting may delineate maxillofacial fractures when there is uncertainty.

Management

1. **Soft-tissue injury.** Wounds are thoroughly cleaned and any foreign body removed. Appropriate antibiotic and antitetanus cover should be given. Abrasions are best left open. Small lacerations can be closed with Steristrips, but larger lacerations should be closed with fine monofilament sutures.

2. **Nasal fracture.** Treatment is not required in some patients because there is no fracture or bony deformity. These patients should be reassured and reviewed again when swelling has subsided. It is also inappropriate to try and manipulate a long-standing deformity as this will inevitably result in failure. It is possible to reduce a simple class 1 fracture under local anaesthetic before any swelling appears if it is seen early enough. Disimpaction and realignment can usually be achieved with laterally applied digital pressure and Walsham's forceps, one blade in the nasal cavity and the other outside. If the fracture is seen later and there is much swelling, manipulation should be delayed for 5–7 days. Manipulation should never be delayed for more than 2 weeks post injury because the nasal bones will fix and reduction will be difficult if not impossible. Class 2 fractures have a propensity to redisplace owing to overlapping of the fractured ends of the septal cartilage and the perpendicular plate of the ethmoid. The manipulation of the nasal bone should be accompanied by an excision of the septal fracture and overlapping segments through a Killian incision. A class 3 fracture will require an open reduction. The depressed nasal bones need to be elevated out of the face and supported with wires via an incision over the nasofrontal angle. The septum is approached through a Killian incision with the aim of pulling the rotated septal cartilage forwards and downwards. Malunion following nasal trauma will require treatment by a formal septorhinoplasty procedure.

3. **Septal haematoma.** This is due to a collection of blood beneath the mucoperichondrium of the nasal septum. It may follow nasal trauma, but it can also occur as a complication of septal surgery (e.g. submucosal resection (SMR)) and, rarely, blood dyscrasias. There is usually complete bilateral nasal obstruction caused by a soft swelling. If this is missed or not treated correctly, a septal abscess, cartilage necrosis and nasal saddle deformity may ensue. Aspiration may suffice if the haematoma is small, but incision and drainage with quilt suturing (to obliterate the dead space) is required if the collection reaccumulates. The patient should be given a course of antibiotics to reduce the risk of local and systemic infection.

4. **Cerebrospinal fluid leaks.** The presence of clear rhinorrhoea at any stage following nasal trauma should raise the suspicion of a CSF leak. The cribriform plate is extremely thin and is the commonest area of fracture. Confirmation of the diagnosis is obtained by checking the glucose content of the rhinorrhoea, which will approach

that of serum levels, or alternatively β_2-transferrin assays (this is a protein present in perilymph and CSF) can be used. Fluorescein injected into the CSF via a lumbar puncture can be collected from the leak in the nose. High-resolution CT scan may delineate the fracture. Until the leak ceases the patient is at risk of pneumococcal meningitis and most advocate oral penicillin and sulphadimidine as antibiotic prophylaxis. Some suggest that antibiotic prophylaxis is not required. Many leaks will close spontaneously, but some will require surgical repair with temporalis fascia, fascia lata or a mucosal flap from the nasal septum. Repair can be approached by an external ethmoidectomy, a trans-septal route, by an intranasal endoscopic approach or by a frontal craniotomy and repair with reduction of the bony fragments.

Further reading

Gleeson M. Fractures of the facial skeleton. In: Mackay IS, Bull TR (eds), *Scott-Brown's Otolaryngology*, Vol. 4, 6th edn. London: Butterworth, 1997, 1–36.
Vuilleriun T, Imola M. Nasal and sinus trauma. *Current Opinion in Otolaryngology and Head and Neck Surgery*, 1994; **2**: 37–41.

Related topics of interest

Examination of the nose, p. 84; Septal perforation, p. 278.

NASOPHARYNGEAL TUMOURS

There are four important groups:

a) Nasopharyngeal carcinoma (NPC).
b) Other nasopharyngeal tumours.
c) Angiofibroma.
d) Adenoids (see Related topics).

Nasopharyngeal carcinoma

Pathology

NPC can be divided into three subtypes based on the World Health Organization (WHO) classification. It divides the cancer on the basis of its light microscopy appearance.

- WHO type 1 is keratinizing squamous cell carcinoma.
- WHO type 2a is nonkeratinizing squamous cell carcinoma.
- WHO type 2b is undifferentiated carcinoma.

The latter has a predilection for those of Southern Chinese or Hong Kong extraction forming 20% of all malignancies in these people and 80% of their head and neck cancers.

Aetiology

The consensus view supports the proposal that in the genetically predisposed a carcinogen is triggered by an environmental co-factor to transform nasopharyngeal epithelial cells. The environmental factor most widely implicated is salted preserved fish, a staple diet of the Hong Kong boat people, the male population of which comprise the world's highest at risk population group. Latent Epstein-Barr virus (EBV) infection is endemic in this group and the evidence for EBV being the carcinogen is compelling. In particular:

1. Southern Blot and Polymerase Chain Reaction consistently detect DNA sequences of EBV in NPC cells.
2. NPC cells consistently express two species of EBV proteins; EB nuclear antigen 1 and latent membrane protein 1 detectable by immunofluorescence.
3. Plasma antibodies to *viral capsid antigen* and to *early antigens* (one of which is an EBV DNAse) are seen, titres of the latter being a significant predictor of tumour relapse after radiotherapy.

It has recently been shown that EBV is associated with all WHO types of NPC.

Genetic factors

The human leucocyte antigen allele A2 without BW46 or B17 is associated with long term survival. The A2 BW46 allele combination is associated with intermediate term survival while the occurrence of B17 is associated with short term survival.

Clinical features

The majority of patients present with a history of epistaxis, nasal obstruction, a neck lump or referred otalgia. Seventy per cent of patients will have metastatic lymph node involvement at presentation and in a large Hong Kong series this was the mode of presentation in 40% of patients. NPC usually arises from the fossa of Rosenmuller and may spread by direct extension to involve:

- Anteriorly to the Eustachian tube causing a serous otitis media.
- Postero-laterally through the pharyngobasilar fascia to the parapharyngeal and retrostyloid space. Involvement of the former space causes mandibular nerve paralysis with partial loss of facial, palatal and pharyngeal sensation and involvement of the pterygoid musculature causing trismus. Involvement of the latter space containing the cervical sympathetic trunk and the IX–XII cranial nerves causes Horner's syndrome, vocal cord, pharyngeal, palatal, shoulder and tongue paralysis and pain.
- Superiorly through the foramen lacerum to cause paralysis of the 3rd, 4th and upper two divisions of the 5th cranial nerves causing diplopia, facial hypoaesthesia and headaches.

Investigations

The diagnosis is made from the history, examination and special investigations. NPC often spreads submucosally from the fossa of Rosenmüller so that no nasopharyngeal abnormality is visible although there may be metastatic lymph node disease. Fibreoptic pharyngoscopy is probably the most reliable method of examining the nasopharynx and should be used if a biopsy of the fossa of Rosenmüller is to be obtained under a local anaesthetic. A 'blind' biopsy is not recommended as the specimen obtained may be non-representative.

The polymerase chain reaction to EB virus genome has been used to diagnose NPC in patients with a malignant neck node with an occult primary. CT is the investigation of choice to assess skull base and paranasal sinus involvement. MRI imaging including a short tau inversion recovery (STIR) sequence to suppress fat clearly defines the tumour margins in soft tissue and will best define the presence and extent of metastatic neck disease. A chest radiograph, liver ultrasound and, if symptoms dictate, a bone scan are useful screening tools in the search for distant metastases.

Staging

Several staging systems have been developed for NPC which has made it difficult to compare treatment results using differing modalities and results between centres. Europe had traditionally used the UICC system, North America the AJCC system and Asia, including Hong Kong, the Ho system. In 1997 the 5th Edition of the AJCC Cancer Staging Manual brought the AJCC into line with the UICC and their staging is:

T1   Tumour confined to the nasopharynx.
T2   Tumour extends to soft tissue of oropharynx and/or nasal fossa.
      T2a: without parapharyngeal extension.
      T2b: with parapharyngeal extension (parapharyngeal extension denotes postero-lateral infiltration of tumour beyond the pharyngo-basilar fascia).

T3   Tumour invades bony structures and/or paranasal sinuses.

T4   Tumour with intracranial extension and/or involvement of cranial nerves, infratemporal fossa, hypopharynx or orbit.

NX   Regional lymph nodes cannot be assessed.

N0   No regional lymph node metastasis.

N1   Unilateral metastasis in lymph node(s) measuring 6 cm or less in greatest dimension above the supraclavicular fossa.

N2   Bilateral metastasis in lymph node(s) measuring 6 cm or less in greatest dimension above the supraclavicular fossa.

N3a   Metastasis in lymph node(s) greater than 6 cm in diameter.

N3b   Metastasis in lymph node(s) in the supraclavicular fossa.

Management

Radiotherapy using a field which includes the nasopharynx, skull-base, the sphenoid and posterior ethmoid sinuses, and posterior orbit is the treatment of choice. The consensus view now is to irradiate the neck bilaterally to reduce the incidence of future neck node metastases. NPC and in particular undifferentiated NPC is highly radiosensitive so a neck dissection is indicated only for radiotherapy failures even if patients present with N3 disease. The 5-year actuarial survival is greater stage for stage in WHO type 2a and 2b patients compared to those with WHO type 1 histology.

There is evidence that adjuvant chemotherapy reduces loco-regional relapse and significantly improves prognosis in NPC (actuarial five year survival 64% v 42% in radiation alone group).

Surgery plays a limited role in the treatment of NPC. Radical neck dissection may control radio-resistant nodes and post-radiation cervical node recurrence. In selected patients, salvage surgery may be indicated for nasopharyngeal recurrence.

Prevention

1. EBV infection of the nasopharynx is not a regular feature in healthy EBV virus carriers. In high risk areas screening nasopharyngeal biopsies for viral genomes is useful for determination of high risk individuals. Counselling this group on their diet and the need for frequent regular follow-up is recommended.

2. A vaccine based on the EBV envelope glycoprotein GP340, a major target for the virus-neutralizing antibody response, is currently undergoing Phase 1 trials.

Follow-up and aftercare

All patients with treated head and neck cancer must be reviewed monthly for the first year, bimonthly for the second year, every three months for the third year and six monthly for the fourth and fifth years post treatment. If they are disease free then for most cancers they may be considered cured (adenoid cystic carcinoma and malignant melanoma are notable exceptions). Many head and neck units will continue to follow patients annually for another five years because such patients are at significant risk of developing a second primary cancer.

Other EBV associated disease

- Burkitt's lymphoma (a monoclonal B cell non-Hodgkin's lymphoma).
- T-cell lymphoma.
- Hodgkin's lymphoma.
- Infectious mononucleosis.

Other nasopharyngeal tumours

- Non-Hodgkin's lymphoma.
- Extramedullary plasmacytoma (predilection for the nasopharynx and paranasal sinuses).
- Paediatric nasopharyngeal tumours: ectodermal (dermoids, teratomas); neuroectodermal (encephalocele, meningocele); dysontogenetic (craniopharyngeoma, chordoma).

Angiofibroma

This histologically benign tumour comprising fibrous tissue with a variable proportion of vascular tissue, often with large endothelial spaces, arises from the posterolateral wall of the nasal cavity and the superolateral nasopharyngeal wall. The sphenopalatine foramen is always involved and may be the specific site of tumour origin. It occurs predominantly and perhaps exclusively in young adult males.

Clinical features

The tumour expands to erode or compress surrounding fissures, foramina and tissues. The commonest symptoms are epistaxis and nasal obstruction. It may expand laterally into the pterygopalatine fossa, through the pterygomaxillary fissure and into the infratemporal fossa, expanding superiorly to erode the pterygoid plates, the greater wing of the sphenoid and the skull base foramen. Anterosuperior expansion into the nasal cavity, paranasal sinuses, parasellar region, cavernous sinus and orbit may also occur. Presenting signs are similar to NPC except there is a smooth mass filling the nasopharynx on endoscopic or mirror examination. A high index of suspicion for any nasopharyngeal mass is essential because angiofibroma should not as a rule be biopsied. In particular it must not be confused with a large adenoid pad.

Investigations and treatment

An MRI scan with a STIR sequence is the investigation of choice to define the extent and vascularity of the tumour. Surgery is the treatment of choice for all but the smallest tumours as they may continue to expand and are typically poorly radiosensitive. Large vascular tumours require digital subtraction angiography to define the important feeding vessels. These should be embolized 1–2 days pre-operatively. *Depending on tumour extent* a mid-facial degloving or, if the cribriform plate is involved, a craniofacial approach are those most widely advocated and these may need to be combined with an infratemporal approach. For tumours where involvement is limited to the nasal cavity, nasopharynx, ethmoid and sphenoid sinus endoscopic approaches compare favourably with external approaches with significantly reduced morbidity.

Further reading

Sam CK, Prasad U, Pathmanathan R. Serological markers in the diagnosis of histopathological types of nasopharyngeal carcinoma. *European Journal of Surgical Oncology*, 1989; **15**: 357–360.

Reddy SP, Raslan WF, Gooneratne S *et al.* Prognostic significance of keratinization in nasopharyngeal carcinoma. *American Journal of Otolaryngology*, 1995; **16**: 103–108.

Geara FB, Glisson BS, Sanguineti G *et al.* Induction chemotherapy followed by radiotherapy versus radiotherapy alone in patients with advanced nasopharyngeal carcinoma: results of a matched cohort study. *Cancer*, 1997; **79**: 1279–1286.

Fagan JJ, Snyderman CH, Carrau RL, Janecka IP. Nasopharyngeal angiofibromas: selecting a surgical approach. *Head Neck*, 1997; **19**: 39–399.

Wilson J (ed). *Effective Head and Neck Cancer Management. Second Consensus.* British Association of Otolaryngologists, Head and Neck Surgeons, 2000.

Related topics of interest

Adenoids, p. 8; Cervical lymphadenopathy, p. 29.

NECK DISSECTION

A primary carcinoma arising from the upper aerodigestive tract may ultimately drain into the lymph nodes of the neck, which form an efficient barrier to the further spread of the disease. The prognosis for the patient regardless of the site of the primary tumour is worse if there are cervical lymph nodes involved at presentation. Only 30–40% of such patients will survive longer than 5 years. The oncologist has two effective treatment modalities for neck node metastases in radiotherapy and surgery. Broadly speaking, radiotherapy will only be effective in the curative treatment of cervical lymph node metastases if they are less than 2 cm in diameter. The advantage of using radiotherapy in these cases is that it precludes the need for surgery, which can be kept in reserve for the treatment of any recurrence. Patients who have larger nodes are less likely to be cured by radiotherapy and must be treated surgically. The operation may be required to remove the nodes alone, or it can be performed in continuity with removal of the primary tumour as an *en bloc* resection.

Classification

The classification below is suggested by the American Academy's Committee for Head and Neck Surgery and Oncology. Radical neck dissection is considered to be the standard basic procedure, and all others represent one or more alterations to this procedure. Modified radical neck dissection involves the preservation of one or more non-lymphatic structures routinely removed in radical neck dissection. It is suggested that this term be used in preference to functional neck dissection, which should be abandoned. However, for the foreseeable future it is likely that both these terms will continue to be used. Selective neck dissection involves the preservation of one or more lymph node groups routinely removed in radical neck dissection. Extended radical neck dissection involves removal of additional lymph node groups or non-lymphatic structures relative to the radical neck dissection (i.e. a superior mediastinal dissection in patients with subglottic or cervical oesophageal tumours).

1. *Radical neck dissection.*
2. *Modified radical neck dissection.*
3. *Selective neck dissection.*
    (a) Supraomohyoid neck dissection.
    (b) Posterolateral neck dissection.
    (c) Lateral neck dissection.
    (d) Anterior compartment neck dissection.
4. *Extended radical neck dissection.*

Radical neck dissection

This operation refers to the removal of lymph nodes in the anterior and posterior triangles extending from the inferior border of the mandible superiorly to the clavicle inferiorly, the midline anteriorly and the anterior border of the trapezius muscle posteriorly. The cervical lymph node groups routinely removed are as follows: submental and submandibular; upper, middle and lower jugular (deep cervical); and the posterior triangle group. The submandibular gland, spinal accessory nerve, internal jugular vein and sternocleidomastoid muscle are also removed.

Complications of radical neck dissection

1. Immediate.

- Haemorrhage (from either end of the internal jugular vein or other ligated vessel).
- Chyle leak (if the thoracic duct has been inadvertently damaged).
- Nerve palsies (phrenic, vagus, marginal mandibular branch of the facial, lingual, hypoglossal, sympathetic trunk, brachial plexus).

2. Intermediate.

- Facial oedema.
- Cerebral oedema (after a synchronous or staged bilateral neck dissection).
- Wound infection.
- Wound breakdown (poor surgical technique, previous radiotherapy, diabetes, poor nutritional status).
- Rupture of the carotid artery (may be a sequel to wound breakdown).

3. Late.

- Frozen shoulder (less likely to occur if the cervical nerve branches of C3 and C4 are preserved as they pass under the fascia of the floor of the posterior triangle).
- Recurrence in the glands or skin.

Modified radical neck dissection

This operation consists of a *monobloc* removal of the cervical lymph nodes from levels I through to V as with a radical neck dissection. There is preservation of any one or all of the following structures: internal jugular vein, the accessory nerve or the sternocleidomastoid muscle. The jugular vein preservation is of great importance when bilateral neck dissections need to be performed, but the main advantage from this procedure is that the risk of frozen shoulder (due to accessory nerve resection) is avoided. Modified radical neck dissection is considered to result in regional control rates similar to those achieved by radical neck dissection as long as patients are carefully selected (patients with mobile nodes not greater than 3 cm in diameter and no more than 3 in number).

Selective neck dissection

The selective neck dissections are based on a knowledge of the distribution of nodal metastases in the different primary sites. Thus for patients with N0 disease the following procedures remain an option:

1. Supraomohyoid neck dissection. Oral cavity tumours commonly metastasize to levels I, II and III.

2. Lateral neck dissection. For cancers of the larynx and hypopharynx the commonest node levels are II, III and IV.

3. Posterolateral neck dissection. Usually applied for skin tumours such as melanoma and skin adnexal tumours (levels II, III, IV and V).

4. _Anterior compartment neck dissection._ Removes the nodes around the visceral structures in the midline (level VI) and is usually indicated for thyroid cancer.

Bilateral neck dissection

The presence of bilateral neck nodes is not an independent poor prognostic sign, but univariate analysis demonstrates a reduced 5-year survival to around 5%. This is because when bilateral disease is present at least one set of nodes is usually of greater diameter than 6 cm and fixed. Surgery probably does not influence the natural history of the disease. Supraglottic carcinoma with bilateral glands is an exception and can still have a reasonable prognosis. Bilateral synchronous neck dissection carries a significant morbidity and a mortality of about 3%. Many of the complications can be reduced by either staging the procedure with an interval of 6 weeks or longer or performing a modified procedure on the opposite side to preserve the internal jugular vein. The most serious complication is that of raised intracranial pressure. Ligation of one internal jugular vein results in a threefold increase in the intracranial pressure, but when the second side is tied there is a tenfold increase in pressure. The patient should have a temporary tracheostomy, be nursed propped up in the bed, and may require an infusion of mannitol (500 ml of 10% mannitol over 4 hours). The most critical period is the first 12 hours postoperatively. Over the following 8–10 days after the operation, the intracranial pressure tends to fall, though it never returns to its normal level.

Further reading

Robbins TK. Neck dissection. *Current Opinion in Otolaryngology and Head and Neck Surgery*, 1993; **1**: 114–119.

Robbins TK *et al*. Standardising neck dissection terminology. *Archives of Otolaryngology and Head and Neck Surgery*, 1991; **117**: 601–605.

Wilson J (ed). *Effective Head and Neck Cancer Management. Second Consensus.* British Association of Otolaryngologists, Head and Neck Surgeons, 2000.

Related topics of interest

Cervical lymphadenopathy, p. 29; Hypopharyngeal carcinoma, p. 124; Laryngeal carcinoma, p. 138; Oral cavity carcinoma, p. 197; Oropharyngeal carcinoma, p. 203.

NECK SPACE INFECTION

Anatomy

Understanding neck space infections is straightforward but requires some anatomical knowledge.

1. The pre-vertebral fascia arises from the base of skull in front of the atlas and inserts into the body of T3. An abscess behind this fascia cannot extend below this level unless the fascia is breached.

2. Immediately anterior to the pre-vertebral fascia is a potential space extending from the skull base to the diaphragm. That portion behind the pharynx is the retropharyngeal space. It is emphasized there is no anatomical barrier preventing an abscess tracking inferiorly into the superior and posterior mediastinum, although the inflammatory reaction usually localizes the abscess to the retropharyngeal space.

3. The parapharyngeal space is a potential space immediately lateral to the oropharynx and nasopharynx, the styloid process dividing it into an anterior or pre-styloid and a posterior or post-styloid compartment. The latter contains the carotid sheath, which is firmly attached on its lateral aspect to the investing layer of deep fascia on the deep aspect of sternomastoid but has only loose areolar tissue lying medially and posteriorly. Infection may therefore spread from the pre-styloid to the post-styloid compartment by passing medial to the carotid sheath or from the retropharyngeal space to the post styloid compartment (and vice versa) by passing posterior to the carotid sheath. An abscess in the post-styloid compartment may track further laterally to point just behind the posterior aspect of sternomastoid. In the pre-styloid compartment a collection may extend as far forward as the fascia surrounding the submandibular gland, just anterior to the sternomastoid but above the hyoid bone.

4. The infratemporal fossa lies beneath the base of skull between the side wall of the pharynx and the ascending ramus of the mandible. It is bounded posteriorly by the styloid process and the anterior wall of the carotid sheath, anteriorly by the posterior wall of the maxilla and superiorly by the infratemporal surface of the greater wing of the sphenoid. The infratemporal fossa therefore is equivalent to the pre-styloid compartment of the parapharyngeal space.

5. The submandibular space is bound by the mucosa of the floor of the mouth superiorly and by the mylohyoid muscle and deep fascia investing the submandibular gland inferiorly.

Neck space infections

Citelli's abscess and *Bezold's abscess*, both complications of acute suppurative otitis media, have been previously described as has *peritonsillar abscess* (see Related topics).

Prevertebral abscess

This is rare today and occurs in adults from tuberculosis of the cervical spine. The attachment of the fascia limits the inferior extent to the vertebral body of T3. A progressively painful and tender neck with limitation of movement is the usual presentation. A lateral neck radiograph shows prevertebral soft tissue shadowing and a rarified vertebral body which may be wedge shaped through collapse. Occasionally collapse will cause acute spinal cord compression, requiring urgent drainage of the abscess and cord decompression. Aspirating the abscess allows a sample to be subjected to a Z-N stain. A positive result does not distinguish between tuberculosis and atypical mycobacterial infection, but it may allow empirical anti-tuberculosis treatment to be instigated while the culture and sensitivity result is awaited.

Retropharyngeal abscess

The overwhelming majority of cases arise in children less than four years old. Older children have fewer retropharyngeal nodes and adults have only the node of Rouviere. The condition occurs in adults when a prevertebral TB abscess ruptures *through* the prevertebral fascia. Suppuration of retropharyngeal nodes occurs after an upper respiratory tract infection (URTI) from lymphatics draining infected tonsils, teeth, pharynx or paranasal sinuses although occasionally the source is an unsuspected foreign body. The child becomes increasingly toxic and may dribble, have stertor or dysphagia. The neck is held rigidly and may become hyperextended. Symptoms mimic laryngotracheobronchitis and acute epiglottitis, although in the latter case the history is longer. It is safer therefore not to examine the throat which, even with a correct diagnosis, might cause rupture of the abscess with inhalation or tracking of the abscess into the mediastinum.

Investigations

An inspiratory lateral soft tissue neck radiograph, the neck extended to prevent the retropharyngeal soft tissues causing a pseudomass, will show the widened retropharyngeal space and narrow oropharyngeal airway. An increase in the retropharyngeal soft tissue density of more than 7 mm or 14 mm in the retrotracheal area, is highly suspicious of a retropharyngeal or retrotracheal abscess. An expiratory radiograph in a normal child can also cause widening of the retropharyngeal soft tissues so the X-ray must be interpreted as part of the overall clinical picture before treatment decisions are made.

Treatment

It has been suggested that in the absence of airway distress, intravenous antibiotics and close observation may obviate the need for incision and drainage of the abscess in the tonsillectomy position. The child may need to remain on ICU for 24–48 hours until the retropharyngeal soft tissue swelling settles.

Parapharyngeal abscess

Sixty percent arise from tonsillitis or peritonsillitis and thirty percent from an abscess of the root of the lower third molar which lies below the mylohyoid line. Mastoiditis or a pharyngeal foreign body are unusual causes. It has potentially life threatening complications including internal carotid artery rupture, internal jugular vein thrombosis and mediastinitis.

Clinical features

These are similar to a peritonsillar abscess. There is trismus, soft palate oedema, often torticollis, and the tonsil is pushed medially. There is a hot, red, tender swelling which may be firm or fluctuant or diffuse. It lies most commonly behind the posterior aspect of the upper or middle third of the sternomastoid because infection most commonly drains from the pre-styloid to the post-styloid compartment and thereafter laterally.

Treatment

Repeat fine needle aspiration of the abscess and intravenous antibiotics, either co-amoxyclav or a broad spectrum penicillin/cephalosporin and metronidazole are the combination of choice. These may obviate the need for formal incision and drainage.

Submandibular abscess (Ludwig's angina)

In over 80% of patients infection arises from a root abscess of the lower premolars or the first and second molars. There may be no history of dental pain if the root is close to the inner table of mandible which gives way early. The remaining cases are secondary to tonsillitis. A mixed population of aerobic and anaerobic organisms are usually present, the choice of antibiotics being similar to retropharyngeal and parapharyngeal abscess.

Clinical features

Floor of mouth oedema secondary to cellulitis can progress rapidly to endanger the airway. The tongue is pushed posteriosuperiorly and there is trismus and dribbling. The submandibular region is red, hot, swollen and tender.

Treatment

If the airway is not in immediate danger fine-needle aspiration of the abscess and intravenous antibiotics are usually adequate. Incision and drainage is necessary if there is not a rapid response to intravenous antibiotics or if the airway is becoming precarious. This is usually preceded by the insertion of a nasopharyngeal tube to secure the airway.

Further reading

Last RJ. *Anatomy: regional and applied*, 7th edn. London: Longman, 1999.

Gidley PW, Ghorayeb BY, Stiernberg CM. Contemporary management of deep space neck infections. *Otolaryngology and Head and Neck Surgery*, 1997; **116**: 16–22.

Flanary VA, Conley SF. Pediatric deep neck space infections: the Medical College of Wisconsin experience. *International Journal of Pediatric Otorhinolaryngology*, 1997; **38**: 263–271.

Related topics of interest

Acute otitis media, p. 5; Tonsil diseases, p. 330; Paediatric airway conditions, p. 232; Stridor and stertor, p. 311.

NOISE-INDUCED HEARING LOSS

Aetiology and background

The ear is a sound-sensitive organ but can be damaged by excessive noise levels. Excessive noise can arise from a variety of sources: occupational, such as factory machinery, building sites and high-impact tools; recreational, such as shooting, home power tools, discos and personal stereos. Motorcycling and car air-bags are both recently recognized causes of noise-induced hearing loss (NIHL). Occupational deafness is a compensable disease and legislation exists to protect the employee (Health and Safety at Work Act). In the UK the first action level is 85 dB(A) for an 8-hour working day, at which point an employer is obliged to monitor the hearing levels of his work force and to monitor noise levels at the work place. At the second action level of 90 dB(A), he is statutorily obliged to provide a hearing protection programme to include hearing protection, monitoring and efforts to reduce sound levels at source.

Pathology

Biological variability means that individuals are not affected equally by the same noise exposure. Gender and increasing age appear to have an influence on susceptibility. However, with increasing noise levels above 90 dB(A), a greater proportion of the exposed population will exhibit pathological changes. Initially noise exposure will lead to temporary threshold shift (TTS), a recoverable phenomena. There are no obvious pathological changes in TTS and the problem is probably due to metabolic 'exhaustion' of the hair cells of the cochlea. With increasing and repeated noise exposure there is permanent direct mechanical and metabolic damage, initially to the outer hair cells (OHCs) of row 1, and subsequently to the OHCs in rows 2 and 3 and the inner hair cells. Damage also occurs to the supporting pillar cells and the stria vascularis. The audiometric hearing loss tends to parallel the loss of hair cells. A doubling in sound intensity corresponds to an increase of only 3 dB, while a 10-fold increase in intensity corresponds to an increase of 10 dB. Therefore small increases in noise exposure recorded in dB expose the cochlea to large increases in sound energy.

Clinical features

TTS may be perceived as ringing in the ears (tinnitus) following excessive noise exposure. Permanent threshold shift (PTS) is frequently asymptomatic initially and is often found on routine screening audiometry carried out in the workplace. Such screening is a requirement of any hearing protection programme. When PTS becomes symptomatic the first complaint is usually reduced understanding for speech, especially when there is background noise. As it becomes more severe the patient complains more of being hard of hearing. Unfortunately tinnitus is a frequent accompanying symptom in noise induced hearing loss.

Examination will reveal normal tympanic membranes (unless the patient has had previous middle-ear disease) and the audiogram will often show a dip at around

4–6 kHz in the early stages. This may become exaggerated as exposure continues, until eventually there is flattening of the audiogram as sensorineural damage progresses.

Investigations

A good history is the key to diagnosis and is essential in personal injury medicolegal cases in order to provide apportionment of disability if more than one type of noise exposure has occurred. It is also essential when assessing any claimant with NIHL to consider alternative explanations for the hearing loss; non-syndromic hereditary and degenerative causes are not uncommon. Cerebellopontine angle tumours may produce a unilateral asymmetrical, high-tone sensorineural hearing loss or intermittent tinnitus, so investigation to exclude this cause is sometimes necessary.

Management

Damage to the cochlea caused by noise is cumulative so that, once diagnosed, further deterioration must be prevented by adequate protective measures or better still, avoidance of further noise exposure. Counselling is helpful, preferably from a hearing therapist, regarding the hearing loss and frequent tinnitus, to minimize disability. A hearing aid may be required. Awareness of the potential hazards of noise will allow prophylactic measures to be taken both at work and recreationally, e.g. the use of earplugs and muffs. There are increasing research reports of the use of pharmacological agents to protect the cochlea metabolically from the effects of noise.

Management: medicolegal

Occupational noise-induced hearing loss (NIHL) became a compensable disorder in 1975, and as such a scheme exists to calculate the disability and hence the amount of compensation. In essence this involves averaging the hearing thresholds for each ear for the frequencies of 1, 2 and 3 kHz. Allowance is then made for any difference between the two ears, age, any conductive loss and the type of audiogram, and a figure for the disability is finally reached. Personal injury cases are argued on their individual merits.

Follow-up and aftercare

Continuing advice and review by a hearing therapist is recommended to minimize disability.

Further reading

King PF, Coles RRA, Lutman ME, Robinson DW. *Assessment of Hearing Disability. Guidelines for Medicolegal Practice.* London: Whurr, 1992.
McFadden SL, Henderson D. Recent advances in understanding and preventing noise-induced hearing loss. *Current Opinion in Otolaryngology Head and Neck Surgery,* 1999; **7**: 266–273.

Related topics of interest

Acoustic neuroma, p. 1; Impedance audiometry, p. 128; Non-organic hearing loss, p. 194; Pure tone audiogram, p. 254.

NON-ORGANIC HEARING LOSS

Non-organic hearing loss (NOHL) is a condition in which a patient consistently displays an apparent auditory deficit, when no true hearing loss exists, or exaggerates a real hearing loss.

This condition is usually encountered either in an adult, in whom there is an ongoing claim for compensation as a result of ototrauma (hearing loss from noise exposure, ototoxic drugs or trauma), or in a child with psychological disturbance. In the former group the patient usually exaggerates an existing hearing loss in an effort to improve any compensatory payment. In the latter group this psychosomatic symptom represents a cry for help in response to some current stressful event, although it may not always be possible to identify the stressor. In the child, the underlying hearing is usually normal.

Clinical assessment

The diagnosis of NOHL depends primarily on a high index of clinical suspicion, particularly financial claims and in children without obvious pathology. The prelimin-ary clinical investigation may reveal some inconsistencies which suggest the diagnosis. The patient appears to hear much better than the subsequent audiogram would suggest (but beware of lip readers). The pure tone audiogram itself may be performed in an erratic and hesitant fashion. Patients complaining of a unilateral hearing loss may deny any hearing of a tuning fork placed on the mastoid process of the affected side. A patient with a genuine unilateral hearing loss would perceive the bone-conducted stimulus in the normal cochlea and report the perception of sound. Those patients who have some degree of psychological upset often appear completely unconcerned about the hearing loss but are very often accompanied by an extremely concerned carer.

Unfortunately, in all patients who are pursuing a financial claim, a non-organic component must be excluded; it has been estimated to occur in up to 25% of cases.

Investigations

A plethora of tests exist to try and distinguish non-organic from organic hearing loss.

1. Tuning forks. These can be used as part of the clinical assessment in cases of apparent unilateral hearing loss, e.g. the Stenger test (see Clinical assessment of hearing, p. 45), which can also be performed using an audiometer.

2. Pure tone audiometry. In the truly deaf patient pure tone audiometry reveals consistent results. One should suspect a NOHL when pure tone responses are inconsistent or when the patient denies hearing, in the good ear, a sound over 70 dB above the threshold applied to the bad ear.

3. Impedance audiometry. The stapedius reflex threshold normally varies from 70 to 95 dB above the pure tone threshold. There may be recruitment, so this is not invariably the case. Even then there is usually at least 20 dB between the reflex threshold and the pure tone threshold. If the thresholds are within 20 dB or less than a NOHL is likely.

4. *Speech audiometry.* This is often useful in making the diagnosis. Patients often find it more difficult to exaggerate their impairment to the same extent in speech as in pure tone audiometry.

5. *Delayed speech feedback.* The patient is asked to read aloud from a book. The voice is recorded and played back into the bad ear via headphones, the recording being delayed by milliseconds. If there is a genuine deafness the patient will be able to read without pausing. If the patient is feigning deafness then the delayed speech feedback will alter the reading pattern causing the patient to stammer, slow down or shout.

6. *Evoked response audiometry.* If knowledge of the auditory thresholds is required with some precision, as in medicolegal cases, electric response audiometry will be required. Cortical responses are preferred to brainstem evoked responses as they provide precise threshold levels and establish integrity of the entire auditory pathway. Electrocochleography can be used, but this technique is invasive and gives no information about the central auditory pathways.

Management

The aims in management are first to recognize that there is a non-organic hearing loss and thereafter to ascertain the true auditory thresholds.

Patients pursuing a financial claim are well aware of their actions. Once it is indicated to a patient that the true thresholds are suspected, and an honourable escape route is provided, the NOHL will often disappear on repetition of testing. Any true hearing loss can then be treated on its merits, including the provision of a hearing aid if required, and compensated accordingly.

Fortunately, in the younger, disturbed, group the condition is usually short lived, rarely lasting more than a few weeks or months, as the stressing event disappears or the patient develops appropriate coping strategies. Confrontation is rarely, if ever, successful. Strong reassurance that there is nothing serious present and that the hearing will improve in time is usually all that is required. A hearing aid may be provided for its placebo effect when there is great distress on the part of the patient or carers.

Follow-up and aftercare

In severe or prolonged cases (up to 20%) appropriate psychiatric referral may be required. Follow-up is only required to document the return of normal hearing.

Further reading

Alberti P. Non-organic hearing loss in adults. In: Beagley HA (ed.) *Audiology and Audiological Medicine*, Vol. 2. Oxford: Oxford University Press, 1981, 910–931.

Brooks DN, Geoghegan PM. Non-organic hearing loss in young persons: transient episode or indicator of deep-seated difficulty. *British Journal of Audiology*, 1992; **26**: 347–350.

Northern JL, Downs MP. *Hearing in Children*, 3rd edn. Baltimore: Williams & Wilkins, 1984.

Related topics of interest

Clinical assessment of hearing, p. 45; Evoked response audiometry, p. 78; Impedance audiometry, p. 128; Noise-induced hearing loss, p. 192; Pure tone audiogram, p. 254; Speech audiometry, p. 301.

ORAL CAVITY CARCINOMA

The oral cavity consists of the buccal mucosa, the upper and lower alveoli, the hard palate, the anterior two-thirds of the tongue and the floor of the mouth to the anterior tonsillar pillars. It does not include the posterior third of the tongue, soft palate or tonsils, which are in the oropharynx.

Pathology

Although benign tumours of epithelial, salivary gland and connective tissue origin occur in the oral cavity, the majority are malignant. Over 90% of the malignant tumours are squamous cell carcinoma. The remainder include adenoid cystic carcinoma, mucoepidermoid tumours, sarcomas and melanomas.

The incidence of squamous cell carcinoma of the oral cavity varies worldwide. In the UK it accounts for less than 2% of all malignancies, but in India it accounts for more than 40% because of the common practice of chewing betel quid containing tobacco. Other aetiological factors include smoking tobacco, particularly in a pipe, and high alcohol consumption. There is also an increased incidence in patients with cirrhosis of the liver. Most patients are over the age of 40 years with a peak incidence in the sixth and seventh decades. The male to female ratio is 2:1.

The commonest sites are the lateral border of the tongue and the floor of the mouth. They usually present as an ulcer but may protrude as an exophytic-type lesion. Tumours of the anterior floor of mouth and alveoli tend to spread to the submandibular nodes, and those from the posterior oral cavity tend to metastasize to the jugulodigastric nodes. The tongue has a well-developed lymphatic drainage. Tongue tip tumours spread to the submental lymph nodes first, tumours of the lateral border of the tongue spread to the jugulodigastric nodes, but some anterior tumours may spread directly to the jugulo-omohyoid nodes. Some tumours present with no nodes palpable (N0), but the incidence of occult metastases is high (35%). Second primary tumours occur in up to 30% of patients with oral cavity carcinoma. They are most commonly found in the oral cavity, but also occur in other sites in the head and neck, the oesophagus and in the lungs.

Clinical features

The patient may complain of a painful ulcer, a warty growth, halitosis and, later, difficulty in eating and speaking. Alveolar tumours may interfere with dentures. On examination the site, size and extent of the tumour should be assessed. Tongue mobility and dental hygiene should also be noted. The neck should be examined for nodal metastases, which are present in nearly a third of patients at the time of presentation.

Investigations

An orthopantomogram may demonstrate involvement of the lower alveolus by the appearance of a moth-eaten rim or an opacity of the normal lucent dental canal. A CT scan is also useful to delineate the extent and local spread of these tumours.

Isotope bone scans are very sensitive for the presence of mandible invasion. However, they are not specific and consequently there is a significant false positive rate. MRI scans are not good for illustrating bone invasion but they are particularly useful in the soft tissue delineation of tongue tumours. A chest radiograph is mandatory to exclude lung metastases. All patients should have an examination under anaesthetic to obtain a biopsy, evaluate the tumour, exclude a second primary, check the neck for nodes and stage the disease. Therapy, including the feasibility and nature of a surgical resection, can then be planned.

TNM classification

Tis   Carcinoma *in situ.*
T1   Tumour 2 cm or less in its greatest dimension.
T2   Tumour more than 2 cm but less than 4 cm in its greatest dimension.
T3   Tumour more than 4 cm in its greatest dimension.
T4   Tumour with extension to bone, muscle, skin, etc.

Management

The management of all patients depends on the site and size of their tumour, the extent of local and distant spread, the presence of any intercurrent disease and their general condition. The aim of surgery is to resect the disease while maintaining maximal function and cosmesis. It is important to remember that the surgery required can impair the functions of swallowing and speech besides its effect on the appearance of the patient. Prior to treatment all patients should see a dentist/prosthodontist to assess the status of the teeth. They should also be referred to a speech therapist for counselling in respect of their postoperative speech and swallowing rehabilitation. Nutritional status and the need for percutaneous gastrostomy should be assessed.

1.   T1 and T2 tumours.   Surgery is as efficient as radiotherapy in the treatment of T1 and T2 tumours. Small tumours can be resected transorally using a cutting diathermy or CO_2 or KTP laser with primary closure or closure with a quilted split-skin graft. With some of the larger T2 tumours a radial forearm free flap may be necessary. Oromandibular function impairment is often quoted as an argument against surgery, but some quality of life studies support surgery as the primary modality for these lesions. Radiotherapy can also be used for T1 and small T2 tumours. A combination of external beam and implants can be used. The patient is spared the ordeal of surgery and maintains good oral function. The disadvantages of external beam radiotherapy are: it cannot be used again at the same site, salvage surgery for radiotherapy failure has a low survival and high morbidity, xerostomia, loss of taste and mucositis can be troublesome side-effects, and patients may require a full dental extraction prior to treatment. Primary radiotherapy should not be used to treat tumours involving the mandible as later excision of the bone may lead to osteoradionecrosis.

2.   T3 and T4 tumours.   Larger tumours of the tongue need a partial or total glossectomy. A partial glossectomy, removing up to half of the tongue, can be repaired with a radial forearm free flap. If more than half of the tongue is removed it should be reconstructed by a pectoralis major myocutaneous flap or a rectus abdominus free flap. Small tumours of the alveolar margin can be treated by a marginal mandibulectomy, preserving the outer cortex of the mandible, but a partial mandibulectomy may be required. If much of the anterior segment of the mandible is removed the soft-tissue and bony defect should be reconstructed with a composite osteocutaneous free flap. The radial forearm or composite fibula flap are usually used. T3 and T4 lesions do badly when treated by radiotherapy alone.

3.   Neck nodes.   In some cases no nodes are palpable (N0) but the incidence of occult metastases is high (35%). Therefore in all (but the very smallest T1 tumours) cases of oral cancer, elective treatment to the first echelon nodes should be given either by radiotherapy or selective neck dissection. A supra-omohyoid neck dissection (levels I, II and III) is the usual procedure. Tongue lesions seem to metastasise to levels II and III more often. Level IV should therefore be resected for these tumours ('extended' supra-omohyoid neck dissection). Because of lymphatic crossover, especially with anterior oral cavity lesions and those located in the midline, consideration should be given to treatment of both sides of the neck. If the patient has palpable neck node metastases, surgical excision of the primary tumour and modified radical (preferable) or radical neck dissection is the treatment of choice. If the patient has bilateral neck node disease, the prognosis is poor. Irradiation to both sides of the neck or bilateral neck dissections with preservation of one internal jugular vein are possible, but the decision to treat other than for palliation should be carefully considered.

4.   Postoperative radiotherapy.   This is effective in reducing primary recurrence and has been shown to improve survival when: there are positive margins, large primary tumours (large T2, T3 and T4), perineural or intravascular invasion, poor histological differentiation, two or more positive nodes and whenever there is extracapsular spread. Most surgeons advocate the use of postoperative radiotherapy, to be given within 6 weeks of surgery.

5.   Palliative treatment.   Some patients who have a large tumour with advanced local spread or with distant metastases will not be suitable for curative treatment. In addition, it may be inappropriate to subject elderly, infirm patients who are in poor general condition, or who have severe intercurrent disease, to radical treatment. These patients should have supportive nursing care and when necessary adequate analgesisa for pain relief.

Follow-up and aftercare

The highest mortality is in the first 2 years after diagnosis. If there is going to be a recurrence it is likely to be in the first year. Patients should have a monthly outpatient review for the first 6 months and then every 2 months for 6 months, then three monthly for the second year. The oral cavity and neck should be carefully examined for signs of recurrent disease. The risk of a second primary tumour should be remembered. The donor sites of grafts and flaps should be checked until they have healed. The nutritional status and weight of the patient should be monitored, and speech therapy may be appropriate in some cases. Intense prosthodontic rehabilitation should be given where appropriate.

Further reading

Wildt J, *et al.* Squamous cell carcinoma of the oral cavity: a retrospective analysis of treatment and prognosis. *Clinical Otolaryngology*, 1989; **14**: 10–13.

Zaretsky L, Shindo ML. Soft tissue reconstruction of the oral cavity and pharynx. *Current Opinion in Otolaryngology and Head and Neck Surgery*, 1994; **2**: 343–347.

DeLacure M. Special considerations in management of the mandible for cancer of the oral cavity. *Current Opinion in Otolaryngology and Head and Neck Surgery*, 1996; **4**: 98–105.

Wilson J (ed). *Effective Head and Neck Cancer Management. Second Consensus.* British Association of Otolaryngologists, Head and Neck Surgeons, 2000.

Related topics of interest

Oropharyngeal carcinoma, p. 203; Reconstructive surgery, p. 267; Radiotherapy, p. 264.

OROANTRAL FISTULA

Definition

A fistula is an abnormal communication between two epithelial-lined surfaces. An oroantral fistula is a communication between the oral cavity and maxillary antrum. Its incidence is probably higher than is recognized because many fistulae escape diagnosis following dental extraction and heal spontaneously without complications.

Aetiology

1. Dental extraction. The fistula forms through the tooth socket following a dental extraction, particularly of the first upper molar and second premolar teeth, the roots of which may penetrate the floor of the antrum. A fistula may also follow the search for retained root fragments after a tooth has been broken.

2. Caldwell–Luc operation. The incision line fails to heal.

3. Trauma. Fractures of the maxilla or penetrating wounds such as a gunshot injury of the hard palate.

4. Neoplasm. Malignant disease of the antrum may occasionally cause erosion into the oral cavity.

Clinical features

The patient may complain of symptoms of chronic maxillary sinusitis. Purulent discharge may collect in the nose or mouth and a foul smell or taste is often noticed. A patient who has previously had inferior meatal antrostomies may notice that air or fluid and food particles can be sucked through the fistula into the nose. The diagnosis can be established by passing a probe through the fistula into the antrum.

Investigations

Radiological examination by sinus radiography and orthopantomogram may show retained root fragments, foreign bodies, signs of erosion by neoplastic disease or infections of the maxillary sinus. A CT scan will improve delineation, especially in the cases of neoplasia. The injection of a contrast medium into the defect is helpful in confirming the presence of a fistula in doubtful cases. Biopsy is needed if neoplastic disease is suspected.

Treatment

The important factors determining treatment are the length of time the fistula has been present and the presence or absence of infection.

For those following dental extraction the most satisfactory treatment is immediate suture at the time of the dental treatment. If there is a retained root, this must be removed or treatment will be unsuccessful. When a fistula is discovered later there will nearly always be friable granulation tissue in the tract and possibly an antral infection. The infection should be treated first. Pus should be sent for culture and sensitivity and a generous meatal antrostomy carried out under antibiotic cover in order to aerate the sinus and allow drainage of pus or secretions. The patient should be reviewed 4 weeks later. If the fistula has not healed it will need formal surgical closure.

Any foreign body must be removed and the bony edges of the alveolus reduced. The fistula tract is incised circumferentially around the margins of the fistula and turned inwards. The bare area is then covered by a mucoperiosteal flap. The adjacent buccal mucosa or a palatal flap based on the greater palatine artery may be used. If adjacent teeth cause a problem in closure they should be removed. The patient should give consent for this. If there is evidence of chronic sinus infection an antrostomy, if not present, should be fashioned at the same time as the fistula closure.

Follow-up and aftercare

Decongestant nose drops and a broad-spectrum antibiotic should be prescribed for the first postoperative week and the choice revised according to culture results. The patient should be reviewed in the outpatient department monthly until healing is complete.

Further reading

Snow GB, Van Der Waal. Diseases of the oral cavity. In: Maran AGD, Stell PM (eds) *Clinical Otolaryngology*. Oxford: Blackwell Scientific Publications, 1979; 363–365.

Related topics of interest

Pharyngocutaneous fistula, p. 249; Sinonasal tumours, p. 280.

OROPHARYNGEAL CARCINOMA

Boundaries
- Roof: oral surface of the soft palate and uvula.
- Posterior wall: from the level of the hard palate to the aryepiglottic folds.
- Lateral wall: anterior and posterior tonsillar pillars and the palatine tonsil.
- Anterior wall: posterior third of tongue and vallecula. The lingual surface of the epiglottis is now classified as being a subsite of the supraglottis (UICC 1997).

Pathology
- 85%: Squamous cell carcinoma (SCC).
- 10%: Non-Hodgkin's lymphoma (NHL).
- 2%: Minor salivary gland carcinoma (MSGC).
- 3%: Others e.g. rhabdomyosarcoma.

Ninety-five per cent of NHL involves the palatine or lingual tonsil. Most MSGC arises from the lateral wall, of these 50% are adenoid cystic. Most soft palate MSG tumours are pleomorphic adenomas. Thirty per cent of SCC patients will have either a synchronous second primary or will develop a metachronous second primary within 10 years of presentation. There is a male : female ratio of 5:1 for SCC. Betel nut chewing, smoking and in smokers alcohol (not proven to be a risk factor alone) are risk factors. Leukoplakia and in particular erythroplakia are pre-malignant.

Staging summary
Tx   Tumour cannot be assessed.
Tis   Carcinoma *in-situ*.
T0   No primary evident.
T1   Carcinoma < 2 cm at largest dimension.
T2   Carcinoma >2 < 4 cm at largest dimension.
T3   Carcinoma > 4 cm at largest dimension.
T4   Carcinoma extending beyond oropharynx, e.g. into the pterygoid muscles, mandible, hard palate, deep muscle of tongue or/and larynx.

Clinical features
Twenty per cent of patients present with a neck lump as the only symptom. Sore throat, referred otalgia, odynophagia and muffled speech are common. Trismus is a late symptom and suggests pterygoid involvement. A full head and neck examination is mandatory because of the high incidence of a second primary. SCC is either exophytic or ulcerative but with NHL the tonsil is either large and vascular or small and shrivelled, looking abnormal compared to its partner. Palpating the tumour and the neck is important to assess the extent of infiltration of the primary and to assess the size, level, number and fixation of any palpable neck lump(s). NHL requires assessment by an oncologist to properly stage the disease.

Investigations

1. An MRI scan with a STIR sequence will accurately define the extent of soft tissue invasion and neck node involvement. It is preferred to CT scanning. A chest X-ray and liver ultrasound are performed as these are the commonest sites for distant metastases.

2. Fine needle aspiration cytology (FNAC) of any palpable neck lump.

3. If a neck lump is not palpable but is defined on MRI or CT imaging FNAC should be performed under either ultrasound or preferably CT guidance.

4. A panendoscopy under general anaesthesia is necessary to properly assess the hypopharynx, oesophagus, trachea and bronchi for synchronous disease. If disease is limited to the tonsil a tonsillectomy is performed in order to obtain macroscopic clearance. Suspicious tongue base lesions always require a deep biopsy as the cancer may be submucosal.

Management

Most oncologists treat medium and high grade NHL as a disseminated disease and the CHOP regime (cyclophosphamide, hydroxydaunorubicin, oncovine (vincristine) and prednisolone) is the most commonly favoured. VAPEL-B (vincristine, adreomycin, prednisolone, etoposide, cyclophosphamide and bleomycin) is a more recent regime favoured by some oncologists. In the relatively unusual event that the lymphoma is very localized, radiotherapy may be used.

MSGC and SCC require a macroscopic margin of 1–2 cm and clearance must be confirmed by frozen section. T1 and small T2 stage SCC can be treated with radiotherapy as can N1 neck disease. Large T2 and T3 stage disease is treated with surgery. With many T4s macroscopic clearance is not possible. Chemotherapy or radiotherapy may reduce tumour size for clearance to be attempted but this will depend on the patient's age, fitness and wishes.

To obtain adequate exposure of the lateral oropharynx, a stepped paramedian mandibulotomy is necessary in order to preserve the inferior dental nerve. The exact site is determined after assessing an orthopantomogram as the incisor and canine roots are often not parallel. One canine and an incisor may need to be extracted at mandibulotomy to ensure the plating screws do not impinge on a root thereby predisposing to a root abscess, osteomyelitis and non-union of the plated mandible. If involvement up to and including the mandibular periosteum has occurred an inner table mandibulectomy is performed. Should the dental canal be involved a partial mandibulectomy is performed with reconstruction using a composite radial forearm (if less than 10 cm of mandible is taken), a composite fibula or a composite deep circumflex iliac microvascular free flap. T2 tongue base SCC may be excised after a paramedian mandibulotomy by a midline tongue split or via a lateral pharyngotomy after exposing the structures in the post-styloid compartment of the parapharyngeal space. The pre-epiglottic space in large tongue base cancer is almost certain to be invaded so that the only oncologically safe procedure is a total glossolaryngectomy with oral and pharyngeal reconstruction with a pectoralis major myocutaneous flap.

Soft palate oropharyngeal cancer should be irradiated if small but larger tumours require a partial soft palatectomy with reconstruction using a radial forearm fasciocutaneous microvascular free flap which gives the best result in terms of function and cosmesis. T1 and small T2 posterior wall SCC can be irradiated. If a recurrence occurs, excision with at least a 1 cm margin may allow reconstruction of the posterior wall with a radial forearm fasciocutaneous microvascular free flap allowing the patient to keep their larynx. Large posterior wall SCC is rare and is probably best treated by a total laryngopharyngo-oesophagectomy and reconstruction with a stomach transposition.

Management of the neck

In the N0 neck, consideration should be given to elective neck therapy as there is a high risk of occult neck involvement in oropharyngeal disease. Bilateral elective neck irradiation or bilateral selective neck dissection (levels I–IV) should be considered. The neck and primary site may be irradiated in N1 neck disease with a small primary. A modified radical neck dissection is used for N1 and some N2 neck disease when surgery is the treatment of choice for the primary. A radical neck dissection is required for N3 disease. Postoperative radiotherapy may be required (more than one node involved, extracapsular rupture or positive margins).

Follow-up and aftercare

After surgery swallowing is frequently seriously impaired. Swallowing rehabilitation should be instituted by a speech therapist with a special interest in swallowing as soon as nourishment is allowed by mouth, normally on around the 10th postoperative day. Rehabilitation so that sufficient fluid and nourishment can be swallowed to maintain homeostasis can take many weeks and in these a percutaneous gastrostomy is preferable to nasogastric feeding. Strictures at the anastomosic line in those who have had a stomach transposition are unusual but may require repeated dilation. Any mucosal irregularity in this region must be biopsied in case there is underlying recurrent disease is. The regularity of follow-up is the same for any head and neck cancer and is outlined elsewhere (see Related topics of interest).

Further reading

Million RR, Cassisi NJ. Oropharynx. In: Million RR, Cassisi NJ (eds) *Management of Head and Neck Cancer*, 2nd edn. Philadelphia, JB Lippincott, 1994; 401–431.

Teknos TN. Oropharyngeal reconstruction. *Current Opinion in Otolaryngology and Head and Neck Surgery*, 1998; **6**: 268–271.

Wilson J (ed). *Effective Head and Neck Cancer Management. Second Consensus.* British Association of Otolaryngologists, Head and Neck Surgeons, 2000.

Related topics of interest

Hypopharyngeal carcinoma, p. 124; Laryngeal carcinoma, p. 138; Oral cavity carcinoma, p. 197; Radiotherapy, p. 264; Reconstructive surgery, p. 267.

OTALGIA

Otalgia is pain in the ear (earache). It is a symptom not a diagnosis. It may be caused by primary disorders of the ear (otological in origin) or may be secondary to disease from other sites in the head and neck which share the same sensory innervation (referred pain).

Anatomy

The sensory nerve supply of the external and middle ears arises from many sources. The lower half of the pinna receives its sensory supply from the great auricular nerve via the cervical plexus, predominantly C2 and C3. The upper half receives its supply from the lesser occipital nerve (C2) medially and the auriculotemporal nerve laterally (mandibular branch of Vth cranial nerve). The external auditory meatus and lateral tympanic membrane receive their supply from the auriculotemporal nerve and branches of the facial and vagus nerves (Arnolds nerve). The medial aspect of the tympanic membrane and middle ear is supplied through the tympanic plexus by the facial and glossopharyngeal nerves (Jacobsens nerve).

Primary otalgia

Primary otalgia arises as a result of direct stimulation of the sensory nerves due to otogenic pathology. The pain may emanate from the pinna, the external meatus or middle ear.

1. Pinna. Haematoma, perichondritis, lacerations, neoplasms, chondrodermatitis nodularis helicis.

2. External auditory meatus. Trauma from ear cleaning, otitis externa, furuncles, shingles. Malignant otitis externa (pseudomonas infection) and tumours, by virtue of involving bone, may also produce severe pain.

3. Middle ear. Traumatic perforation of the tympanic membrane, acute otitis media, myringitis bullosa (Coxsackie B virus infection), acute mastoiditis, neoplasms.

Secondary (referred) otalgia

Referred otalgia may arise from disease in any peripheral territory supplied by the nerves. It is important to remember that otalgia may arise from a primary neuralgia of any of the sensory nerves, although it is most common in the glossopharyngeal nerve. This condition gives rise to severe lancinating pain arising in the tonsillar fossa or tongue base and radiating deeply in the ear, often induced by talking or swallowing. Less commonly the pain may be centred in the external auditory meatus and not be induced by throat movement. Shingles of the ear (herpes zoster oticus – VII, IX and Xth cranial nerves) also causes neuralgic type pain.

Causes

A brief list and system of classification for the commoner causes of referred otalgia is given below.

1. **Second and third cervical nerves** (C2 and C3).
- Arthritis/cervical spondylosis.
- Soft tissue injury.

2. **Trigeminal nerve** (Vth cranial nerve).
- Dental disease such as tooth impaction, caries and abscess, particularly of posterior teeth, and temporomandibular joint dysfunction are probably the commonest non-otological causes of otalgia.
- Nasopharyngeal disease such as viral infection, tumour or post adenoidectomy.
- Sinonasal disease and salivary gland disease are uncommon causes of referred otalgia.

3. **Glossopharyngeal nerve** (IX cranial nerve).
- Almost any oropharyngeal infective process may lead to otalgia, such as pharyngitis, tonsillitis and quinsy. Otalgia is common following tonsillectomy.
- Tumours of the tongue base.

4. **Vagus** (Xth cranial nerve).
- Carcinoma of the larynx and hypopharynx.

Assessment

A full history and examination will normally direct attention to the offending part of the head and neck. The examination should include the ears, the temporomandibular joints, the neck and the oral cavity. Particular attention should be paid to the tongue base, pharynx and larynx, as pathology here can be catastrophic if overlooked. In cases where doubt exists, scans may be appropriate (e.g. a small adenoid cystic carcinoma of the tongue base may not be apparent on examination, but obvious on an MRI scan).

Management

Appropriate treatment should then be directed at the underlying cause. Occasionally, no abnormality can be found even after a thorough examination and further investigation, except perhaps some mild clunking of the temporomandibular joint. It is not uncommon to find a small group of patients with otalgia shuttling back and forth between ENT and oral surgeons, with both claiming the symptom is in the other's department. In such cases, and in those in whom there are absolutely no abnormal findings, it is worth reconsidering a neuralgia (e.g. glossopharyngeal neuralgia). A trial of carbamazepine or amitriptyline may benefit the patient. This condition may be successfully treated by tympanotomy and section of the tympanic plexus.

Further reading

Cook JA, Irving RM. Role of tympanic neurectomy in otalgia. *Journal of Laryngology and Otology*, 1990; **104**: 114–117.

Related topics of interest

Acute suppurative otitis media, p. 5; Facial pain, p. 97; Otitis externa, p. 209.

OTITIS EXTERNA

Definition

Otitis externa is an inflammation of the skin of the external auditory meatus (EAM).

Pathology

The skin of the EAM comprises in the outer third an epithelial layer containing hair follicles, ceruminous glands and sebaceous glands, lying on a thin dermal bed containing sweat glands. The skin of the bony ear canal lacks appendages and thins from without in. The secretions of the sebaceous glands keep the stratum corneum watertight and supple. Sweat gland secretions keep the secretion at a pH between three and five which is lethal for most human pathogens. Usually the EAM is sterile or contains *Staphylococcus albus* commensals. *Staphylococcus aureus* and non-haemolytic streptococci are unusual.

In the acute phase of otitis externa there are dilated dermal blood vessels of increased permeability which cause signs of a red, hot, oedematous and tender ear canal. The epithelial reaction consists of vesication, parakeratosis and spongeosis.

Predisposing factors

- Heat, humidity, bathing, swimming.
- Trauma, especially from dirty fingernails, cotton buds and hairgrips.
- Inherited – narrow ear canals and non-atopic eczema.

Classification

1. Infective

(a) Bacterial   Diffuse otitis externa commonly caused by *Pseudomonas aeruginosa, S. aureus* and *Proteus.*
Furunculosis, usually caused by *S. aureus.*
Malignant otitis externa, usually caused by *P. aeruginosa* or occasionally *S. aureus.*
Erysipelas caused by *Streptococcus pyogenes.*
Perichondritis.
Impetigo, an infection of the superficial layers of the epidermis, usually by *S. aureus* or occasionally *S. pyogenes.*
Secondary to an acute or chronic otitis media.

(b) Fungal   *Aspergillus niger*
Aspergillus fumigatus
Candida albicans

(c) Viral   Herpes simplex
Herpes zoster
Presumptive in otitis externa haemorrhagica.

2. **Reactive.**   Eczema.
Seborrhoeic dermatitis.
Neurodermatitis.
Keratitis obturans.
Psoriasis.

Clinical features

Otitis externa may be confined to the meatus (localized) or involve other areas of skin (generalized). Localized infection can be circumscribed or diffuse while generalized infection can be either primary otological or primarily dermatological.

Inquiries regarding direct trauma to the ear canal, swimming habits, atopic tendency and previous otological problems should be made. Symptoms of infection elsewhere in the head and neck, for example tonsillitis and sinusitis and preceding symptoms of otitis media should be sought. Conditions affecting the ear canal are limited and a diagnosis can usually be made on examination. Although the history may provide a pointer towards the diagnosis, severe itching suggests eczema, neurodermatitis or mycotic infection. Otalgia occurs with furunculosis, diffuse otitis externa and herpes infections.

On examination erythema is a feature of eczema, seborrhoeic dermatitis, mycosis or acute trauma. Vesication occurs in eczema, and herpetic infection, excess squamous debris suggests chronic eczema or mycosis and hypertrophic meatal skin suggest chronic disease

It is not uncommon to find the ear canal occluded by oedema in a patient with acute otalgia. Careful examination will usually distinguish furunculosis (common) from acute mastoiditis (now much less common). In the former there is post-auricular tenderness localized to a palpable lymph node. Exceptionally this node may break down to cause diffuse tenderness and oedema which may displace the pinna slightly forwards and there is always pain on moving the pinna. A patient with acute mastoiditis will have a more marked post-auricular swelling which may be fluctuant, displacing the pinna down as well as forwards. There is no pain on moving the pinna and there will be a preceding history of acute suppurative otitis media. Plain lateral-oblique and Towne's projection mastoid radiographs may show mastoid air cell coalescence in acute mastoiditis but in this and furunculosis the mastoid air cells may be cloudy on the lateral view. In furunculosis this is because post auricular oedema is superimposed on the plate.

Investigations

A culture swab should be taken for microbiological culture, including fungal culture, and antibiotic/antimycotic sensitivity.

Management

1. Meticulous and regular aural toilet paying particular attention to the antero-inferior meatal recess.
2. Splinting the meatus. The two recommended choices are 12 millimetre ribbon gauze, impregnated with 10% ichthammol in glycerine, the hygroscopic action of which reduces meatal swelling or a pope's sponge earwick onto which

eardrops containing an antibiotic and steroid mixture are applied. In resistant cases, 8% aluminium acetate ear drops which act as an astringent may be considered. Its low pH is lethal for many bacteria including pseudomonas. Splinting will be necessary when there is EAM oedema preventing an adequate view of the tympanic membrane on otoscopy implying that ear drops will not reach the deeper recesses of the ear canal. The dressing should be changed at least every 48 hours until the canal swelling has settled sufficiently to allow any applied drops to reach the anteroinferior recess directly.

3. The ears should be kept scrupulously dry until resolution. Swimming is inadvisable and precautions taken when bathing to prevent water entering the ear canal.

In most reactive conditions the above regime is also recommended in order to prevent secondary infection of a raw ear canal surface.

Follow-up and aftercare

Treatment should continue for at least one week after resolution because of the tendency to recurrence particularly in otomycosis. Itchy reactive conditions may benefit from a course of beclomethasone ear drops and an 8% solution of aluminium acetate or acetic acid ear spray is recommended in patients with chronic otitis externa after the acute infection has been eradicated.

Malignant otitis externa

This condition describes an otitis externa which progresses to an osteomyelitis initially of the tympanic plate which then may spread to involve the skull base and petrous portion of the temporal bone. It is most common after middle age, in diabetics and is usually caused by *P. aeruginosa*. The overwhelming symptom is a constant deep otalgia and it may cause 7–12th cranial nerve palsies, meningitis, sigmoid sinus thrombosis, brain abscess and death.

The condition should be suspected in a patient with granulation tissue deep in the external meatus which does not settle with the usual treatment. The diagnosis is often not considered until a cranial nerve palsy has developed. When such a patient develops a facial nerve palsy the differential diagnosis is between the ASOM (almost always secondary to a dehiscent horizontal portion of the facial nerve), CSOM, malignancy of the EAM or middle ear and malignant otitis externa. Histological and microbiological examination of granulation tissue, and a high definition CT scan of the petrous temporal bone are required to make the diagnosis.

Treatment

Appropriate intravenous antibiotics as gleaned from the culture and sensitivity results should be commenced. The dose and duration of treatment is decided after discussion with a senior microbiologist and by monitoring clinical response but often therapy has to be continued for six weeks or more. Even with aggressive treatment there is still a significant mortality. Opiate analgesia may be required to control the deep otalgia.

Further reading

Hammond V. Diseases of the external ear. In: Booth JB (ed.), *Scott-Brown's Otolaryngology*, Vol. 3, 6th edn. London: Butterworth, 1997.

Related topics of interest

External ear conditions, p. 89; Acute otitis media, p. 5; Chronic otitis media, p. 38.

OTITIS MEDIA WITH EFFUSION (GLUE EAR)

Aetiology

The fundamental pathology is Eustachian tube dysfunction. The exact cause for this remains in doubt, but there are associations with recurrent upper respiratory tract infections, parental smoking, allergy and reduced overall nasopharyngeal dimensions. The adenoid is recognized as an important contributor to otitis media with effusion (OME) because it is a source of pathological bacteria, and not because it mechanically obstructs the orifice of the Eustachian tube. There is no difference in effusion rates between those children who have large versus small adenoids.

Pathology

The prevalence of OME is highest in young children (40% at 2 years) and decreases with age so that it is uncommon in teenagers (1% at 11 years). The prevalence is also higher in the winter months, in boys, in children with cleft palate or Down's syndrome, in those with allergy and in the children of parents who smoke. The underlying Eustachian tube dysfunction leads to a chronic reduction in middle-ear pressure. This ultimately causes an inflammatory response in the middle-ear mucosa and the production of glue: thick, tenacious mucus rich in glyco- and mucoproteins and containing inflammatory cells which fill the middle-ear cleft. In most cases (90%) spontaneous resolution is the rule, punctuated by numerous remissions and relapses. In a small number of persistent and severe cases there is progressive atrophy and retraction of the tympanic membrane. Sequalae such as retraction pockets and even cholesteatoma may ultimately develop.

Clinical features

The presence of fluid in the middle-ear cleft leads to a conductive hearing loss of variable severity and is responsible for most of the clinical features. Hearing impairment, whether persistent or intermittent, noticed by parents, relatives or teachers or picked up at routine screening is the presenting symptom in over 80% of cases. Learning difficulties and speech delay account for the bulk of the remainder, and recurrent infections and otalgia are uncommon features of this condition (1–2%) although they are common complaints in childhood. Most cases present between the age of 3 and 6 years, with the more severe cases tending to present earlier. Examination may or may not reveal a middle-ear effusion depending on the activity of the process at consultation. The otoscopic appearance of the effusion varies. The tympanic membrane can look dull red, grey or an amber yellow colour. It can bulge forward or be retracted. Attic and posterior retraction pockets may occur, but bony erosion is relatively unusual. Air bubbles or a fluid level can occasionally be seen.

Investigation

An audiogram appropriate to age and impedance audiometry are all that is required. Pure tone audiometry if feasible will show a conductive hearing loss. Impedance audiometry will show a flat tympanogram (type b) which is typical of otitis media with effusion and helps distinguish the disease from Eustachian tube dysfunction and otosclerosis.

Management

Management should be appropriate to the severity of the symptoms and should always take account of the natural history of the condition towards spontaneous resolution. For many children explanation and reassurance to the parents are all that is required. A review visit after 3 months is useful to establish the persistent nature of the patient's condition, in particular a persistent hearing loss.

Medical treatment has little role to play in this condition: antihistamines and decongestants have no useful effects and antibiotics produce short-term improvements, but do not affect the long-term course. Auto inflation of the Eustachian tube using the Otovent device has been shown to give useful results, but is significantly less effective than grommets. Compliance can also be a problem.

In the more severe cases the insertion of ventilation tubes improves hearing and shortens the overall duration of the condition. The benefits of ventilation tubes may be augmented by combination with adenoidectomy. The benefits of adenoidectomy are greatest between the ages of 4 and 8 years. Tonsillectomy does not seem to influence the condition. Grommets should be used rather than T-tubes, which are associated with an unacceptably high rate of residual perforation (up to 50%). The main complications of grommets are infections and the development of tympanosclerosis (which is found in 30–40% of children 1 year after grommet insertion). Tympanosclerosis is associated with multiple episodes of grommet insertion and intratympanic bleeding at myringotomy; mini-grommets seem to cause less but tend to extrude sooner. Infections should be treated by aural toilet and antibiotic/steroid ear drops in the first instance, but grommet removal may be required if the condition fails to settle.

Follow-up and aftercare

Grommets require little aftercare. There is no good evidence that swimming with unoccluded ears increases the risk of infection, although some form of ear plug should be worn when shampooing (soap reduces the surface tension of the water). Grommets extrude after approximately 9–12 months following which some form of review is required to recheck the hearing. A sizeable proportion of affected children (25%) will require further subsequent grommet insertion.

Further reading

Maw AR, Bawden R. Spontaneous resolution of severe chronic glue ear in children and the effect of adenoidectomy, tonsillectomy and insertion of ventilation tubes (grommets). *British Medical Journal,* 1993; **306**: 756–760.

Maw AR, Tiwari RS. Children with glue ear: how do they present? *Clinical Otolaryngology,* 1988; **13**: 171–177.

Related topics of interest

Impedance audiometry, p. 128; Paediatric hearing assessment, p. 239; Tympanosclerosis, p. 344.

OTOACOUSTIC EMISSIONS

Using modern computing technology and signal averaging techniques, outer hair cell vibrations can be detected in the external auditory meatus as otoacoustic emissions (OAEs). They were first described by David Kemp in 1978 and represent an objective measure of cochlear function. Acoustically evoked OAEs are almost never found in ears with a hearing level worse than 40 dB.

Physiology

The cochlea provides an elegant mechanism for transforming the physical properties of sound into electrical neural impulses. Sound vibrations pass from the environment through the external and middle-ear systems to cause vibrations of the cochlear perilymph. These vibrations produce travelling waves in the basilar membrane. As a result of the gradient of width, thickness and consequently stiffness of the basilar membrane, these travelling waves reach maximal amplitude at specific points along the cochlea. High frequencies are represented at the basal turn and low frequencies at the apical portion. These vibrations are detected as a result of shearing forces on two separate hair cell systems in the organ of Corti: the inner (IHCs) and outer (OHCs) hair cells. The inner hair cells are purely sensory and are responsible for detecting these vibrations and producing neural impulses to allow them to be perceived by the central nervous system as sound. The outer hair cells also detect these vibrations but, in contrast, have a motor function. The outer hair cells at the region of maximal travelling wave amplitude vibrate in synchrony with the stimulating signal while the OHCs on either side of this region suppress vibration of the basilar membrane. This mechanism allows the fine-tuning found in the healthy cochlea. These outer hair cell vibrations can be detected in the external auditory meatus as otoacoustic emissions.

Types of otoacoustic emissions

Four classes of OAE exist:

1. **Spontaneous OAEs (SOAEs).** These are low-level signals which occur without external acoustic stimulation in about 40–50% of the normal hearing population. Although they are relatively constant in frequency, they vary in terms of occurrence and intensity and consequently have little use in clinical monitoring.

2. **Stimulus-frequency OAEs.** These are recorded at the frequency of a stimulating pure tone. They appear to have little clinical or research use.

3. **Transient evoked OAEs (TEOAEs).** These signals, usually between 0.7 and 4 kHz, occur in response to short-lasting stimulatory acoustic signals (usually clicks or tone bursts). The signal is very different for each individual but remains fairly constant for any given ear. TEOAEs occur in almost all human ears with hearing levels better than 40 dB, but are of greater amplitude and wider frequency range in children. As they are relatively quick and easy to measure, they are finding increasing use for clinical screening and research.

4. *Distortion-product OAE (DPOAE).* Stimulation with two pure tones of specific frequency and intensity ratios gives rise to DPOAEs. They are nearly always present in normal hearing ears and can be measured in the 6–8 kHz range. These characteristics make them an ideal tool for investigating frequency-specific cochlear function.

OAE measurement. An OAE analyser consists of a mobile probe which contains a sound emitter and microphone for recording. Unlike a tympanometer, an airtight seal is not required. The acoustic stimuli are usually broadband clicks, at a maximal rate of 50/s. The stimulated signals are then received and fed to a signal processor where, by the use of appropriate frequency filters and time window averaging, OAEs can be demonstrated on either a visual or print-out display. Research is still being undertaken into the optimal method of producing and subsequently analysing OAEs.

Clinical uses

Although still a research tool for the investigation of cochlear function, the use of evoked OAEs has now found a place in clinical practice in the screening of neonates and high-risk infants for hearing loss. Evoked OAEs are quick, easy to test and do not require an anaesthetic, in contrast to electrical evoked response audiometry. The sensitivity and specificity of the test is sufficiently good that there are widespread recommendations that all newborn infants are screened for hearing loss by OAE prior to discharge from hospital.

Further reading

3rd International symposium on cochlear mechanisms and otoacoustic emissions, 1992. *British Journal of Audiology*, 1993; **27**(2): 71–159.
Probst R, Harris FP. Otoacoustic emissions. *Advances in Oto-Rhino-laryngology*, 1997; **53:** 182–204.

Related topics of interest

Evoked response audiometry, p. 78; Paediatric hearing assessment, p. 239.

OTOLOGICAL ASPECTS OF HEAD INJURY

A blow to the side of the head by a blunt or sharp instrument may cause injury to the external, middle or inner ear in isolation or in combination. There may be a fracture of the temporal bone and other skull base fractures. Conditions caused by such trauma are described below.

External ear
- Subperichondrial haematoma.
- Perichondritis.
- Loss of pinna tissue, including degloving injuries.
- Otitis externa.
- External auditory meatus stenosis.
- Occlusion of the external canal by clot.

Middle ear
- Tympanic membrane haematoma and petechiae.
- Tympanic membrane rupture with or without the deposition of squamous epithelium within the middle ear.
- Ossicular chain discontinuity.
- Facial nerve injury.
- Haemotympanum and acute non-suppurative otitis media.
- Acute suppurative otitis media.

Inner ear
- Perilymph fistula from either a round window rupture or from the oval window.
- Serous or a purulent labyrinthitis.
- Labyrinthine 'concussion'.
- Intracranial complications – lateral sinus thrombosis, meningitis, extradural, subdural, intracerebral (cerebellar and temporal lobe) abscess or haematoma and otitic hydrocephalus.

Temporal bone fractures
These are classified into longitudinal, transverse and mixed, depending on the orientation of the fracture line to the long axis of the petrous temporal bone. Occasionally with a fracture of the squamous temporal bone, a type of longitudinal fracture, the only sign will be bruising of the postauricular skin (Battle's sign).

Over 80% of temporal bone fractures involve a combination of both longitudinal and transverse fractures. An isolated longitudinal or transverse fracture is unusual.

1. Longitudinal fractures. In 80% of temporal bone fractures a longitudinal fracture is the dominant fracture and usually arises from a lateral blow to the skull. The fracture extends from the squamous temporal bone in the roof of the bony external auditory meatus to the tympanic membrane and the roof of the middle ear before turning anterior to the labyrinth where it may involve the carotid canal.

2. *Transverse fractures.* This is the dominant fracture in 20% of temporal bone fractures and usually arises from a blow to the front or back of the skull. The fracture extends across the long axis of the petrous bone through the labyrinthine capsule and is demonstrated with plain temporal bone radiographs in 50% of cases.

Clinical features

Longitudinal fractures tear the skin of the external auditory meatus and tympanic membrane to cause swelling of the canal skin and bleeding from the ear. These findings should be presumed to indicate such a fracture following a head injury. A haemotympanum and ruptured tympanic membrane will occur if the fracture line extends to the middle ear cleft. This usually heals without residual conductive deafness if infection is prevented. A sensorineural hearing loss is usually secondary to inner ear concussion and therefore temporary. Facial nerve injuries are uncommon although CSF otorrhoea is more common with this fracture. The latter is suspected when an initial serosanguinous aural discharge becomes clear.

In a pure *transverse fracture* there is a haemotympanum but no bleeding from the ear because the tympanic membrane remains intact. Facial nerve injury occurs immediately in half of these fractures. Labyrinthine capsule disruption causes an irreversible sensory hearing loss, usually a dead ear, severe vertigo, nystagmus to the opposite ear, IXth to XIIth cranial nerve injury, raised intracranial pressure and focal neurological signs. These fractures occur with a more severe head injury so otological symptoms may not become apparent until recovery from the acute head injury. Symptoms of secondary endolymphatic hydrops may be caused by involvement of the vestibular aqueduct in the fracture line.

Temporal bone fractures often have a mixed longitudinal and transverse component and this will be suspected from combined clinical features.

Management

The general management of the head injury takes precedence but it is important to avoid introducing infection into the ear so prophylactic antibiotics are often indicated. In the absence of a facial palsy the ear should be left untouched in the early post injury period. Sequelae are unusual in longitudinal fractures and a conductive hearing loss is unlikely to be due to a traumatic ossicular discontinuity. It should resolve when the ear canal skin and tympanic membrane heal.

Management of a facial palsy following a head injury

It is unusual for otolaryngologists to see a patient with a significant head injury soon after the injury as they will have been managed by neurosurgeons. If such a patient is seen soon after the injury and there is a clear history of an immediate and total lower motor neurone facial palsy, this suggests a severe injury to the nerve (it may be caught in a fracture line or be compressed by a fracture, a bony spicule may be impinging on the nerve or there may be complete transection of the nerve). A high definition CT scan of the temporal bone on bone setting with fine (1 mm) cuts is required. No matter what the finding of the scan such a case should be discussed with an expert otoneurosurgeon. If there is a fracture in the tympanomastoid segment, many otoneurosurgeons would advocate a complete decompression of the nerve from the internal auditory meatus to the stylomastoid foramen. A fracture of the labyrinthine segment requires, as a minimum, decompression of the horizontal and labyrinthine segments of the nerve and this requires otoneurosurgical input. If no fracture is seen on a CT scan many otoneurosurgeons would still advocate complete decompression of the nerve from the IAM to the stylomastoid foramen. The scan may have missed a bone splinter impinging on the nerve and waiting at least 14 days for nerve conduction studies may result in irreparable damage to the nerve. Even if there was no fracture then a neuropraxia or axonotmesis may have occurred and early decompression may prevent further injury to the nerve. Others argue that a high quality scan is unlikely to miss a fracture and that exploring the nerve in such circumstances may further traumatize the nerve. The decision therefore depends on the surgeon's experience and expertise.

In patients who develop a facial palsy hours or days after injury or in whom the palsy is partial, the injury is likely to be secondary to a neuropraxia and a conservative policy should be adopted. Electromyography will provide an indication of the severity of the injury and the prognosis in those patients where the history is not clear. If the summating potential is more than 10% of normal after 14 days the prognosis is good, with about 90% recovery to House and Brackmann grade I or II. If it is less than 10% after 14 days then the consensus view is to explore the nerve, decompressing the tympanomastoid segment and the labyrinthine segment. The latter segment is important as it is in this region where the bony canal is narrowest and the nerve most susceptible to injury from oedema. It therefore follows that an otoneurosurgeon should be contacted if decompression of the nerve is contemplated.

CSF otorrhoea is confirmed by the presence of glucose and $\beta2$ transferrin. A policy of bed rest but sitting up to reduce intracranial CSF pressure and antibiotic cover to prevent intracranial infection usually allows resolution to occur after about ten days. Should the leak persist a CT scan using intrathecal metrisamide may identify the site of the leak, usually from the middle fossa and allow exploration by an otoneurosurgeon. Traumatic perilymph fistula is discussed elsewhere.

Further reading

Bassiouny M, Hirsch BE, Kelly RH *et al.* β2 transferrin application in otology. *American Journal of Otolaryngology*, 1992; **13**: 552–555.

Related topics of interest

Facial nerve palsy, p. 92; Perilymph fistula, p. 244.

OTORRHOEA

Definition

Otorrhoea is the discharge of material from the external auditory meatus. It is both a symptom and a sign. It is not a diagnosis.

Causes

Otitis externa and active suppurative otitis media are the commonest diseases causing this problem. Other causes include: wax, debris, blood (acute otitis media, trauma, neoplasm), and CSF (usually following a fracture).

Clinical features

The character of the discharge depends on (and therefore gives clues to) its source.

1. External ear. There are no mucinous glands in the external canal. Acute inflammatory conditions of the external meatus therefore tend to produce a watery, serous exudate or transudate. In addition, they tend to provoke a hyperkeratosis. This combination generally leads to soggy white debris collecting in the canal and a thin white watery discharge from the ear. The cardinal symptom of otitis externa is itchiness, in addition to the discharge, pain and tenderness. The external canal may also be the subject of trauma, which may lead to bleeding from the ear.

2. Middle ear. The middle-ear cleft is well endowed with mucous glands. Thus, if there is a mucoid component to the discharge it usually arises from the middle ear via a perforation of the tympanic membrane. Trapped keratin is offensive; if a cholesteatoma should become infected the discharge tends to be particularly unpleasant and once smelt is never forgotten. A serosanguinous discharge is common with chronic otitis media when the middle-ear mucosa has become granular and polypoid; there is glandular hyperplasia and there may be blood as the mucosa bleeds easily. Blood stained discharge is also a feature of carcinoma of the middle ear. Chronic otitis media is not typically characterized by pain, so in patients where chronic otorrhoea becomes painful and fails to respond to the usual conservative measures, it is wise to consider a carcinoma.

3. Cerebrospinal fluid. CSF rarely discharges from the ears spontaneously but may do so following skull base surgery or more commonly trauma, when it will develop in about 5% of cases. In both cases the fluid may initially be mixed with blood and may be recognized by the halo sign in which there is a clear ring of moisture surrounding the blood after absorption on to blotting paper. This is due to the faster diffusion of the less viscous CSF. Differentiation of CSF from thin serous discharge from a middle-ear cavity may be more difficult but can be done by estimation of the glucose content or by confirming the presence of $\beta2$-transferrin in CSF. If the tympanic membrane is intact CSF may still leak from the ear should there be a fracture in the roof of the ear canal. Otherwise it may pass down the Eustachian tube and become evident as rhinorrhoea or post-nasal drip.

Management

Optimum management depends on making an accurate diagnosis. Although the history will give many clues, the diagnosis is usually not made until the tympanic membrane has been visualized. This may not be possible at the initial consultation owing to swelling and debris in the external auditory meatus. A swab should be taken for culture and sensitivity (bacteria/fungi). This is especially important in patients who have already been on treatments which have not worked. Any granulation type tissue removed should be sent for histology. The mainstay of therapy is aural toilet, ideally by microsuction clearance. This enables a thorough assessment, diagnosis of cause, and allows better penetration of any topical treatments.

Treatment will often commence on the basis of a best guess diagnosis. This will invariably require attention to the primary or secondary otitis externa by thorough aural toilet and possibly the insertion of a wick. At the time of definitive diagnosis more appropriate treatment can be continued. Treatment of the otitis externa will be sufficient if this is the diagnosis. Middle-ear disease will demand treatment on its own merits.

Patients with CSF otorrhoea should be initially covered with prophylactic antibiotics to reduce the risk of meningitis. Post-traumatic leaks usually resolve spontaneously within a short period, but surgical repair will be required if they continue beyond 14 days. Iatrogenic leaks should hopefully be recognized and repaired at the time of surgery. If this is not the case, conservative management is reasonable for the first few postoperative days but surgical repair will be required if the leak fails to settle.

Conservative management includes sitting upright in bed and avoidance of manoeuvres that raise intracranial pressure (e.g. coughing, straining). Prior to any surgical exploration a thorough radiological assessment of the temporal bone should be undertaken to try to establish the site of the leak. This is best achieved with high-resolution CT scanning and the subarachnoid injection of Omnopaque 500. Fluorescein injected by lumbar puncture may be helpful in finding the site of the leak at the time of surgery.

The type and method of repair employed will depend on the site and cause of the leak and to some extent the state of the middle ear and the patient's hearing; it would be inappropriate to obliterate the middle ear of an individual with normal hearing, for instance.

Further reading

Applebaum EL, Chow JM. CSF leaks. In: Cummings CW *et al.* (eds), *Otolaryngology, Head and Neck Surgery*, vol. 1, 2nd edn, St. Louis: Mosby, 1993; 965–974.

Related topics of interest

Acute suppurative otitis media, p. 5; Cholesteatoma, p. 35; Chronic suppurative otitis media, p. 38; Otitis externa, p. 209; Otological aspects of head injury, p. 218.

OTOSCLEROSIS

Definition

Otosclerosis is an autosomal dominant disease of incomplete penetrance affecting bone derived from the otic capsule in which mature lamellar bone is replaced by woven bone of greater cellularity and vascularity featuring large Haversian canals, lacunae, canaliculi and marrow spaces.

Pathogenesis

Otosclerotic foci are most commonly located just anterior to the oval window in the region of the fissula ante fenestram. Symptoms occur when these foci fix the stapedial footplate and encroach upon the labyrinth. It is uncertain whether cochleovestibular symptoms arise directly from this encroachment or from factors released by the plaque or from both. Foci have also been noted in the region of the fissula post fenestram, the semicircular canals, the round window, the base of the styloid process, the petrosquamous suture and in the cochlea.

The three main theories of pathogenesis are:

1. It is an expression of a genetic mutation in collagen metabolism which is only phenotypically expressed in bone derived from the otic capsule.
2. It is an expression of humoral autoimmunity to type II collagen.
3. It is an expression of persistent measles virus infection of otic capsule-derived bone.

Prevalence and incidence

The clinical disease has been estimated to effect 0.5–2% of the population (the prevalence) and the sub-clinical disease affects about 10% of the population. The incidence of clinical disease (number of new cases per year) is much lower. The average consultant/trainee team in the UK perform on average eight stapedectomies per year (range 0–30), but not all consultants perform stapedectomy. The incidence of stapedectomy, even if we were to assume every consultant performed eight stapedectomies per year, would be approximately 4000 per 60 million or 0.0067%. The incidence of otosclerosis is higher, perhaps 0.05% as we would not expect all subjects with clinical otosclerosis to have a stapedectomy, but will nowhere near approach the 1% incidence that is often quoted in major texts. Eighty-five per cent of otosclerotics have bilateral disease.

Otosclerosis is more common in Caucasians. A female:male ratio of 2:1 has been noted, perhaps because women are more likely to seek advice because pregnancy, menstruation and the menopause may cause the disease to progress rapidly. Women are more likely to have bilateral clinical disease.

Clinical features

The main symptoms are:

1. ***Deafness.*** Noticed in most cases before the age of thirty. Better hearing in noisy surroundings is often described – paracusis Willisi.

2. **Tinnitus.** Present in 75% of patients especially when there is a cochlear element to the deafness.

3. **Vertigo.** Mild and usually transient. Symptoms may mimic benign paroxysmal positional vertigo.

Ten per cent of ears display Schwartze's sign, a pink tinge of the tympanic membrane imparted from dilated blood vessels on the mucous membrane of the promontory. It causes no other otoscopic signs. Rinne's test usually suggests a conductive hearing loss. The Weber may be referred to either ear depending on whether disease is unilateral or bilateral, and on the cochlear reserve.

Investigations

1. **Pure tone audiometry (PTA).** In addition to a conductive hearing loss there may be cochlear impairment. Masked air conduction typically shows a loss which is greater at low frequencies when there is minimal cochlear impairment but the frequency response curve flattens and then shows a predominantly high frequency loss as cochlear impairment progresses. The masked bone conduction curve typically shows a dip at 2000 Hz which may be small or exaggerated particularly when there is only a slight cochlear loss (Carhart's notch). The curve shows a predominately high tone loss when there is severe cochlear impairment.

2. **Speech audiometry.** With amplification the score approaches one hundred with normal cochlear function but the score falls according to the severity of the cochlear loss.

3. **Impedance audiometry.** Unreliable as a diagnostic aid although it may be useful in selecting the more suitable ear for surgery in bilateral otosclerosis with a symmetrical PTA by suggesting the more rigid stapes.

Differential diagnosis

- Fibro-osseous foot plate fixation.
- Congenital foot plate fixation.
- Ossicular discontinuity.
- Fixed malleous-incus syndrome.
- Crural atrophy.
- Congenital cholesteatoma.
- Paget's disease (usually produces a mixed hearing loss).
- Osteogenesis imperfecta.

Management

1. **Sodium fluoride.** No major randomized prospective double blind trial has been performed to assess its effectiveness. Its use remains controversial.

2. **A hearing aid.**

3. **Stapedectomy.** The minimum requirements are at least a 15 dB conductive hearing loss with 60% speech discrimination. The ear including the external ear canal should be dry. It is contraindicated in pregnancy. If both ears are suitable for

surgery in bilateral disease the poorer hearing ear should be chosen. Second ear stapedectomy is still controversial but is advocated by many who perform the small fenestra procedure.

Preoperative counselling
- A hearing aid is an alternative method of treatment.
- A dead ear may occur with stapedectomy. The incidence reported by expert otologists varies from less than 1–4% and a further 10% may have no better or worse hearing than pre-operatively.
- Tinnitus may not improve and may be more intense after surgery.
- Vertigo may be present immediately postoperatively and in a minority there may be a permanent sense of imbalance.
- Taste may alter or be lost on one side of the tongue (damage to chorda tympani).
- There is a very small chance that the facial nerve will run an anomalous course either splitting around or coursing inferior to the oval window and may be injured.

Postoperative advice
- Avoid diving when swimming, lifting heavy objects and aggressive nose blowing.
- Open the mouth on coughing or sneezing.
- Avoid flying for the first three weeks post-operatively.

Technique
1. *Small fenestra.*   A micro drill, a stapedotomy needle, or an argon or KTP laser is used to create the fenestra in the stapes footplate. The smaller the fenestra, the smaller the risk of a high tone cochlear hearing loss. A 0.6 mm fenestra drill piece and 0.4 mm prosthesis are popular. The Causse technique comprises a 0.8 mm fenestra over which a vein graft is placed and a 0.4 mm prosthesis.

2. *Large fenestra.*   A portion of the footplate is removed with picks and fine right angle hooks. An attempt is usually made to seal the oval window with a vein or fat graft prior to prosthesis insertion.

The otologist aims to get complete or over-closure of the air bone gap. Over-closure is possible because of the Carhart effect and is greatest at 2000 Hz (see audiometry chapter).

Complications of stapedectomy
1. *Peroperative.*
- Tympanic membrane tear.
- Chorda injury.
- Overhanging facial nerve.
- Persistent stapedial artery.
- Tympanosclerosis arthrodesing the incudostapedial joint.
- Perilymph flooding.
- Floating footplate.
- Depressed footplate.

- Injury to the saccule. This lies as close as 0.4 mm beneath the footplate, but is usually 1–2 mm beneath. It is easily disturbed when performing the stapedotomy or inserting the prosthesis. It may be the cause of a dead ear from an apparently uncomplicated procedure.

An immediate dead ear may arise from the footplate problems noted above, probably because of injury to the saccule with each of these events.

2. **Early.**
- Detachment of prosthesis from incus.
- Displacement of prosthesis from oval window.
- Loose attachment of incus and prosthesis.
- Footplate granuloma.
- Persisting primary perilymph fistula.

3. **Late.**
- Secondary perilymph fistula.
- Necrosis of the long process of the incus.
- Late detachment or displacement of the prosthesis.

Cochlear otosclerosis

Consider when there is a family history of otosclerosis and progressive sensorineural hearing loss in early adult life of no apparent cause. Look for Schwartze's sign on otoscopy. A high definition CT scan may detect an otosclerotic plaque.

Revision stapedectomy

There are three main groups who should be considered for revision stapedectomy:

(a) Patients who have redeveloped a conductive hearing loss after stapedectomy. The commonest causes are a dislocated prosthesis (from either the oval window or from the incus), or erosion of the long process of the incus due to pressure necrosis from the loop of the prosthesis.

(b) Patients who have had no closure of the air-bone gap following stapedectomy. The commonest causes of a persistent conductive hearing loss are a dislocated prosthesis, a prosthesis which is too short or a dislocated malleo-incudal joint .

(c) If vertigo persists or develops several weeks after stapedectomy, particularly if associated with loud noises or with applying pressure to the external ear canal. This is due to too long a prosthesis irritating the saccule. An immediate dead ear may occur if too long a prosthesis injures the saccule.

The overall results of revision surgery are not as good as primary surgery. Reported post-operative sensorineural loss in a number of series varies from 0.7 to 20%.

Further reading

Altermatt HJ, Gerber HA, Gaeng D *et al.* Immunohistochemical findings in otosclerotic lesions. *HNO*, 1992; **40**: 476–479.

Hammerschlag PE, Fishman A, Scheer AA. A review of 308 cases of revision stapedectomy. *Laryngoscope*, 1998; **108**: 1794–1800.

Han WW, Incesulu A, McKenna MJ *et al.* Revision stapedectomy: intraoperative findings, results and review of the literature. *Laryngoscope*, 1997; **107**: 1185–1192.

Related topics of interest

Labyrinthitis, p. 134; Perilymph fistula, p. 244; Speech audiometry, p. 301.

OTOTOXICITY

Ototoxicity is the partial or total reduction in cochleovestibular function caused by the interaction of chemicals, commonly therapeutic agents, with the vestibule, cochlea or the vestibulocochlear nerve.

There are over 200 ototoxic substances but only a small group of drugs in common therapeutic use are regularly associated with ototoxicity.

Aminoglycosides

All aminoglycoside antibiotics have a tendency to be predominantly either cochleotoxic (e.g. neomycin and kanamycin) or vestibulotoxic (e.g. gentamicin and tobramycin). The former relates to the number of free amino groups ($-NH_2$), the latter the number of free methylamine groups ($-NHCH_3$).

Mechanism of action

Current opinion holds that secretion of aminoglycoside from the stria vascularis into the endolymph and perhaps from the vessels of the spiral ligament into the perilymph occurs with active uptake of antibiotic from the perilymph into the endolymph. Resorption by the stria clears the endolymph of aminoglycoside. The concentration in the endolymph therefore depends on the ratio of secretion to resorption which in turn depends on the drug's serum concentration.

Findings in animals suggest an elimination half-life of 6 months within the outer hair cells. This may explain the cumulative ototoxic effects of aminoglycosides and why some patients develop ototoxicity only after a prolonged course or repeated courses of aminoglycosides.

Geneticists have found that susceptibility to aminoglycoside ototoxicity is transmitted exclusively by women. It is not X-linked but can be explained by mitochondrial inheritance. Mitochondrial DNA is inherited maternally because the tiny amount of cytoplasm in spermatozoa cannot transmit mitochondrial DNA. Aminoglycosides cause mitochondrial dysfunction in susceptible patients so that there is inhibition of translation or mistranslation of mitochondrial protein synthesis. This in turn causes a reduction in intracellular adenosine triphosphate (ATP) production with a resultant toxic accumulation of ions such as calcium and potassium within the cytoplasm and ultimately cell death.

Light microscopy shows destruction of the sensory cells of the organ of Corti, the ampullary cristae and the maculae of the saccule and utricle. Electron microscopy confirms that injury to the first row of the outer hair cells, particularly at the basal turn of the cochlea and to spiral ganglion neurons occurs with cochleotoxicity.

It is important to note the damage to the vestibular and cochlea sensory cells is greatly enhanced by the synchronous use of a loop diuretic.

Studies with preloading antioxidants (in particular glutathione and vitamin C) prior to aminoglycoside exposure have shown a significant protective effect. The mechanism is thought to be that antioxidants prevent aminoglycosides being converted enzymatically within the cell to a cytotoxin that causes mitochondrial dysfunction. Neurotrophins such as brain-derived neurotrophic factor protect the spiral ganglion neurons but do not prevent outer hair cell degeneration. Gentamicin in the presence of iron salts produces peroxidation of arachidonic acid *in vitro* so aminoglycoside ototoxicity may be caused by free radical formation in the presence of iron salts. It is of note that two iron chelators, desferoxamine and 2,3-dihydroxybenzoate reduce gentamicin ototoxicity in guinea pigs *in vivo* and iron chelators may have a clinical role to play in reducing aminoglycoside ototoxicity in the future.

Aminoglycosides are excreted by the kidney and the administered dose must be reduced in renal failure. A pyrexia, a large total dose (in gentamicin's case >1 g) and a subject aged over 60 all increase the chances of ototoxicity. Hypoproteinaemia also increases the chances of cytotoxicity but this can be overcome by administering large doses of glutathione with vitamin C.

Clinical features

1. ***Tinnitus*** may occur during or after withdrawing treatment. It may become more intense and persistent in spite of drug withdrawal.

2. ***Hearing loss*** is principally high frequency and sensorineural, presenting some days into treatment and is usually progressive. Withdrawing therapy may prevent further significant deterioration provided renal function is adequate.

3. ***Vertigo*** is characteristically a bobbing oscillopsia whereby distant objects appear to jump about on head movement. Nystagmus may not be demonstrable but caloric testing shows a bilateral decline in labyrinthine function.

Investigations

Monitoring of patients taking these antibiotics by regular inquiring of otological symptoms and by the regular measurement of serum peak and trough levels are necessary to reduce the incidence of ototoxicity and to allow early withdrawal of therapy should they arise. Preloading with glutathione and vitamin C may become standard practice to minimize ototoxicity.

Loop diuretics

Frusemide, bumetamide and ethacrynic acid in high doses may produce a reversible high tone sensorineural hearing loss. Light microscopy shows the stria vascularis to be grossly oedematous but the organ of Corti remains essentially normal. A permanent hearing loss is unusual but has been described in renal dialysis and transplant patients. Since 5% of this group become deaf purely as a result of their disease the contribution of the diuretic to the deafness is, in many cases, uncertain.

Cytotoxic agents

Cisplatin is the most important drug in this group as for many it is the drug of choice in palliating head and neck cancer. It and nitrogen mustard have a similar cochleotoxic effect to the aminoglycosides in causing greatest injury to the first row of outer hair cells particularly at the basal turn of the cochlea but inner hair cells are also injured. There is degeneration of spiral ganglion neurons, particularly towards the apex, and degeneration of the stria vascularis. These ototoxic effects are potentiated by hypoproteinaemia and anaemia. Pre- and post-dose audiometry is necessary to monitor cochleotoxicity which may be partially reversible on withdrawal of treatment. *In vivo* studies in humans have suggested that preloading with diethyldithiocarbamate and an agent known only as WR2721 prior to cisplatin delivery significantly reduces not only ototoxicity but also toxic effects on the gastrointestinal tract, bone marrow and kidney. Ongoing studies are taking place to confirm this and also to demonstrate whether the agent affects the tumouricidal effects of cisplatin.

Beta blockers

A mixed deafness has been described, the conductive element being secondary to a middle ear effusion. The pathogenesis of both the cochleotoxicity and the effusion is unknown. The cochleotoxic effects are generally mild and reversible.

Salicylates

Aspirin in overdose may induce tinnitus and a flat pure tone hearing loss of up to 60 dB. This is usually reversible on withdrawing the drug. The vestibular apparatus is undisturbed and recent work has suggested a direct effect of salicylates on the outer hair cells of the cochlea. Aspirin is cleared rapidly by the kidney so that treatment comprises adequate hydration and the use of an H_2 antagonist e.g. cimetidine or a proton pump inhibitor e.g. omeprazole to prevent upper GI complications.

Quinine

Formerly used in the treatment of malaria and still used today to control night leg cramps, quinine has cochleotoxic effects similar to aspirin except hearing loss may progress after withdrawing therapy and is more likely to be permanent. In a minority, hypersensitivity occurs whereby cochleotoxicity develops at therapeutic plasma levels. As most of the drug is bound to plasma proteins, plasmaphoresis is an effective therapy in massive overdose.

Anticonvulsants

Vestibulotoxicity has been described with phenytoin and ethosuximide. The vertigo may be either acute and reversible on withdrawing treatment or more commonly chronic. In those where phenytoin must be used to control the disorder careful monitoring of the serum levels are necessary.

Aftercare and follow-up

Cochleotoxic symptoms require regular pure tone audiometric monitoring until thresholds are stable or improve (temporary threshold shift) in order to quantify the disability. Vestibulotoxic recovery can be symptomatically monitored by outpatient assessment and if necessary quantified by ENG caloric measurements. Vestibulosedative medication and rehabilitation exercises, e.g. Cooksey-Cawthorne exercises, minimize morbidity and may aid symptomatic recovery by accelerating compensation.

Further reading

Rybak LP, Ravi R, Somani S. Mechanism of protection by diethyldithiocarbamate against cisplatin ototoxicity: antioxidant system. *Fundamentals of Applied Toxicology*, 1995; **26**: 293–300.

Lautermann J, McLaren J, Schacht J. Glutathione protection against gentamicin ototoxicity depends on nutritional status. *Hearing Research*, 1995; **86**: 15–24.

Song B, Schacht J. Variable efficacy of radical scavengers and iron chelators to attenuate gentamicin ototoxicity in guinea pigs *in vivo*. *Hearing Research*, 1996; **94**: 87–93.

Related topics of interest

Sudden hearing loss, p. 314; Vertigo, p. 346; Tinnitus, p. 327; Caloric tests, p. 27.

PAEDIATRIC AIRWAY PROBLEMS

Introduction

Paediatric airway problems are different from adult problems because congenital abnormalities manifest themselves early in life and the airway is significantly narrower. Any factor which reduces the size of the lumen will therefore have a greater effect in the neonate and child. There are many diseases which can cause paediatric airway problems, but this topic confines itself to the following conditions:

- Laryngotracheobronchitis.
- Laryngomalacia.
- Vocal fold paralysis.
- Subglottic stenosis.
- Vascular ring.
- Miscellaneous conditions (papillomata, cysts, webs, gastro-oesophageal reflux).

Problems will nearly always produce noisy breathing (stridor/stertor) or affect the voice (hoarseness), and individual conditions are best discussed through these symptoms.

Stridor

Abnormal noise during breathing may emanate from the chest, the neck or the mouth and nose. Noisy breathing from the chest is usually expiratory, is known as wheezing and is the result of an asthma-like condition. Noise from the neck region is known as stridor and is caused by narrowing of the respiratory lumen in the upper trachea or larynx. It may be expiratory or inspiratory. A laryngeal lesion is usually characterized by inspiratory stridor and a tracheal lesion by expiratory stridor, although if high in the trachea it may be 'biphasic'. Wheezing is the province of the respiratory physician and will not be discussed here.

Stertor

Stertor is noise originating from the back of the mouth or nose. Bilateral choanal atresia can cause such symptoms but there are other more serious problems in this condition and surgical relief is provided as a matter of urgency. Choanal stenosis, enlarged adenoids (or tonsils), rhinitis and muscular incoordination can all be responsible and each condition should be treated on its merits. Children with Down's syndrome and cerebral palsy are particularly prone to trouble. The insertion of a nasopharyngeal tube which projects just beyond the soft palate is helpful in most refractory cases.

Hoarseness

Hoarseness indicates an abnormality of the vocal cord. It is temporary in laryngitis and is the presenting symptom with papillomata. The commonest cause of persistent hoarseness is the presence of vocal nodules. These are unlikely to be caused by misuse of the voice as they have been described in the neonate, but they do respond to speech therapy. Removal with the laser is only indicated when they are large. Unilateral vocal cord palsy can also produce a weak or hoarse voice and is seen following cardiac operations.

Laryngo-tracheo-bronchitis

This is a very common cause of stridor, and most of the milder cases will not reach the hospital. The inspiratory stridor accompanied by a harsh cough will usually follow a throat infection. Infective oedema will narrow the lumen, particularly in the subglottic area, where the airway in the child is narrowest and the submucosal tissue lax. Since the diameter of the subglottis in the normal population follows a normal distribution curve, it is self-evident that those who have a small glottis initially will be more affected. The condition follows a self-limiting course, and many patients can be treated at home with antibiotics and humidity in the form of steam. If the symptoms get worse, admission to hospital, preferably to an intensive therapy unit, becomes necessary. The child is closely observed after treatment with humidity, antibiotics, oxygen, dexamethasone and sometimes an adrenaline nebulizer.

If further deterioration occurs, intubation is carried out. This is best done by a paediatric intensivist or anaesthetist and as small a tube as possible is used. As the condition improves a leak appears around the tube and the child is extubated. On those unusual occasions when extubation is not possible a tracheostomy will be necessary.

Endoscopy should be avoided in the acute period (as it increases oedema) but should be done to identify an underlying abnormality if attacks recur. The usual finding is a relatively narrow subglottis which will widen with growth. Allergic oedema produces similar symptoms, and they appear more quickly and clear equally rapidly. Epiglottitis produces more severe symptoms which are discussed elsewhere.

Laryngomalacia

This condition may appear within an hour or two of birth and is the commonest cause of stridor in infants. It is characterized by an intermittent stridulous squeak of varying severity. It is due to an indrawing of floppy supraglottic structures (particularly the arytenoids and aryepiglottic folds) during inspiration. It may only be slight and present in certain positions, but at worst there would be recession of the chest and suprasternal region and interference with feeding. If slight and parental anxiety is absent, nothing need to be done apart from a 3-monthly follow-up with advice to return in the interim if symptoms worsen. If severe or if there is parental anxiety, a direct laryngoscopy is carried out. The diagnosis is confirmed and, if symptoms are marked, the surplus lax mucosa can be excised from the superior border of the aryepiglottic fold under the microscope or a laser aryepiglottoplasty can be performed. The symptoms gradually improve with time but may take several years to stop.

Tracheostomy is virtually unknown for laryngomalacia and, if considered, an associated vocal cord palsy should be suspected and excluded.

Vocal cord paralysis

A unilateral vocal cord paralysis will usually produce no symptoms apart from some weakness of the voice, but a bilateral vocal cord paralysis produces a stridor which is very similar to that found with laryngomalacia. However, with vocal cord paralysis the symptoms and signs become worse with time as the baby makes stronger inspiratory effort. The cry is usually normal as adduction is not affected. The diagnosis is made by laryngoscopy and it is sometimes possible to see the larynx in the awake patient with a transnasal fibreoptic endoscope. More commonly it is necessary to perform direct laryngoscopy with the baby anaesthetized but maintaining vocal cord function. In order to exclude the diagnosis, wide abduction of the cords must be seen.

Adduction and passive movements of the cords with respiration can easily be mistaken for normal function and there are occasions when a diagnosis cannot be made with certainty. It is useful to reach a consensus by inviting the anaesthetist and any available surgeon present to make an assessment as there is a considerable subjective element. In many cases the cause is unknown, although a significant number have other abnormalities.

An attempt should be made to treat the condition conservatively, as most will recover within 2–3 years. The baby should be seen at regular intervals and the movement reassessed every 6 months. The parents will require support and must have easy access to the hospital if they are worried. In some cases the stridor is so bad and indrawing so severe that tracheostomy is the only treatment. Decannualation should occur as soon as normal function returns. The decision to treat the vocal cord surgically should be left for several years and should be made only after thorough and informed consultation with the child and parents.

Subglottic stenosis

The subglottis is the narrowest portion of the paediatric airway, and any additional narrowing due to oedema or scar tissue will tend to cause stridor. The stridor of laryngo-tracheitis is due to temporary oedematous stenosis and a relatively small cricoid ring may first manifest itself with these symptoms. The most severe cases, however, follow trauma, and in the neonate prolonged intubation associated with prematurity is the usual cause. It may be impossible to extubate the infant; sometimes a progressive stridor develops weeks or months after extubation. A large tube predisposes to stenosis, but a constitutional tendency to fibrosis is the only explanation for those who develop stenosis after only 2 or 3 days of small tube intubation.

If extubation is impossible, the cricoid can be split in the neonate and a temporary stent inserted. More often, however, a tracheostomy becomes necessary. The size of the subglottis is then assessed under general anaesthesia every few months by passing endotracheal tubes until a snug fit is obtained. If the lumen is obviously enlarging, the child can be left until there is an adequate airway and then decannulated. If there is total stenosis or if a pin-hole lumen persists, surgery is necessary, although this is best left until the age of 2 years.

Splitting of the cricoid and upper trachea with insertion of costal cartilage into the split is the standard surgical approach. More severe cases will require an anterior and posterior split, but an anterior split will suffice in milder cases. A stent is usually introduced for a few weeks, but this is not mandatory. This operation, known as laryngotracheoplasty, may need to be repeated before an adequate airway and decannulation is achieved.

Vascular ring

Abnormal blood vessels in the chest may compress the trachea and oesophagus and classically produce an inspiratory and expiratory stridor associated with feeding difficulties. Every neonate with no obvious cause for the stridor should therefore have a barium swallow, which will demonstrate the oesophageal narrowing.

Endoscopy will show a pulsatile narrowing of the trachea and correction is carried out by the chest surgeons. Even after correction there may still be narrowing due to tracheomalacia, which is believed to be caused by softening of the tracheal rings by the pulsatile vessel. There is little to be gained from consideration of the vascular abnormalities as these are complex and often confusing to the chest surgeons themselves.

Miscellaneous

Numerous lesions in the laryngeal region will encroach upon the airway and cause stridor.

1. Papillomata are viral warts which vary greatly in virulence. They usually disappear when immunity develops, but in the interim laser removal is required and certain individuals do not develop immunity. If very virulent and florid, a tracheostomy may become necessary. Hoarseness and airway problems occur as a result of scarring and can require reconstructive surgery.

2. Cysts, haemangiomata and lymphangiomata can occur in the subglottis and less often in the glottis and supraglottis. Subglottic haemangioma is the most common neoplasm of the infant airway. A conservative approach can often be taken as many lesions involute as the infant grows, but the laser has made early removal possible. Cysts can also be aspirated and sometimes removed.

3. Laryngeal webs may be congenital or acquired. If they are small and only produce minimal symptoms they are best left alone. Larger webs may be opened with the laser, but reconstructive surgery with stenting can be necessary.

4. Micrognathia or a large tongue can narrow the upper airway, as in the Pierre–Robin syndrome. Nursing in the prone position is helpful, but even a tracheostomy is considered in the worse cases.

5. Gastro-oesophageal reflux is widely accepted as an important factor in all sorts of paediatric airway problems. As many as 80% of laryngomalacia babies are said to have reflux and it is suggested that these be treated empirically with anti-reflux medication. Reflux has been implicated in the cause and exacerbation of laryngo-tracheal stenosis and if there is evidence that effective management of reflux improves the primary pathology of even laryngeal papillomatosis. Where there is no obvious anatomical cause for stridor, reflux oesophagitis needs to be excluded by investigation.

Related topics of interest

Epiglottitis, p. 70; Laryngeal carcinoma, p. 138; Paediatric endoscopy, p. 237; Stridor and stertor, p. 311; Tracheostomy, p. 336.

PAEDIATRIC ENDOSCOPY

Endoscopy of the respiratory tract is commonly carried out by the otolaryngologist, although subsequent treatment is often the province of the chest surgeon, physician or anaesthetist. Paediatric oesophagoscopy is also commonly performed by the paediatric surgeon.

Fibreoptic examination of the nose, postnasal space and larynx can be done in the child or infant, but it can be difficult owing to lack of cooperation in the awake patient. The fibreoptic endoscope can be passed through the nose or through a laryngeal mask and the latter procedure is very useful in the diagnosis of vocal cord paralysis.

In most cases, paediatric endoscopy involves the use of a rigid laryngoscope or bronchoscope (with a telescope incorporated). This gives a better view and suction is available. There is an increasing use of Hopkin rod telescopes with video and still documentation facilities. These are excellent for teaching purposes, clinical record and follow-up comparisons.

Endoscopy is best avoided within a week following infection and oedema should first be allowed to subside. Essentially, paediatric endoscopy is indicated to provide a diagnosis in the presence of hoarseness and stridor.

Laryngoscopy

Adult laryngoscopes such as the Kleinsasser range can be safely used for children, and the smaller ones can even be used for neonates. As large a size as possible is advantageous in order to obtain the widest view of the larynx. It is important that the lower lip is not pinched between the instrument and the teeth (or gums) and the upper teeth should be protected. An endotracheal tube is in place for the induction of anaesthesia, but this is withdrawn into the hypopharynx during laryngoscopy and the patient breathes spontaneously.

For the purpose of identifying a lesion in the glottis or subglottis, the tip of the laryngoscope is passed posteriorly to the epiglottis as this structure may obstruct the view. If vocal cord movement or laryngomalacia is being assessed, the tip of the laryngoscope is best placed in the vallecula to avoid fixation of the glottic and supra-glottic structures. When a tracheoscopy or bronchoscopy is also to be performed, it is best to watch glottic and supraglottic movement at the end of the procedure while the patient is regaining consciousness and producing more movement.

Laryngomalacia is easily distinguished by the indrawing of the arytenoids, but normal vocal cord movement is more difficult to identify. A wide abduction of the cords must be seen before normal cord movement is diagnosed.

Subglottic stenosis is identified on laryngoscopy if the vocal cords are not in spasm. Where a full examination of the respiratory tract is required, the hypo-pharynx, oropharynx and mouth are examined with the laryngoscope at the same time and both oesophagoscopy and examination under anaesthetic of the nose may be indicated.

Bronchoscopy

A rigid telescope and bronchoscope of suitable size is introduced into the larynx with the help of McGill's anaesthetic laryngoscope. The vocal cords are examined before passing the instrument gently through the glottis, and anaesthesia is then administered via the laryngoscope. This may not be possible if there is a high subglottic stenosis.

In the normal patient the carina can be seen as soon as the instrument passes through the glottis. An inability to see the carina when the lumen is apparently clear should raise suspicions of a vascular ring, tracheomalacia or some other source of extrinsic pressure. The bronchoscope is passed down to the carina with examination of the walls to exclude a tracheo-oesophageal fistula. The main bronchus should be entered, but more extensive investigation of the bronchial tree is necessary if a foreign body is suspected. If there is a tracheostomy present, suprastomal granulations will nearly always be seen, but it is often possible to pass the bronchoscope past the tube. If not, the tube is removed. During the removal of the endoscope the surgeon should continue to visualize the respiratory tract as damage is avoided and rarely a lesion is seen which had previously been missed.

Related topics of interest

Laryngeal carcinoma, p. 138; Paediatric airway problems, p. 232; Stridor and stertor, p. 311; Tracheostomy, p. 336.

PAEDIATRIC HEARING ASSESSMENT

The assessment of hearing in children demands a variety of approaches which vary with the age of the child. The choice of test will depend on the child's age, intellect and motor abilities. Screening tests, subjective hearing tests and objective tests are all available. Nearly all subjective testing will require two testers. The best results are achieved in multidisciplinary paediatric assessment centres where the environment and organization are geared for children. A thorough history from the parent or regular carer and a clinical examination are essential parts of the assessment.

Screening tests

Hearing is important for normal speech development, and it is important that moderate and severe hearing losses are diagnosed early. This will allow the provision of suitable support and aids, which will help facilitate the development of speech and communication. In an effort to achieve this aim, children in the UK have been subject to regular screening tests, at 7 months, 2–4 years and again shortly after school entry. Recent evidence has suggested that waiting until 7 months of age for a first screening test is too late; 0.1% of live-born babies will have a severe hearing impairment. So called 'Universal neonatal screening' has therefore been proposed as a better solution. This involves otoacoustic emission testing shortly after birth (the failure rate is reduced by waiting until after 48 hours of age). Any failures are then subject to automated brainstem evoked audiometry. Children failing both tests are referred for a more thorough audiological assessment, as will any child who persistently fails a screening test at any stage. In addition, children may be referred for assessment from other sources because of concern about their hearing, e.g. parental concern, post meningitis, family history, intensive care units (1–2% will have a severe hearing loss). Most health authorities maintain an at-risk register of families in whom possible prenatal and perinatal causes exist.

Listed below are the current screening methods of choice for the various age groups at which testing occurs.

1. **Neonatal:** Universal screening (OAEs with BERA if indicated).

2. **7 months:** distraction test (see below).

3. **2–4 years:** distraction tests or conditioned response audiometry.

4. **5 years and over:** pure tone audiometry.

Subjective hearing tests

1. **Behavioural techniques (0–6 months).** This method is based on the presentation of a loud sound and observation of the baby's response. Some experience is needed in interpreting the variety of possible responses, which include startle, blinking, crying or the cessation of activity. A positive response is one in which there is a significant alteration in activity. This area of testing has been largely superseded by otoacoustic emissions.

2. Distraction techniques (6–18 months). With the child sitting comfortably on his or her mother's lap, an assistant attracts the attention of the child. The tester then distracts the child by making sounds of various intensity, behind and to one side of the child, without giving any visual cues. A positive response is when the child turns to the sound. The procedure is repeated on both sides. Test sounds include conversational voice for low frequency, sibilant s for higher frequency or a high-frequency rattle in younger children. A hand-held audiometer may be used with older children.

3. Visual reinforcement audiometry (9–36 months). This technique is relatively uncommon in the UK but more frequently used in USA and Australia. In essence it is a free-field audiogram. The child sits in an acoustic room at a table (usually with a parent) and is allowed to play with some toys. Sounds (warbles or pure tones) are produced from one of two loudspeakers placed at 30° either side of the child. If the child turns to the correct speaker at signal presentation a visual (reinforcing) stimulus is presented adjacent to the speaker (e.g. a flashing light) to reinforce the turning response. The tester sits outside the test room and observes the procedure through a one-way mirror. In this way a reasonably accurate free field audiogram may be obtained.

4. Conditioned reflex (performance testing) audiology (24–60 months). This technique involves training the child to perform a specific task such as putting a marble in a cup, or giving a toy to the mother, after hearing a specific auditory stimulus. The stimulus may be the spoken word or a tone produced by a hand-held audiometer. With this method it is important to avoid any visual cues. This technique may also be used with older children to obtain a pure tone audiogram.

5. Speech discrimination tests (24–60 months). These tests involve asking the child to point to or handle a variety of toys. The toys are selected so that their names cover a range of speech patterns. In the McCormick toy test there are seven pairs with names that are acoustically very similar, e.g. cup/duck, key/tree. Only those toys that are recognized by the child are used and the aim is to establish the speech level that gives an 80% correct response rate.

6. Pure tone audiogram (60 months+). This technique is discussed in detail elsewhere (pure tone audiometry). Most children of around 5 years can with a little encouragement be persuaded to perform an audiogram, even if only at three frequencies in each ear.

Objective hearing tests

1. Auditory response cradle (0–6 months). This device monitors four behavioural responses to the production of sound. Head turning, startle responses and body movements are recorded by pressure transducers in the head rest and mattress. Respiratory changes are monitored by a transducer in a band around the baby's chest. The stimulus is 5-second bursts of 85 dB sound pressure level (SPL) sound made into earphones. A microprocessor analyses the responses to the sound stimuli, taking account of the baby's overall level of arousal, and makes an objective verdict of pass or fail.

2. *Otoacoustic emissions (0–12 months).* Much of the recent work with oto-acoustic emissions is related to their feasibility as a screening tool for sensory hearing loss. Distortion-product otoacoustic emissions have been shown to be particularly effective at 4 and 8 kHz. The use of evoked otoacoustic emissions has been recommended as a mainstay of universal screening programmes.

3. *Evoked response audiometry.* This is indicated if there is any difficulty or uncertainty in the results of conventional distraction techniques, or if the child is too young for conventional testing and there are doubts as to the child's hearing ability. Its use is also suggested for neonatal screening in infants failing an OAE screen.

Further reading

McCormick B. *Paediatric Audiology 0–5 Years.* London: Whurr, 1992.
Culpepper B. Universal newborn hearing screening programs. *Current Opinion in Otolaryngology and Head and Neck Surgery*, 1998; **6**: 346–351.

Related topics of interest

Evoked response audiometry, p. 78; Impedance audiometry, p. 128; Otoacoustic emissions, p. 216; Pure tone audiogram, p. 254.

PAPILLOMA OF THE LARYNX

Squamous cell papilloma is by far the commonest benign tumour of the larynx. Adenomas, chondromas, fibromas, haemangiomas and other neurogenic and mesodermal benign tumours are all rare and will not be considered further.

Aetiology

The aetiology of laryngeal papillomas is now known to be infection of the epithelial cells with human papillomavirus (HPV), particularly HPV types 6 and 11. It is thought that in some patients the disease is transmitted at the time of delivery from a mother infected with genital warts. Electron microscopy and immunofluorescent techniques have shown that human papillomavirus DNA is incorporated into the host's cellular DNA. Polymerase chain reaction is now the most sensitive technique available to show evidence of HPV infection. Apparently normal mucosa cells adjacent to the papillomas also contain viral DNA, which may become activated to form a recurrent lesion. This partly explains the difficulty in curing the disease.

Pathology

Squamous papillomas usually occur at any age from birth to 5 years. They may grow anywhere in the respiratory tract from the lips to the lungs, but the vocal cords, anterior commissure and vestibular folds are the commonest sites of involvement. The lesions have a predilection for points of airway constriction, where there is increased airflow, drying, crusting and irritation. Laryngeal mucus is thought to behave as a protective blanket in some sites, for example the interarytenoid area. The growths may present as scattered single lesions or clusters or as a huge exuberant mass. They can be sessile or pedunculated and are characteristically non-keratinizing with a connective tissue core.

Clinical features

Hoarseness of voice or an abnormal cry is the usual presenting symptom. Respiratory obstruction and increasing stridor are late manifestations of the disease process.

Investigations

Endoscopy is required to establish the diagnosis, obtain tissue for confirmatory histology and to assess the extent of the disease and potential risk to the patient's airway. Treatment can also then be initiated.

Treatment

The aim of treatment is to remove the papillomas as they appear, to maintain a safe patent airway and laryngeal function, without damaging the larynx in the process, and to wait for resolution of the condition. Remission can take place at any age and does not seem to be related to treatment. It is most likely to occur if the disease presents between the ages of 6 and 10 years and if the disease is confined to the larynx.

1. *Surgery* is the most satisfactory treatment of this condition. The treatment of choice is the removal of all the lesions using a laser, and repetition of this procedure at intervals. This increases the remission rate to approximately 50% in patients below 16 years of age. If disease is found to involve the anterior commissure, two operations 4 weeks apart are required to avoid web formation, treating first one cord then the other. Tracheostomy should be avoided if possible as the papillomas can become implanted into the trachea and bronchi.

2. *Medical treatment.* Alpha interferon has been shown to significantly reduce the growth rate of papillomas in one-third of patients. Isotretinoin (13-cis-retinoic acid) produces a significant response in about two-thirds of patients. Because of treatment side-effects and uncertain response these treatments should be reserved for cases requiring frequent (i.e. more than 1–2 monthly) laser treatment, or if the trachea and bronchi become involved. It has been claimed that the antiviral drug ribavirin is a useful adjuvant to surgery, but further trials are required to substantiate this. Radiotherapy was used in the past, but should be avoided as it predisposes to malignant change. Squamous cell carcinoma and verrucous carcinoma are also more likely to occur in adults if the patient smokes.

Single papilloma

Single papillomas are usually seen in adults, arising from the free edge of a vocal cord. It is liable to recurrence and malignant degeneration. The papilloma should be removed at direct laryngoscopy. The patients should be followed up for 5 years because of the risk of recurrence and malignant change.

Follow-up and aftercare

Laser laryngoscopy is repeated as often as necessary to preserve the airway and the voice in those cases which do recur.

Further reading

Eicher SA, Taylor-Cooley LD, Donovan DT. Isotretinoin therapy for recurrent respiratory papillomatosis. *Archives of Otolaryngology and Head and Neck Surgery*, 1994; **120**: 405–409.

Leuenthal BG, Kashima HK, Mounts P *et al*. Long term response of recurrent respiratory papillomatosis to treatment with lymphoblastoid interferon alpha-n1. *New England Journal of Medicine*, 1991; **325**: 613–617.

McGlennen RC *et al*. Pilot trial of ribavirin for the treatment of laryngeal papillomatosis. *Head and Neck*, 1993; **15**: 504–513.

Terry RM *et al*. Demonstration of human papillomavirus types 6 and 11 in juvenile laryngeal papillometosis by in situ hybridisation. *Journal of Pathology*, 1987; **153**: 245–248.

Wilson J (ed). *Effective Head and Neck Cancer Management. Second Consensus.* British Association of Otolaryngologists, Head and Neck Surgeons, 2000.

Related topics of interest

Lasers in ENT, p. 147; Paediatric airway problems, p. 232; Paediatric endoscopy, p. 237; Stridor and stertor, p. 311.

PERILYMPH FISTULA

Definition

A perilymph leak into the middle ear arising from a defect of the oval and/or round window. It should not be confused with labyrinthine fistula, which is a fistula in the cortical labyrinthine bone secondary to CSOM. It may or may not have eroded through the endosteum to cause a perilymph leak.

Aetiology

1. *Congenital middle and inner ear deformities*, in particular Mondini's dysplasia or when there is a malformed stapes superstructure.
2. *Head injury.*
3. *Barotrauma.*
4. *Iatrogenic*, in particular following stapedectomy.

Clinical features

A congenital perilymph fistula (PLF) should be suspected in children with an unexplained fluctuating or progressive sensorineural hearing loss with or without vertiginous symptoms. An external ear deformity may occur with the middle and inner ear malformation. A similar history following a head injury, barotrauma or middle ear surgery should be regarded as secondary to a PLF until proven otherwise. Shea's series of iatrogenic post-stapedectomy PLFs presented with a mild mixed hearing loss and occasional dizzy spells but in over 36 000 otological operations he has not seen a spontaneous PLF. Schuknecht has never seen temporal bone evidence of a spontaneous PLF including the review of the temporal bones of patients reported by Kohut as having a PLF. The current consensus view now holds that a spontaneous PLF does not occur in an otherwise normal ear without the above risk factors.

Investigations

A high definition CT scan of the petrous temporal bone is mandatory in suspected congenital PLF. Many subjects demonstrate a minor or major aplasia (see congenital hearing disorders chapter), in particular an enlarged vestibular aquaduct or Mondini's dysplasia. Eighty-five per cent of congenital PLFs will have anomalies of the stapes superstructure, incus, promontory or round window demonstrable on CT. It has recently been shown that β2 transferrin is found in all human CSF and perilymph but in the serum of only 1 in a 100 subjects. In those where a PLF is suspected from the history but not confirmed by a tympanotomy, washings of the middle ear for β2 transferrin can be made. Difficulty arises in deciding whether CSF or perilymph is the responsible agent in head injury patients with a positive β2 transferrin test. Hazel has noted that positioning a patient with a suspected PLF with the affected ear uppermost often improves hearing thresholds presumably because little perilymph escapes due to gravity.

Management

The diagnosis of PLF can only be made at tympanotomy. Sixty per cent arise from the oval window, 20% from the round window, 20% both windows, and 20% are bilateral. The oval or round window should be plugged with a fat graft, temporalis fascia or a vein graft. This is held in position in oval window PLF with a stapes prosthesis provided the incus superstructure is not malformed. Fibrin glue and more recently the KTP laser have been suggested to properly anchor an oval or round window graft in position. Temporalis muscle may be used to splint a round window graft reinforced by fibrin glue.

Follow-up and aftercare

Bed rest in the sitting-up position for 2–6 weeks is recommended as is avoiding straining or flying for three months. Diving is contraindicated. The patient is advised to cough or sneeze with the mouth open to reduce the chance of air entering the Eustachian tube and displacing the graft. One week of antibiotic cover is recommended.

Further reading

Shea JJ. The myth of spontaneous perilymph fistula (Editorial). *Otolaryngology Head and Neck Surgery,* 1992; **107**: 613–616.

Schuknecht HF. Myths in neurotology. *American Journal of Otolaryngology,* 1992; **13**: 124–126.

Kohut RI, Hinojosa R, Ryu JH. Perilymphatic fistulae: a single-blind clinical histopathologic study. *Advances in Otorhinolaryngology,* 1988; **42**: 148–152.

Bassiouny M, Hirsch BE, Kelly RH, *et al.* β2 transferrin application in otology. *American Journal of Otolaryngology,* 1992; **13**: 552–555.

Related topics of interest

Labyrinthitis, p. 134; Chronic suppurative otitis media, p. 38; Cholesteatoma, p. 35; Osteosclerosis, p. 223.

PHARYNGEAL POUCH

Diverticula of the pharynx are uncommon. The term pharyngeal pouch refers to a posterior pharyngeal pulsion (Zenker's) diverticulum, and this has an incidence of approximately 1 case per 200 000 population per year. Other diverticula are very rare but include congenital lateral diverticulae, pharyngoceles and posterolateral pharyngeal diverticula.

Aetiology and pathogenesis

The cause of pulsion diverticulae is unknown. They arise posteriorly by herniation of the pharyngeal mucosa through a relatively unsupported part of the posterior pharyngeal wall known as Killian's dehiscence. This weak area is at the lower part of the inferior constrictor muscle and is bound superiorly by the thyropharyngeal fibres and inferiorly by the cricopharyngeal fibres of this muscle. The pathogenesis is probably multifactorial, in part the result of a weakness at Killian's dehiscence, incoordination of the pharyngeal phase of swallowing and cricopharyngeal spasm causing high intrapharyngeal pressure. A hiatus hernia and gastro-oesophageal reflux are sometimes present. Once a pouch is formed, food enters it and stretches it even more so that it enlarges. It may remain static for many years or slowly increase in size until it eventually passes into the posterior mediastinum. When the pouch reaches a moderate size it lies in line with the oesophagus and food may enter it preferentially. Pressure from the pouch may then be exerted on the oesophagus from behind to cause dysphagia.

Clinical features

Pharyngeal pouches are most frequently seen in the elderly. They cause a sensation of a lump in the throat, long-standing dysphagia, regurgitation of undigested food, halitosis, weight loss and recurrent chest infections due to aspiration. Hoarseness is unusual, but may occur as a result of irritation of the vocal cords from repeated aspiration or more rarely as a result of involvement of the recurrent laryngeal nerve by a carcinoma arising in the pouch. Rarely, a pouche may have an invasive squamous cell carcinoma in its wall. Swelling in the neck may be present and is nearly always on the left side. It may gurgle on palpation (Boyce's sign) and empty on external pressure.

1. Radiology. A lateral plain film of the neck may reveal an air bubble in the pouch, but the definitive investigation is a barium swallow, which demonstrates the pouch.

2. Endoscopy. Oesophagoscopy should be carried out to exclude the presence of carcinoma. The instrument usually enters the pouch and an anterior bar may be seen separating it from the oesophagus. This investigation is often performed immediately prior to surgical excision of the pouch. In such instances a naso-gastric tube is passed and the pouch is packed with proflavine gauze after any debris has been sucked clear. This will aid identification of the pouch during surgery.

Management

1. **No treatment.** Each case must be judged on its individual merits, with the patient being fully aware of the possible complications and potential benefits of operation. No treatment is indicated for a diverticulum which is causing few symptoms or in patients who are old, infirm and in poor general condition.

2. **Endoscopic dilatation** of the cricopharyngeal sphincter with bougies is only temporarily effective in relieving symptoms. It does not remove the diverticulum, which results in an eventual recurrence, and there is a risk of perforating the sac.

3. **Endoscopic division** of the bar between the pouch and the oesophagus. This can be performed with scissors or diathermy (Dohlman's procedure). It is a quick procedure and a reasonable treatment for the frail and the elderly. The procedure does not remove the pouch, but it relieves the symptoms and restores swallowing by dividing the cricopharyngeus and widening the mouth of the diverticulum. The major risks are haemorrhage, mediastinitis, surgical emphysema and later stenosis. Amendments to the approach include the introduction of a specialized endoscope with a split beak. Endoscopic staple guns (which divide the wall and staple it synchronously) are now commonly used. This is the treatment of choice in nearly all pouches as results are good, morbidity low, and hospital stay short.

4. **Pouch inversion.** In this procedure a cricopharyngeal myotomy is performed and the pouch is mobilized, and then invaginated into the oesophagus and its neck oversewn with vicryl sutures. This operation avoids the risks of opening the sac, has a low complication rate and requires only a short hospital stay. This is the preferred treatment for small pouches.

5. **Diverticulectomy.** Excision of the diverticulum combined with a cricopharyngeal myotomy has remained a treatment of choice for many years. It now tends to be used for the very large pouches or when one of the other approaches has failed. The operation is performed in two stages, the first of which is the oesophagoscopy and the second the external approach to excise the pouch. Nasogastric feeding is continued for 5–7 days postoperatively, after which fluids are given. If there are no problems the tube is removed and a soft diet can be commenced the next day.

Complications

1. **Immediate.**
- Primary haemorrhage.
- Surgical emphysema (mucosal tear or incomplete suture line).
- Pneumothorax.

2. **Intermediate.**
- Secondary haemorrhage (infection).
- Hoarseness (recurrent laryngeal nerve damage).
- Wound infection.
- Fistula (usually the result of infection).
- Mediastinitis (leak tracking downwards).

3. *Late.*
    - Persistent hoarseness (recurrent laryngeal nerve divided).
    - Stricture (too much mucosa excised when dividing the neck of the sac).
    - Recurrence (endoscopic diathermy 7%, diverticulectomy 2–3%).

Further reading

Bowdler DA. Pharyngeal pouches. In: *Scott-Brown's Otolaryngology*, vol. 5, 6th edn. Hibbert (ed.) London: Butterworths, 1997: Chapter 10.

Parker AJ, Hawthorne MR. Endoscopic diverticulotomy versus external diverticulotomy in the treatment of pharyngeal pouch. *Journal of the Royal College of Surgeons of Edinburgh*, 1988; **33**: 62–64.

Related topics of interest

Globus pharyngeus, p. 113; Hypopharyngeal carcinoma, p. 124.

PHARYNGOCUTANEOUS FISTULA

Definition

A fistula is an abnormal communication between two epithelial-lined surfaces. A pharyngocutaneous fistula is an abnormal tract joining the pharynx to the skin of the neck.

Pathology

Fistulae are unlikely after closed pharyngeal surgery but may occur following open surgery to the head and neck in which the pharyngeal mucosa has also been damaged. Consequently, laryngectomy is the most commonly associated procedure, but it may occur after pharyngeal pouch surgery, partial pharyngectomy or major oropharyngeal procedures (e.g. commando operation). Risk factors are:

- Previous radiotherapy.
- Infection (a persistent cough from a chest infection will put strain on the repair, and infection of the operated site will cause necrosis of the affected tissue with a leak through this defect).
- Postoperative haematoma/chylous fistula/seroma.
- Residual disease.
- Poor nutritional status.
- Poor surgical technique.

Clinical features

The patient most commonly develops a pyrexia 3 or 4 days postoperatively, associated with cellulitis of the neck wound. A swinging pyrexia and abscess formation may ensue. Typically on the seventh day the collection will rupture and a fistula will form. At this stage there will be a discharge of mucopus and the patient's general condition will improve. In time, the discharge will become more mucoid than purulent and ultimately saliva alone is discharged. In many cases spontaneous resolution will occur, usually within 6 weeks. In persistent cases, especially in those having residual tumour or previous radiotherapy, there is the uncommon but ever present spectre of a carotid blow-out.

Investigation

The diagnosis will be strongly suspected from the clinical features, especially from a red fluctuant swelling in the neck. After rupture, if the tract is small, the diagnosis may be confirmed by a gastrograffin swallow. With persistent and profuse discharge from a fistula, the urea, electrolytes and serum proteins should be checked regularly and the haemoglobin kept above 10 g/dl. Occasionally a fistula occurs several days after commencing oral feeding in patients who have had an apparently uncomplicated postoperative course. A gastrograffin swallow performed on the 10th to 12th postoperative day will show an anterior sinus in about 15% of patients, and it is this group who are at a significantly higher risk of developing such a fistula. It is suggested that nasogastric feeding be continued in this group for a further week and the gastrograffin swallow thereafter repeated. In most cases the sinus will have resolved, but if not the process is repeated until healing is complete.

Management

A pharyngocutaneous fistula is initially managed conservatively. Nasogastric or gastrostomy feeding continues until the fistula has healed. The wound should be cleaned regularly and absorbent dressings used to avoid maceration of the surrounding skin until all necrotic tissue has separated and healing has started, this initial stage taking 2 or 3 weeks. The size of the external opening of the fistula should thereafter be measured weekly. The fistula may take many weeks to close spontaneously, and if personal and home circumstances are suitable the patient can be allowed home and reviewed regularly in outpatients. Provided that the fistula continues to reduce in size, no surgical intervention is necessary, although granulation tissue should be biopsied to exclude recurrent disease in cancer patients. If the size does not reduce over any 2-week period after the initial separation stage, a prudent plan would be to endoscope the patient under a general anaesthetic to exclude recurrent disease then to proceed with a repair. If the fistula opening is less than 1 cm diameter, a local rotation skin flap should be considered in the first instance. These often fail, however, because local tissue is relatively ischaemic either as a result of previous radiotherapy or because of scar tissue formation during healing. If a local flap fails or the defect is too large to consider this, the repair method of choice is, depending on the surgeon's experience and microvascular training, a choice of: a pectoralis major myocutaneous flap, a deltopectoral flap or a radial forearm fasciocutaneous microvascular flap. Two flaps are often needed because it is important to line the mucosal and cutaneous surfaces with skin.

Follow-up and aftercare

Patients who have had surgery for a fistula are followed up at the same interval as those who did not develop a fistula, although they are at a higher risk of developing a stenosis at the level of the fistula. This may settle after several dilations, but occasionally the stenosis recurs persistently and frequently so that excision of the affected segment with reconstruction is indicated. The repair method of choice is a microvascular jejunal loop because of its low morbidity and mortality compared with a gastric transposition. Those who have had surgery for benign disease are unlikely to develop a stenosis, but follow-up for a year to exclude a late onset would seem sensible.

Further reading

Stringer, SP. Flaps and grafts for reconstruction. In: Million RR, Cassisi NJ (eds). *Management of Head and Neck Cancer*, 2nd edn. Philadelphia: J.B. Lippincott, 1994: 157–169.

McCombe AW, Jones AS. Radiotherapy and complications of laryngectomy. *Journal of Laryngology and Otology*, 1993; **107**: 130–132.

Related topics of interest

Hypopharyngeal carcinoma, p. 124; Laryngectomy, p. 143; Oropharyngeal carcinoma, p. 203; Radiotherapy, p. 264; Reconstructive surgery, p. 267.

PRESBYACUSIS

As with all sensory systems in the human body, there is a progressive degeneration in the auditory system with ageing, which leads to hearing impairment in the affected individual. Presbyacusis is defined as the lessening of the acuteness of hearing that characterizes old age.

Pathophysiology

Both the sensory peripheral (cochlea) and central (neural) components of the auditory system are affected and the deterioration appears to become more rapid with increasing age. Peripheral degeneration is reported to be responsible for at least two-thirds of the clinical features of presbyacusis. A variety of possible mechanisms exist. Cellular degeneration gives rise to a reduction in the numbers of inner and outer hair cells, particularly at the basal end of the cochlea. This can lead to secondary neural degeneration in the spiral ganglion. Circulatory changes such as arteriosclerosis, atrophy of the stria vascularis and microangiopathy can lead to metabolic upset and further cell death. This leads to an elevation of hearing thresholds and a loss of frequency selectivity. Degeneration in the central pathways leads to a reduction in performance in terms of signal processing. The end result in most instances will be a combined sensorineural, rather than a sensory or neural, impairment.

Clinical features

Moderate hearing impairment (45 dB hearing level averaged over 0.5, 1, 2 and 4 kHz) occurs in 4% of the age group 51–60 but in 18% of those aged 71–80. Men and women are both affected, although men tend to have a slightly worse loss for the same age group. Patients typically complain of difficulty in hearing which is worse in the presence of background noise, so that they find conversations difficult to follow. Recruitment is a frequent problem and adds to the distortion. Many patients eventually become socially isolated and even depressed. In the absence of any other otological pathology the clinical examination is normal bar the hearing loss.

Investigations

In the presence of an appropriate history and a symmetrical sensorineural hearing loss on pure tone audiometry, little further investigation is required. Hearing loss in a young patient, asymmetry on a pure tone audiogram, unilateral tinnitus or a conductive component to the audiogram will require investigation in its own right. MRI scanning may be necessary to exclude an acoustic neuroma in any patient thought to be at risk. Although several different audiological patterns of hearing loss have been described, depending on the predominant histological changes, in general a sloping high-frequency loss is the commonest pattern found.

Management

As there is no curative treatment for deafness associated with ageing, the main aims in management are to assess the degree of disability, to provide a hearing aid and rehabilitate the patient.

1. *Hearing aids.* Although about 75% of hearing aid users are over the age of 60, only 18% of the elderly with hearing loss have and use hearing aids. There are several reasons for this, including denial of hearing impairment, vanity, acoustic feedback and difficulty with manipulating the aid. In those with neural presbyacusis poor speech discrimination may limit the benefit of amplification as may the performance of the aid itself. Hearing aid uptake may be improved by the proposed introduction to the NHS and improved performance of digital hearing aids. Some patients have minimal handicap from their hearing difficulty despite a significant loss and therefore do not present themselves to medical services. Obtaining a hearing aid has become less of a problem for many patients since the introduction of direct referral schemes from general practice.

2. *Rehabilitation.* Some patients may be helped by rehabilitation in the form of speech reading or auditory training. The role of rehabilitation and its benefits for the average hearing-impaired individual are not proven.

3. *Accessory aids.* An induction coil fitted to the telephone or television may help some patients. The sound is transmitted by induction from a special attachment and is picked up by the patient's aid when it is switched to the T position. This system is now available in many public places such as churches, concert halls and lecture theatres.

Follow-up and aftercare

Audiological support is initially required to familiarize and rehabilitate the user with the aid. In some centres patients provided with a hearing aid are not seen again. The ENT surgeon or audiologist therefore has no idea if the patient has benefited from the treatment. Many hearing aids dispensed are not used, perhaps because the patient experiences some of the difficulties outlined above. Follow-up and appropriate support for all patients issued with a hearing aid should be mandatory. Any difficulties the patient might have can then be identified and dealt with. It is likely that this aspect is the most important in hearing aid provision. In the longer term, access is required for repairs and replacements, which may be dictated by further hearing deterioration with the passage of time.

Further reading

Browning GG, Davis A. Clinical characterisation of the hearing of the adult British population. *Advances in Otorhinolaryngology*, 1983; **31**: 217–223.
Divenyi PL, Simon HJ. Hearing in ageing: issues old and young. *Current Opinion in Otolaryngology Head and Neck Surgery*, 1999; **7**: 282–289.
Salomon, G. Hearing in the aged. The European Concerted Action Project. *Acta Otolaryngologica*, 1991, Suppl. 476.

Related topics of interest

Evoked response audiometry, p. 78; Hearing aids, p. 117; Noise-induced hearing loss, p. 192; Pure tone audiogram, p. 254.

PURE TONE AUDIOGRAM

The pure tone audiogram is probably the cornerstone of clinical auditory assessment. It is a psychoacoustical test which aims to establish the subject's pure tone hearing threshold, that is the minimum sound level at which a specific response can be obtained.

Introduction

The ear responds equally, not to equal increments, but to equal multiples of sound intensity. In other words, intensity is exponentially related to loudness perception and therefore a logarithmic scale to measure loudness is necessary. The bel is the log to the base 10 of the ratio of the sound intensity being measured to a reference intensity which is constant, and is measured in W/m_2. The decibel is 10 times this ratio. Therefore:

Sound intensity (Ix) in dB $= 10 \log_{10}$ Ix/Io   where Io $= 10^{-12} w/m^2$

Since sound intensity is proportional to the square of the sound pressure then:

Sound intensity in dB $= 10 \log_{10}$ sound pressure^2 or
$= 20 \log_{10}$ sound pressure level

$\log_{10} 2$ is about 0.3, so doubling sound intensity corresponds to a 3 dB increase. Each 10 dB increase represents a 10-fold increase in the intensity of sound ($\log_{10} 10 = 1$), a 3.3-fold increase in sound pressure, but the perception of only doubling the loudness.

Decibel scales

1. **Sound pressure level scale (dB SPL).** In terms of pressure, the threshold of hearing corresponds to a sound pressure level (dB SPL) of approximately 20×10^{-6} pascals and the threshold of pain to a level of 200 pascals. The auditory system is less efficient at detecting sounds at the upper and lower ends of the frequency spectrum than in the middle regions. The detection of sounds in decibels of sound pressure level (dB SPL) produces a pure tone audiogram which in normal circumstances would not be flat. It was considered that the use of a dB SPL scale in pure tone audiometry would make abnormalities difficult to identify.

2. **Hearing level scale (dB HL or dB ISO).** A decibel scale of human hearing was designed so that 0 dB hearing level (HL) would be the expected threshold of detection of a pure tone irrespective of its frequency. The amount of energy at 0 dB HL at each frequency is not the same. It is measured in relative terms (dB ISO), where the reference zero is an internationally agreed standard. This standard represents the thresholds at each test frequency for a group of presumed otologically normal young adults. In the dB HL scale normal hearing individuals would be expected to have a flat audiogram, the mean level being 0 dB HL. The clinical audiogram therefore gives an estimate of the subject's hearing relative to normal.

3. **The A-weighted scale (dB A).** The ear is not equally sensitive to sounds of different frequencies. It is particularly sensitive to sounds in the 'speech frequencies'

(500–4000 Hertz) and progressively less so to sounds of lower and higher frequencies. In addition it appears that the ear is less easily damaged by the sound frequencies to which it is less sensitive. To take account of this an 'A- weighting' is used, which reduces the contribution of very low and very high frequencies to the overall noise level measurement. This dB A scale is used in industrial and other noise exposure settings.

Background

Pure tones of several frequencies are tested, usually 250, 500, 1000, 2000, 4000 and 8000 Hz for air conduction (although 3000 and 6000 Hz will be required for noise-induced hearing loss claims) and 500, 1000, 2000 and sometimes 4000 Hz for bone conduction. The results of bone conduction become less reliable at and above 4000 Hz, and at 250 Hz are often not representative as they may be felt rather than heard.

Bone conduction is taken to give an indication of cochlea function, but because a variety of routes for the transmission of sound to the cochlea exist for bone conduction, it is not an absolute representation of inner ear threshold. When the skull is set in vibration by a bone conduction vibrator, the sounds reach the inner ear by the direct osseous route or via transmission across the middle ear. This causes an artificial depression of the bone conduction thresholds whenever a conductive defect is present. If the middle-ear defect is corrected, then the bone conduction thresholds will appear to improve because of the addition of the middle-ear component. This has become known as the 'Carhart effect' after he described it in patients who had successful fenestration surgery for otosclerosis.

Method

The subject is seated in a soundproof room and the procedure is explained by the examiner. Earphones are used for air conduction and the subject is asked to signal by pressing a small hand-held button as soon as the tone is heard. Pure tones are produced by a calibrated audiometer and are first presented to the subject's better ear. Thresholds are ascertained using a psychophysical method of limits. Tones are first presented at an intensity above the patient's suspected threshold. The intensity is reduced in 10 dB steps until no sound is heard. The signal is then increased in 5 dB steps until half of the tone pips are consistently heard. This continues in the following order: 1000, 2000, 4000, 8000, 500 and 250 Hz. Finally 1000 Hz is tested again to check on subject accuracy and should be within 10 dB of the first result. The second ear is then tested in identical fashion. The timing and duration of signal presentation should be varied and no visual clues should be offered.

With any psychoacoustic test there is a variation in the results obtained in any test–retest situation, with a standard error of 3–5 dB. For this reason 5 dB steps are used for clinical audiometry. Smaller steps could be used (e.g. 2 dB) but the procedure would be markedly prolonged without significantly improving accuracy.

Masking

Masking is the phenomenon by which one sound impairs the perception of another. In the context of pure tone audiometry, masking is used to raise the threshold in the non-test ear using air-conducted sound. This overcomes any cross-hearing (the interaural attenuation for air conduction is of the order of 40–60 dB when wearing headphones) and allows an accurate assessment of the true threshold of the test ear for either air or bone conduction.

As masking is most effective when the frequency of the masking noise overlaps the test tone, narrow band noise with a central frequency identical to the test tone is used. The masking level in the non-test ear is determined by shadow masking and recording the thresholds on a masking chart. The masking noise is delivered by an ear insert for bone conduction and headphones for air conduction.

There are three scenarios when masking is essential:
(a) Masking must be applied to the better ear when testing air conduction in the deafer ear if the difference in unmasked thresholds is found to be 40 dB or more (to prevent interaural attenuation).
(b) Air conduction studies whenever the unmasked bone conduction is 40 dB or more better than the worse air conduction.
(c) Bone conduction testing whenever the unmasked bone conduction is 10 dB or more better than the worse air conduction.

Variations

1.   Computerized pure tone audiometry.   In essence this is identical to the above but a microprocessor presents the tones and analyses the responses against predetermined values. It is useful as a screening test and in very busy clinics, but if the result is unusual it will require manual confirmation.

2.   Bekesy audiometry.   This variant uses a special audiometer which automatically sweeps from low to high frequencies while presenting continuous or pulsed tones. The subject alters the intensity of the tone by pressing a button if the tone is heard which lowers the intensity of the signal. When the signal cannot be perceived the button is released which increases the intensity again. Thus a zig-zag printout is obtained from which thresholds at each frequency can be estimated. As the test can be self-administered and provides an automatic printout, it is ideal for workforce screening. By varying the test technique (e.g. forward/backward sweeps, continuous/pulsed tones) additional diagnostic information about adaptation, recruitment and non-organic hearing loss can be provided. Although still used for screening industrial hearing loss, the method has fallen into disuse for most other problems because it is too unreliable.

Further reading

British Society of Audiology/British Association of Otolaryngologists. Recommended procedures for pure-tone audiometry using a manually operated instrument. *British Journal of Audiology*, 1981; **15**: 213–216.
Browning GG. Audiometric tests. In: *Clinical Otology and Audiology*. London: Butterworths, 1986: 38–47.
Leijon A. Quantization error in clinical pure-tone audiometry. *Scandinavian Audiology*, 1992; **21**: 103–108.

Related topics of interest

Noise-induced hearing loss, p. 192; Non-organic hearing loss, p. 194.

RADIOLOGY IN ENT

H. Lewis-Jones

Diagnostic imaging techniques

Plain films

Following the increased use of complex diagnostic techniques such as CT and MR, plain films are rarely used for diagnostic purposes in ENT. The Royal College of Radiologists' guidelines recommend that 'plain films of the sinuses are not routinely indicated'. The radiation dose of a 4 projection sinus series is equivalent to 25 chest X-ray doses or 10 weeks of background radiation.

Lateral soft tissue views of the neck are of limited value in isolation. They may demonstrate opaque foreign bodies, but many foreign bodies are likely to be non opaque. Contrast swallows are more accurate in this situation.

Contrast swallow

A contrast swallow is indicated in the investigation of dysphagia or symptoms suggestive of motility disorders.

Barium swallows are of superior sensitivity in demonstrating pharyngeal pouches, pharyngeal webs (the web is a line indenting the anterior aspect of the barium column at the level of C5/6) and cricopharyngeus hypertrophy (indents the posterior column of barium at the C6/7 level). Digital screening is preferred to reduce radiation dose. Image acquisition is preferably at the rate of 2 frames per second during a bolus swallow. Motility disorders are best assessed using dynamic video swallow fluoroscopy.

Water soluble contrast swallows (using non ionic relatively inert contrast media) are indicated when the history suggests that aspiration into the lungs is a real risk (if barium is used in these circumstances it may lead to resistant chest infection or permanent lung damage), when perforation of the oesophagus is suspected or a surgical anastamosis is being evaluated (barium used in these circumstances will remain in the soft tissues if a leak is present, obscuring the area for further follow up studies and being a viscous thick suspension it is less likely to demonstrate small oesophageal leaks than water soluble contrast).

Computerized tomography

CT provides vastly improved delineation of bony structures and of soft tissue structures of the head and neck compared with plain films. Unenhanced CT scans are usually performed for the assessment of benign sinus disease prior to functional endoscopic sinus surgery, and of the temporal bone for assessment of bony anatomy. In tumour work it is routine to administer iodine based intravenous contrast, which has the benefit of opacifying blood vessels making lymph node enlargement easier to detect, and also of demonstrating abnormal areas of enhancement. Intravenous contrast usually flows from the vascular compartment into the extra cellular compartment, but not into cells. In abnormal tissues it leaks into the intra cellular compartment, and this causes abnormal tissues to enhance (appear white). The only exception to this rule is in the brain where the blood–brain barrier prevents contrast flowing into the extra-cellular compartment also. Pathological enhancement in the brain is, therefore, more conspicuous. CT is disadvantaged in the densest part of the skull base where artefacts are commonly caused in the adjacent soft tissue due to X-ray absorption in dense bone. Modern multi-slice CT scanners can now acquire data volumetrically allowing multi-planer recontruction of CT images. This is particularly useful in oncology and in complex anatomical evaluation of the temporal bone.

Magnetic resonance imaging

MRI provides markedly superior delineation of soft tissues in any imaging plane. The fundamental imaging unit in MR is the proton or hydrogen nucleus, in abundance in the body, which when placed in a strong magnetic field act like small metallic dipoles and align predominantly in the direction of the magnetic field. Energy in the form of a radio wave is transmitted into the body at a precise frequency causing the protons to resonate, whereupon they realign in a direction against the magnetic field. The resonant radiowave is then turned off and protons gradually relax back into the direction of the magnetic field giving off a radiowave which is detected as the MR signal. The images generated, therefore, represent the biochemical composition of tissues in the body and it is this concept of tissue characterization through MRI that makes soft tissue delineation so superior. The MR signal given off by protons can be detected and resolved into two different components. One of these components, the T1 spin lattice or longitudinal relaxation time, is related to the time taken for excited spinning protons to return to their normal position in the magnetic field.

The second, the T2 spin spin or transverse relaxation time, depends on excited spinning protons moving out of phase with each other as they relax.

These characteristics are represented in T1 or T2 weighted imaging sequences. T1 weighted images provide high resolution of anatomy and excellent soft tissue detail. The T2 weighted images tend to provide lower resolution images in terms of anatomy, but provide better contrast for the detection of abnormal tissues such as tumour or inflamed tissue. The T2 weighted images are good at detecting abnormal biochemistry related to abnormal tissues. *Table 1* below shows patterns of tissue characterization, where observation of signal on T1 and T2 weighted images allows identification of tissue type, and it also relates the MR characterization to CT appearance.

Gadolinium is a paramagnetic contrast agent used in MRI. It behaves in exactly the same way as iodine based contrast media described in the CT section. T1 weighted images are used to demonstrate enhancement (an increase in signal) with gadolinium. Enhancement of an area directly indicates its vascularity and the degree of enhancement shown in MRI is in the range of 50–100 times greater than that shown in CT.

A final, but important, set of MR images is worthy of mention, the STIR sequence. This creates images with a T2 weighting, but with fat signal suppression. This leaves pathology and fluid including oedema as white in the image and more conspicuous than in ordinary T2 weighted images where high signal fat may well obscure the boundaries of a tumour. This sequence is of great value in the delineation of head and neck cancers.

MR cannot be used in patients with cardiac pacemakers, iron containing brain clips, certain cardiac prosthetic valves, in the first trimester of pregnancy, or in patients with cochlear implants.

Table 1. Correlation of MR and CT appearances of tissues

Tissue	MR signal intensity		CT image appearance
	T1 weighted	T2 weighted	
Water (CSF, oedema)	Low (dark) (grey)	High (white)	Dark grey
Fat	High (white)	High (white)	Very dark grey
Malignant/ inflamed tissue	Intermediate (grey)	Intermediate (grey)	Grey
Cortical bone			White
Air	Signal void (black)	Signal void (black)	Black
Fast flowing blood			Grey

Ultrasound

Ultrasound is a very useful technique for the assessment of masses in the neck, thyroid goitres and for suspected salivary gland pathology. It does not involve any radiation exposure and can be linked with ultrasound guided fine needle aspiration, performed as an outpatient procedure at the time of diagnostic scanning. A high frequency (7.5–10 mHz) hand held probe is placed directly on the neck and the fine needle can be visualized directly entering individual lesions as small as 1 cm in diameter. As a technique, however, it is very operator dependent requiring an ultrasonologist with specific technical skills who performs head and neck ultrasound regularly.

ENT pathology

Temporal bone disease

The choice of investigation rests between CT and MRI.

1. *High resolution CT (1 mm slices), bone algorithm.* This provides superb bony detail of both the inner and middle ear structures. It does, however, involve a high radiation dose (100 chest X-ray-equivalents or 1 year background radiation). It is indicated as the first line choice of radiological investigation when chronic middle-ear disease is being investigated, in particular, when the diagnosis of cholesteatoma is suspected, for trauma induced deafness and suspected otosclerosis. It is also used for specific cases following MRI (see below).

2. *MRI.* High resolution T2 weighted MRI of the temporal bone is now the accepted screening tool for patients with suspected acoustic neuromas although gadolinium enhanced MRI remains the gold standard for detection of small acoustic neuromas. The high resolution T2 weighted technique must identify the normal facial and acoustic nerves separately within the internal acoustic meatus to successfully exclude small intracanalicular neuromas. Developmental anomalies including vestibular aqueduct dilatation can usually be identified on a high resolution T2 weighted MRI. This will provide evidence of abnormal appearance at this site. It may be necessary to recall the patient for images in the sagittal plane to allow accurate measurement of the vestibular aqueduct in equivocal cases. Destructive lesions of the temporal bone apex or elsewhere at the skull base should be imaged in all three planes, and supplemented by high resolution CT of the affected area if surgical treatment is contemplated. High resolution T2 weighted MRI is also a useful screening test for evaluating congenital deafness.

Sinus disease

CT is indicated following failure of medical treatment and on consideration of functional endoscopic sinus surgery. High radiation doses is a particular problem with CT of the sinuses and for this reason a low dose protocol is recommended. This involves:

- Coronal images 2 mm cuts every 8 mm from anterior frontal sinus to posterior border of sphenoid sinus.
- Two axial cuts are also performed, one through the frontal sinus to show the posterior sinus wall and the second through the apex of the orbital foramen to show the relationship of sinuses to the optic nerve.

The radiation dose is equivalent to 80 chest X-rays or 10 months of background radiation. The scans would identify the pattern of sinus disease, whether the cause is related to the osteo-meatal complex and its nature (inflammatory sinus disease associated with parallel walled mucosal thickening, allergic sinus disease associated with nodular and irregular mucosal thickening + or – polyposis).

All anatomical variants should be identified, particularly those which place vital structures under increased risk of damage during endoscopy, e.g. low lying or asymmetrical cribriform plate, onodi cells next to the optic nerve, dehiscent roof of carotid canal in the sphenoid sinus. Bone destruction can be seen with polyposis and fungal disease, but a tumour should be excluded. If a tumour is suspected, a contrast enhanced spiral CT or contrast enhanced MRI is indicated.

Head and neck cancer

1. *Skull base and nasopharynx.* This is often clinically occult disease, presenting with cranial nerve palsy or neuralgia. Multi-planar MRI with gadolinium enhancement is the first line investigation supplemented with high resolution CT if focal bone destruction is suspected. MRI is accurate at showing vascular occlusion or encasement by tumour. In equivocal cases MR angiography or venography is indicated. This does not require arterial or venous catheterization or even intravenous contrast. Moving blood can be specifically identified in an ultra fine slice and placed in a 3D matrix representing the vascular tree. This technique is also of value in diagnosing cavernous or lateral sinus thrombosis, secondary to orbital or mastoid infection.

2. *Oral cavity and oropharyngeal tumours.* Gadolinium enhanced MRI provides the superior soft tissue delineation required for defining the extent and spread of these tumours. Differentiating oedema from tumour can be difficult.

Bone destruction of the mandible is best evaluated using a combination of isotope bone scan with plain film. The plain film OPG allows accurate detection of dental caries which can cause increased activity on the isotope bone scan (and otherwise a false positive result). Absence of caries associated with increased activity indicates bone invasion.

3.   Hypopharynx and larynx.   CT and MRI are comparable at staging tumours at this site. Spiral CT is regarded as superior, predominantly as it minimizes movement/swallowing/breathing artefact. CT also appears superior to MRI in the detection of early thyroid cartilage invasion (this is seen initially as some sclerotic change within the cartilage before lysis occurs). Imaging has low specificity levels due to variable ossification of cartilage in normal life. It is superior in the demonstration of small, but enlarged, retro-laryngeal lymph nodes.

4.   Cervical lymph node assessment.   Ultrasound, CT and MRI can demonstrate lymph nodes in the neck. All three imaging modalities use essentially the same criteria for nodal involvement by tumour:

- Jugulo-digastric node with minimum axial diameter greater than 15 mm.
- All other nodes minimum axial diameter greater than 10 mm.
- Grouping of more than three lymph nodes of 5–8 mm in one lymph node level.

These criteria will provide approximately 60% sensitivity and 95% specificity for lymph node involvement by tumour.

- Central necrosis: This is visible as cystic change within the lymph node and can be seen on all three modalities. There is 100% specificity for tumour involvement by squamous cell carcinoma.
- Extracapsular spread: This is shown by attachment or invasion of adjacent structures. MRI is probably superior in this regard as it can reveal oedema in adjacent anatomy, as well as direct spread of tumour.

5.   The N0 neck.   Ultrasound guided fine needle aspiration is the most accurate method of a radiological assessment of the N0 neck. The technique involves identification of the 3 largest lymph nodes in the ipsi-lateral neck, and are biopsied using a fine needle. This gives an 85% sensitivity and 100% specificity for detection of tumour.

Even so, not all involved lymph nodes in an N0 neck will be detected and if neck dissection is routinely planned, then imaging or FNA of the nodes is of little value.

6.   Distant metastases.   Recent studies have shown a high incidence of disease in the thorax, either metastatic or a synchronous primary bronchial neoplasm, which is not detected by a plain radiograph. It is suggested that CT scan of the thorax should be routinely performed in patients with head and neck cancer who have a normal chest X-ray. The incidence of occult disease has been reported as high as 15%. CT of the thorax is probably not indicated for T1 N0 tumours, which by definition are at an early stage.

7. Postoperative assessment. If complex reconstructive procedures have been performed and there is a high likelihood of recurrence (close margins, more than one involved lymph node at pathology unfavourable histology), a baseline post-operative scan at 6 to 8 weeks is helpful. MRI has proven superior in detection of recurrence. Radiotherapy creates a great deal of oedema which can last up to 12 months following treatment, and makes scan interpretation difficult. This is also the case in the post-operative larynx.

Recurrence may take the appearance of a focal occult mass lesion at the site of reconstruction or of clinically occult lymphadenopathy, again masked by post surgical or post radiotherapy fibrosis.

Salivary gland pathology

Control films with contrast sialography is still indicated for intermittent swelling of the major salivary glands. Failed procedures usually in the submandibular area can be referred for isotope sialography. This will provide information regarding gland function and obstruction, although no other specific information will be obtained. Stones and strictures can be treated percutan-eously under imaging guidance using micro angioplasty ballons and micro cages mounted on guide wires.

Salivary gland masses can be assessed, if necessary, by CT, MR or ultrasound. MR can provide superior information re:

(a) Characterization of cysts or lipomas.
(b) The pattern of homogenous enhancement or non-homogenous enhancement.
(c) Extension of the mass into the deep lobe of the parotid gland.

Imaging can usually successfully identify benign salivary gland lesions, allowing prioritization for potentially malignant masses. Imaging should always be combined with clinical assessment and fine needle aspiration of the mass.

Laryngeal nerve palsy

Urgent endoscopy should be co-ordinated with radiological assessment. The PA chest radiograph is the first investigation. If endoscopy and the chest radiograph fail to identify the cause of laryngeal nerve palsy, a spiral CT from skull base to the lower border of the lung hila is required.

Further reading

Valvassori GE, Matee BL, Carter BL. *Imaging of the Head and Neck*. New York: Theime Publishers, 1995.

Vogl TL, Balzer J, Mack M, Steger W. *Differential Diagnosis in Head and Neck Imaging*. New York: Theime Publishers, 1999.

Radiological Clinics of North America. *Imaging of the Paranasal Sinuses and Oro-maxillo-facial Region*. Philadelphia: Saunders, 1993.

Wilson J (ed). *Effective Head and Neck Cancer Management. Second Consensus*. British Association of Otolaryngologists, Head and Neck Surgeons, 2000.

Related topics of interest

Acoustic neuroma, p. 1; FESS, p. 108; Laryngeal carcinoma, p. 138; Oral cavity carcinoma, p. 197; Oropharyngeal carcinoma, p. 203; Hypopharyngeal carcinoma, p. 124; Nasopharyngeal carcinoma, p. 180.

RADIOTHERAPY

A. Shenoy

Radiotherapy is treatment with ionizing radiation. This may consist of high-energy electromagnetic radiation (X-rays and gamma rays) or particulate radiation (electrons (beta particles) or neutrons).

1.   X-rays   X-rays have a smaller wavelength than UV light and have high energy: kilovolts (kV) to megavolts (MeV). They are produced when high-speed electrons expelled by thermionic emission from an electrically heated tungsten filament are arrested by a target anode of high atomic number, usually tungsten, converting their kinetic energy into heat and photons. A photon is a quantum or bundle of electromagnetic radiation. Megavoltage linear acceleration of the electrons produces X-rays in the energy range of 4–20 MeV. Orthovoltage machines produce X-rays of about 300 kV. For treatment of head and neck cancer, energy of 4–6 MeV is used.

2.   Gamma rays   Radioactive atoms disintegrate to form a more stable atom, releasing energy, which may be particulate (usually electrons) or uncharged electromagnetic radiation called gamma rays, having the same wavelength and energy as X-rays.

3.   Electrons   High-speed electrons can be used as an alternative to electromagnetic radiation. They give a uniform dose up to a certain depth which varies depending on the energy of the beam, with a rapid fall-off in dose beyond this. They are used to boost the dose to a neck lump lying in close approximation to the spinal cord. The technique is more skin sparing than orthovoltage radiotherapy and is the treatment of choice for irradiating the nose and pinna.

4.   Neutrons   These are produced by bombarding stable nuclei with electrons in a cyclotron. However, the maximum dose delivered is to the skin, there is a relatively slow fall-off in dose with depth, there is significant scatter and the dose is more difficult to map precisely. Its role in head and neck cancer has yet to be defined but some authorities find it useful in the treatment of sinonasal and advanced salivary tumours.

5.   Energy   The amount of energy of a photon beam is described by the roentgen (R), while the gray (Gy) is the unit of absorbed dose by the tissues.

Biologic principles

Factors that affect the response of cells to a given dose of radiation include:

- *Radiosensitivity* is an inherent characteristic of the cell (e.g., seminoma and leukaemia cells are exquisitely sensitive to radiation whereas glioma and melanoma cells are relatively radio-resistant). This is to a certain extent dependent upon cellular repair mechanisms, which are enhanced in melanoma cells.

- *Oxygen* is a potent sensitizer, due to its ability to form free radicals. Oxygen enhancement ratio (OER) is the ratio between doses in hypoxic and euoxic cells to produce the same biologic effect. OER for low energy X-rays is between 2.5 and 3, meaning the dose to hypoxic cells is three times greater than in oxygenated cells. Many tumours are thought to have hypoxic cores leading to radio-resistance.

- *Linear energy transfer (LET)* is the amount of energy deposited as the X-ray travels through matter. High LET radiation (neutrons) have a more biologic effect than low LET radiation (X-rays).

- *The position a cell occupies in the cell cycle* determines sensitivity to radiation. S phase cells are relatively more resistant than M phase cells. DNA is most susceptible to lethal injury when the cell is dividing and is not able to repair DNA damage. Malignant cells have a greater proportion of actively dividing cells (a larger growth fraction) and so a greater percentage of cells will die. Resting cells may also sustain DNA damage. Normal cells are able to synthesize factors such as p53 protein, prolonging the S-phase (synthesis of DNA), allowing repair of damaged DNA before the next cell division. Resting malignant cells have much less capability to arrest in S-phase, have a shorter cell cycle, are less likely to repair damaged DNA and more likely to undergo apoptosis before entering mitosis. A higher proportion of malignant cells will therefore die from radiotherapy.

Clinical principles

Radiotherapy should be defined in terms of type, method of application, number of fractions, fraction size, interval between fractions and volume treated. The principle is to provide a sufficient dose to the tumour to effect a cure or adequate palliation but provide a minimal dose to the surrounding normal tissue in order to minimize complications. Each tissue has its own tolerance level beyond which radiation toxicity will occur, so that a small increase in dose may greatly increase tissue injury. Omission of one or two fractions of radiotherapy, perhaps because of acute side-effects, can significantly reduce the chances of cure.

There are various methods of application in the head and neck including external beam therapy (teletherapy) using linear accelerators or cobalt isotope machines; interstitial brachytherapy, for example iridium wires placed in flexible plastic tubes; and systemic radioactive isotopes (i.e. iodine-131 for thyroid cancer).

Maximizing the therapeutic ratio is the overriding principle of radiation therapy, and is the ratio between normal tissue complication dose to the tumour control dose. Many manoeuvres are utilized to maximize the ratio including fractionation of dose, multiple fields, use of lead alloy blocks (to reduce normal tissue included within the radiation fields) and use of wedges to alter the dose distribution.

Dose fractionation spares normal tissues because of cellular repair in between fractions and due to repopulation if the treatment time is sufficiently long. There are however more complex differences between various normal tissues and it is important to realise that prolonging treatment time has little effect on late effects, but a large sparing on early effects. As a result, fraction size is the dominant factor in determining late effects in normal tissue, while overall treatment time has little effect. In contrast, both fraction size and treatment time determine response of acutely responding tissues.

Conventional fractionation is defined as treating once daily at a dose of 1.8–2 Gy per fraction, five fractions per week over 5 to 7 weeks. The adoption of fractionation into radiation has led to the concept of four 'Rs' of radiobiology; Repair, Repopulation, Redistribution and Re-oxygenation.

Altered fractionations use more than one fraction per day and are essentially divided into two schedules of accelerated fractionation and hyperfractionation.

Acceleration uses the same or slightly lower dose than conventional therapy with the same number of fractions delivered in a markedly reduced overall time. The intent is to reduce repopulation in tumours. The late effects are not reduced, as the fraction size is similar to conventional treatment. Hyperfractionation uses less than conventional dose fraction in the same overall time, but because multiple fractions are used, the total dose delivered is about 10 to 15% higher than conventional treatment. Various trials have been performed which have demonstrated the clinical effectiveness of the above strategies and radiotherapy treatments using multiple fractions are being increasingly used in clinical practice.

Treatment planning

Examination and CT or MR scanning defines the treatment volume. A variable margin around the tumour is included to allow for microscopic involvement. Accurate targeting is essential due the close proximity of vital but radiation-sensitive structures (cervical spinal cord, eye, pharynx). The patient is immobilized in an individually made plastic head and neck shell. On a simulator (X-ray machine with image intensifier) the field is chosen and lead alloy blocks used to protect vulnerable structures. These blocks are marked on the shell. Two or more beams from different angles may be needed to obtain an adequate radiation dose to the tumour volume while maintaining surrounding tissue tolerance. Use of wedges that attenuate a beam's dose differentially across its width helps this. A computer maps out a plan of the dose applied to the tumour and surrounding structures by calculating the summation of the contributions of the applied beams modified by wedges, blocks and compensators. Verification radiographs are taken during the first fraction dose and compared with the simulation films to ensure that the field is correctly positioned.

Side effects

General side effects include tiredness, lassitude and anorexia. Nausea and vomiting are less common. Local side effects depend on the type of radiotherapy, volume treated, the total dose, the number of fractions and the total treatment time. Typically, radiotherapy can damage skin (erythema, desquamation, and atrophy of sweat glands and other skin appendages); mucous membranes (mucositis, candidiasis and reduced saliva production due to minor salivary gland atrophy); cartilage (perichondritis); brain and spinal cord (transverse myelitis, localized cortical radionecrosis) and bone (osteoradionecrosis).

Further reading

Fu KK, Pajak TF, Trotti A *et al*. A Radiation Therapy Oncology Group(RTOG) phase III randomised study to compare hyperfractionation and two variants of accelerated fractionation to standard fractionation for head and neck squamous cell carcinomas: first report of RTOG 9003. *Int. J. Radiat. Oncol. Biol. Phys.*, 2000; **48**: 7–16.

Related topics of interest

RECONSTRUCTIVE SURGERY

N. Niranjan and R.D.R. McRae

Reconstructive surgery is the surgical technique to replace tissue loss caused by trauma, tumours or congenital deformity.

The advent of antibiotics, refined anaesthesia and microsurgery have allowed more major head and neck resection procedures to be developed. Manchot in 1889 studied the blood supply of the skin and introduced the concept of vascular territories, while in 1936 Salmon confirmed the distribution of the perforating branches from marginal arteries. Although skin cover could be achieved by staged transposition of tubed pedicled fasciocutaneous flaps from distant sites, cosmesis, retention of function and quality of life were usually poor. In addition some procedures took over a year to complete. The development of one-stage pedicled myocutaneous flaps and microvascular free tissue transfer over the last 25 years has largely removed these criticisms with the consequential enormous improvement in the quality of life for head and neck cancer patients. We have classified reconstruction into four levels.

Level 1

Direct closure. It may be desirable to close small defects directly. Excision of a lesion should be planned so skin incisions are in the line of least tension as mapped out by Langer's lines. These lines are usually at right angles to the underlying muscle fibres. Following the excision, undermining should be between tissue planes. The depth of plane varies according to site; for example on the face the level of undermining is very superficial but on the scalp it is deep to the galeoaponeurotica. On the trunk and limbs it lies between the superficial and deep fascia. The skin is able to be stretched but its tolerance varies according to site and age. Skin suturing should be without undue tension.

Level 2

Skin grafts. A skin graft is a segment of epidermis and dermis that has been completely separated from the donor site and thus has no blood supply. They may be classified into split skin grafts (also called partial thickness skin grafts) or full thickness skin grafts (also called Wolfe grafts). The graft has no blood supply and so needs a vascular bed. It will not take on bone without periosteum, cartilage without perichondrium or tendon without paratenon. A skin graft is less likely to take at sites of poor vascularity, for example over fat, heavily irradiated tissue or on infected tissue. The contact between the graft and recipient site is maintained by a pressure dressing or by the exposed method. The pressure dressing could a pressure bandage or a tie over dressing with foam or cotton wool. In exposed wounds one needs to observe for a seroma, haematoma or a collection of pus between the graft and recipient site. If a haematoma or seroma develops, it can be promptly dispersed by making a small nick in the graft and drawing out the collection using a sterile cotton bud.

Split skin grafts. Split skin grafts consist of epidermis and a thin layer of dermis, but the troughs of the rete pegs and epithelium lining the hair follicles are left in situ to allow re-epithelialization of the donor site should be harvested using an electric dermatome set at 3 or 4 on the circular scale corresponding to a thickness of 0.3–0.4 mm. A thicker graft of 0.5 mm is recommended for covering within the oral cavity. It should be noted that the dermatome scale acts as a guide only: other factors such as angle of the dermatome to the skin and skin tension will alter the graft thickness.

Indications

(a) To cover donor sites, for example radial forearm free flaps and deltopectoral flaps. It is recommended that, after taking the graft at operation, it be placed keratin side down on tulle gras, which is rolled, placed in a sterile pot and refrigerated at 4°C. Unroll the graft onto the donor site after 3–5 days when all bleeding and serous ooze from the raw bed has stopped and vascular granulated tissue has started to form.

(b) To cover excised conchal bowl skin and cartilage defect after the excision of a basal cell carcinoma.

(c) To line cavities, for example the inner layer of a maxillectomy cheek flap, to line the orbital cavity after exenteration or as a cover for a floor of mouth or tongue raw surface. Immediate grafting with quilt suturing and cross-hatching of the graft is recommended so that blood and serum can escape and do not lift the graft from its bed. The donor site should be hairless and inconspicuous. The inner aspect of the upper arm or thigh is therefore recommended.

Full-thickness skin graft (Wolfe graft). This consists of the epidermis and the whole of the dermis.

Indications

(a) Nasal tip and conchal bowl defects.

(b) A full-thickness graft with all adipose tissue excised is ideal when performing a septodermaplasty. The postauricular donor site is preferred because primary closure is easy and leaves an inconspicuous scar.

Level 3

Pedicled skin flaps. These are skin flaps that remain attached at their base to provide a blood supply and lymphatic drainage. They can be classified into random, axial and myocutaneous.

Random. Skin gets its blood supply either from direct cutaneous vessels which run superficial to the deep fascia or from indirect vessels which pass from feeding vessels through muscle or fascia to reach the skin. A random flap is one where there is an indirect or an unknown direct blood supply to the skin. When planning such a flap the length of the flap should not exceed the width of the base otherwise the distal portion of the flap may become ischaemic.

Examples of random skin flaps are Z-plasty, rhomboid, advancement, rotation or transposition skin flaps. Although these flaps may be raised anywhere and run in any direction, careful planning is necessary to obtain optimal cosmesis. Where possible, the use of relaxed skin tension lines should be used.

Axial. Examples include deltopectoral and nasolabial flaps. These are fasciocutaneous flaps with a named blood supply running superficial to the deep fascia supplying the overlying skin. The length of the flap corresponds to the area supplied by these vessels. The pectoralis major myocutaneous flap has replaced many of the indications for the deltopectoral flap, which may still occasionally be used to replace lateral neck skin and peristomal skin. The main disadvantage of these flaps is that the patient must submit to a two-stage procedure, the second to return the pedicle to its original site after the distal portion has gained an adequate blood supply at its new site; this normally takes 3–4 weeks. Between stages the patient must endure moist dressings to an unsightly granulating bed from which the flap has been lifted.

Musculocutaneous. A pectoralis major flap is an example. Although a large number of head and neck musculocutaneous flaps have been described, the pectoralis major flap is now by far the most popular. This is a flap of skin, deep fascia and muscle based on the acromiothoracic artery, a branch of the first part of the axillary artery. It runs in a layer between the deep aspect of the muscle and its underlying fascia. The vessels perforate the muscle to supply the overlying skin. Its advantages are that it is straightforward to raise, provides good bulk and is reliable. Its main disadvantage is that its bulk may compromise function, and for this reason the radial forearm fasciocutaneous free flap has taken over much of its previous work. Two important points in technique in raising the flap are:

(a) suture the muscle edge to the subcutaneous edge as the flap is raised to prevent shearing of the perforating vessels;
(b) after measuring the flap allow an extra 1–2 cm of pedicle length as the flap retracts on raising; it is important that the pedicle is not under tension when suturing the flap into position.

Level 4

Free tissue transfer. These flaps provide the gold standard in terms of cosmesis and preservation of function. Good results require sound microvascular training and meticulous attention to detail. Raising the flap and preparing both the donor and recipient vessels and their subsequent anastomosis are critical areas in which small errors may cause the graft to fail. Good results come from expert training in a centre with an interest in such reconstructive surgery and cannot be learned from a book. A take rate of at least 90% should be obtained. Common free tissue transfer flaps in head and neck reconstruction with their main indications are:

(a) Radial forearm fasciocutaneous free flap. Reconstruction of the floor of mouth, tongue, lateral oropharyngeal wall, soft palate and the repair of a pharyngocutaneous fistula.
(b) Jejunal free flap. Reconstruction of a neopharynx after pharyngolaryngectomy.
(c) Composite osteocutaneous radial forearm free flap. Reconstruction of the floor of mouth and mandible after a mandibulectomy of less than about 8–10 cm. The length available depends on the interval between the insertions of pronator teres and pronator quadratus. One should aim to take no more than 40% of the diameter of the radius in the composite flap in order to reduce the risk of a subsequent radial fracture.
(d) Rectus abdominis myocutaneous free flap. Reconstruction following total glossectomy and reconstructing the lateral skull base after petrosectomy. This flap is based on the inferior epigastric vessels.

(e) Iliac crest osteocutaneous free flap based on the deep circumflex iliac vessels. Reconstruction of mandibulectomy greater than 8–10 cm, in particular a hemimandibulectomy with or without floor of mouth reconstruction. The osseous portion of this free flap is very reliable but the skin less so.

Further reading

Shaheen OH. The repair of defects. In: Shaheen OH (ed). *Problems in Head and Neck Surgery*. London: Baillière Tindall, 1984; 70–91.

Related topics of interest

Hypopharyngeal carcinoma, p. 124; Oral cavity carcinoma, p. 197; Oropharyngeal carcinoma, p. 203.

SALIVARY GLAND DISEASES

There are four main salivary glands – two parotids and two submandibular glands – and multiple minor salivary glands which occur throughout the upper respiratory tract, notably in the oral cavity and oropharynx. Patients with enlargement of these glands or sialomegaly can pose an interesting diagnostic dilemma.

Pathology

1. ***Infection.***
   (a) Viral: mumps virus, coxsackie virus, echovirus, human immunodeficiency virus (HIV).
   (b) Bacterial: staphylococcal, actinomycosis, tuberculosis, leprosy.

2. ***Neoplasm.***
   (a) Benign: pleomorphic adenoma, adenolymphoma.
   (b) Malignant: adenoid cystic carcinoma, adenocarcinoma, squamous cell carcinoma.
   (c) Variable: mucoepidermoid carcinoma, acinic cell tumour.
   (d) Non-epithelial: haemangioma, lymphangioma, neurofibroma, lymphoma.

3. ***Inflammatory.*** Sjögren's syndrome is an autoimmune disease which is characterized by periductal lymphocytes in multiple organs. The salivary glands are affected in approximately 40% of all cases. In one in six patients the disease will progress to a lymphoma. Sjögren originally described xerostomia, keratoconjunctivitis sicca and rheumatoid arthritis, with no mention of salivary gland swelling. Now the disease can be classified into:

   (a) Primary Sjögren's syndrome (or sicca complex) consisting of xerostomia and xerophthalmia with no connective tissue component.
   (b) Secondary Sjögren's syndrome, which consists of xerostomia, xerophthalmia and a connective tissue disorder, usually rheumatoid arthritis.

4. ***Metabolic.*** Myxoedema, diabetes, Cushing's disease, cirrhosis, gout, bulimia, alcoholism.

5. ***Drug induced.*** Coproxamol (dextropropoxyphene and paracetamol), oral contraceptive pill, thiouracil, phenylbutazone, isoprenaline.

6. ***Sialectasis.*** Progressive destruction of the alveoli and parenchyma of the gland accompanied by duct stenosis and cyst formation. Many cases are thought to be congenital. Epithelial debris or calculi may be found in the main ducts.

7. ***Pseudoparotomegaly.*** These disorders should be kept in mind as they may mimic sialomegaly: hypertrophic masseter, winged mandible, mandible tumours, dental cyst, branchial cyst, preauricular lymph node, sebaceous cyst, lipoma and neuroma of the facial nerve.

History

The diagnosis is often obvious from the clinical findings. The history should include the age of the patient (think of mumps or congenital sialectasis), the number of glands affected (tumours are unilateral apart from Warthin's on rare occasions), whether the swelling is exacerbated by eating (calculus disease secondary to sialectasis), duration of symptoms (benign tumours grow slowly and malignant ones fairly rapidly) and any related pain (infection, calculus or adenoid cystic carcinoma). There should be a thorough review of systemic symptoms (metabolic causes), and any medication the patient is taking should be noted. The social history including alcohol intake and risk of HIV infection may be relevant in some cases.

Examination

Inspect the enlarged gland and then all the other salivary glands. Inflamed skin over the swelling should make one consider an infection or skin involvement from a malignant lesion. The facial nerve should be tested as facial weakness also raises the suspicion of a malignant lesion. Before palpating the lesion be sure to ask if it is tender; this is kind to the patient and a good habit in clinical medicine – it is essential in an examination! Palpation should determine whether the lesion is local or diffuse, solid or cystic, mobile or fixed and whether or not other glands are affected. Inspect the oral cavity and palpate all of the glands bimanually. In the floor of the mouth a submandibular calculus may be felt or pressure on a parotid gland may express pus from the parotid duct. Then examine the pharynx to look for a parapharyngeal lesion (in particular one arising from the deep lobe of the parotid), which may push the tonsil medially. Complete the ENT examination and perform a general examination if systemic or disseminated neoplastic disease is suspected.

Investigations

1. Blood tests. Rheumatoid factor, antinuclear factor and abnormal electrophoresis are sometimes found in Sjögren's syndrome. Specific Sjögren's antibodies are usually also present (SSrho and SSla). Tests for the relevant endocrine disorders may be appropriate.

2. Radiography. A plain film is useful as it may reveal a radiopaque submandibular calculus. Most submandibular gland calculi are radiopaque, but most parotid calculi are radiolucent. A sialogram is probably the most useful investigation of benign salivary gland disease. Duct stenosis, calculi and sialectasis can all be diagnosed if sialography is possible. MRI scanning is usually the preferred investigation in neoplastic disease to delineate any potential deep lobe involvement and to assess the tumour's relationship to the facial nerve.

3. Biopsy. Incisional and Trucut biopsy should not be performed as there is a risk of seeding neoplastic disease. Fine-needle aspiration biopsy is safe and often useful, but the results have to be interpreted in conjunction with clinical suspicion as incorrect reports are not uncommon, especially with cystic lesions. A parapharyngeal mass should never be biopsied through the pharynx because there may be uncontrollable bleeding if the patient has a vascular lesion. Sublabial biopsy is the definitive investigation to confirm the diagnosis in Sjögren's syndrome (periducatal lymphocytic infiltration found).

Management

The management and specific treatment of the patient depends on the cause of the salivary gland swelling.

Further reading

Maran AGD. Non-neoplastic salivary gland disease. In: Scott-Brown's *Otolaryngology*, Vol. 5, 6th edn. London: Butterworth, 1997; chapter 19.

Related topic of interest

Salivary gland neoplasms, p. 274.

SALIVARY GLAND NEOPLASMS

Pathology

Neoplastic lesions are divided into benign or malignant, and malignant lesions can be primary or secondary. In addition, if one can remember the epithelial and the non-epithelial histology of the organ, an excellent framework for working practice is easily established. Salivary gland tumours are no exception in this respect, except that some such neoplasms have variable biological behaviour.

Classification

The WHO histological classification of salivary tumours now includes over 35 variants and also includes tumour-like lesions (e.g. salivary gland cysts). A simplified classification is presented below:

*1. **Benign.*** Pleomorphic adenoma, Warthin's tumour (papillary cystadenoma lymphomatosum), monomorphic adenoma, oncocytic adenoma, ductal papilloma.

*2. **Malignant.*** Adenoid cystic carcinoma, adenocarcinoma, squamous cell carcinoma, undifferentiated carcinoma, carcinoma expleomorphic adenoma.

*3. **Variable.*** Mucoepidermoid carcinoma, acinic cell carcinoma.

*4. **Non-epithelial.*** Haemangioma, lymphangioma, neurofibroma, lymphoma.

A good approximation to remember is that 80% of all salivary tumours are in the parotid, 80% of parotid tumours are benign and 80% of the benign tumours that arise in the parotid are pleomorphic adenoma. One in three tumours arising in the submandibular gland and one in two tumours that arise in the minor salivary glands are malignant.

Clinical assessment

All patients with a mass in a salivary gland should have: an inspection and palpation of the mass itself, oral examination with particular inspection of the relevant salivary gland duct, peroral palpation, inspection of the oropharynx for parapharyngeal extension assessment, facial nerve assessment and neck node palpation.

Investigations

*1. **Radiography.*** CT scanning of a parotid tumour is useful in the assessment and delineation of anatomical structures, extension to the deep lobe and relation to the facial nerve. MRI has significant advantages. Using STIR sequencing appears to add to the sensitivity in detecting lesions of the parotid gland, delineating the facial nerve and in identifying the tumour edge.

*2. **Fine-needle aspiration biopsy (FNA).*** The role of FNA in the diagnosis of benign and malignant salivary gland disease is a controversial issue. Proponents of the technique argue that FNA provides diagnostic information which may allay a patient's anxiety and aid in preoperative counselling and planning of surgery.

However, those against the routine use of FNA argue that one cannot rely on the sensitivity or specificity of the procedure. This is particularly true in patients with cystic lesions of the parotid, in whom the aspirates often yield straw-coloured fluid, which is almost invariably hypocellular or acellular, and thus non-diagnostic. FNA is a relatively painless procedure, has few complications (seeding of the tumour does not appear to occur) and may prevent an ill-advised and often ill-fated incisional or excisional biopsy of a parotid mass. If the result of FNA is at variance with other findings then clinical judgement should prevail.

Staging

With malignant tumours of the parotid gland, a significant correlation exists between tumour stage and survival. The stage of the disease has been shown to be a more important prognostic parameter than its histological grade. The UICC system is summarized below:

T0   No clinical evidence of tumour.
T1   < 2 cm in diameter, without extraparenchymal extension (skin, soft tissues).
T2   2–4 cm in diameter, without extraparenchymal extension.
T3   4–6 cm in diameter, and/or extraparenchymal extension (but not facial nerve).
T4a   > 6 cm in diameter, and/or base of skull or facial nerve invasion.
T4b   A tumour of any size with significant local extension.

Benign tumours

1. Pleomorphic adenoma   is the commonest benign salivary tumour. The sex distribution is equal and the peak age incidence is in the fifth decade. It has a pseudo-capsule of compressed parotid tissue into which the tumour usually has many protuberances. It arises from intercalated duct cells and myoepithelial cells. Micro-scopically it comprises epithelial and mesodermal elements with a mucopolysaccha-ride stroma giving rise to a characteristic mixed staining pattern. If the capsule is ruptured during removal, then tumour may implant, causing recurrence. They are therefore excised with as large a margin as possible to reduce the risk of capsule rup-ture. Superficial parotidectomy or hemisuperficial parotidectomy when the lesion is small is now the preferred procedure. Management of recurrent tumour is difficult as the facial nerve may be involved and its sheath may need to be stripped. The facial nerve should if at all feasible not be sacrificed; rarely radical surgery is needed with resection of the facial nerve. Many surgeons advocate adjuvant postoperative radio-therapy in these situations.

2. Warthin's tumour (papillary cystadenoma)   is a benign tumour, usually seen in elderly men. The peak incidence is the seventh decade and the male–female ratio is 7:1. They are soft and cystic tumours which are thought to arise from heterotopic parotid tissue in the lymph nodes within the parotid gland. Ten per cent are bilateral, but rarely synchronously. Treatment is by excision and, unlike pleomorphic adenoma, recurrence almost never occurs.

3. Monomorphic adenomas   arise from ductal epithelium and are treated by surgical excision with a cuff of tissue.

4. *Oncocytoma* is a benign eosinophilic tumour (also called oxyphil adenoma) that arises from intralobular ducts or acini. It is usually found in the superficial lobe of the parotid. It can undergo malignant change and treatment is also by excision with a cuff of tissue.

Malignant tumours

1. *Adenoid cystic carcinoma* is the commonest malignant tumour and may arise from any salivary tissue, but is more common in minor than in major salivary glands. The sex incidence is equal and they are seen most often in patients in their sixth decade. The tumour is slow-growing and tends to spread along nerve sheaths. The patients often complain of facial pain and may present with a facial paresis. The incidence of lymph node metastases is low and distant metastases occur late. Treatment is usually by radical excision and adjuvant radiotherapy. If the facial nerve is free of tumour it may be dissected out and left intact. However, it is often involved, and in this situation it needs wide excision and anastomosis with a nerve graft. The sural nerve is preferred as the greater auricular nerve may be involved and should also be excised. Postoperative radiotherapy will not affect the graft. Radiotherapy in the curative and palliative treatment of patients with adenoid cystic carcinoma of salivary gland origin is useful in some cases, but is still being assessed.

2. *Adenocarcinoma* accounts for about 3% of parotid tumours and 10% of submandibular and minor salivary gland tumours.

3. *Squamous cell carcinoma.* Some pathologists doubt their existence, regarding them as high-grade mucoepidermoid tumours; true malignant pleomorphic adenomas are rare.

Tumours with variable behaviour

1. *Mucoepidermoid carcinoma* arises in any salivary tissue but predominantly the parotid gland. It is the commonest salivary neoplasm in children. Low-grade or well-differentiated tumours usually behave in a benign fashion, intermediate ones are more aggressive and high-grade or undifferentiated tumours metastasize early and carry a poor prognosis. However, the behaviour is not always accurately predicted by the histological appearance.

2. *Acinic cell carcinoma* is similarly difficult to classify. They are, however, much more benign than mucoepidermoid tumours.

Further reading

Medina JE. Salivary gland tumours. *Current Opinion in Otolaryngology and Head and Neck Surgery*, 1993; **1**: 91–96.

Roland NJ, Caslin AC, Jones AS. Fine needle aspiration cytology of salivary gland lesions reported immediately in a head and neck clinic. *Journal of Laryngology and Otology*, 1993; **107**: 1025–1028.

Wilson J (ed). *Effective Head and Neck Cancer Management. Second Consensus.* British Association of Otolaryngologists, Head and Neck Surgeons, 2000.

Related topic of interest

Salivary gland diseases, p. 271.

SEPTAL PERFORATION

Perforation of the nasal septum is most common in the anterior cartilaginous part except for that caused by syphilis, which normally involves the bony septum. Most perforations are iatrogenic in origin, usually as a complication of septal surgery, particularly when the Killian incision is used. Many septal perforations that were previously considered to be idiopathic are now thought to be secondary to nose picking. Septal perforations are usually preceded by ulceration except when following a septal haematoma or septal abscess.

Aetiology

1. *Trauma.*
   Iatrogenic (SMR, septoplasty, nasal cautery).
   Self-inflicted (nose picking).
   Injury (assault, road accident, sport injury).

2. *Infection*
   (Syphilis, tuberculosis).

3. *Neoplasm*
   (Squamous cell carcinoma, adenocarcinoma, basal cell carcinoma, T-cell lymphoma).

4. *Inflammatory*
   (Wegener's granulomatosis, polyarteritis nodosa, systemic lupus, chronic relapsing polychondritis).

5. *Inhalation of irritants.*
   Occupational (hexavalent, chrome, arsenic, alkaline dusts).
   Drugs (cocaine, snuff).

6. *Idiopathic.*

Clinical features

The majority of perforations are asymptomatic. The main complaints are recurrent epistaxis, dryness in the nose, crusting and nasal obstruction. The severity of the symptoms depends on the position and the size of the perforation. The larger the perforation and the more anterior its position, the worse the symptoms. A very small perforation may cause whistling on nasal breathing.

Investigations

The history will very often give the diagnosis. In any patient where there is uncertainty about the cause, the following tests should be performed:

- Blood tests should include an FBC, ESR, FTA for syphilis, ANCA for Wegners.
- A chest radiograph may show lesions in tuberculosis, Wegener's granulomatosis or metastases.

- Urinalysis (haematuria or proteinuria may result from nephritis in Wegener's granulomatosis or polyarteritis).
- A biopsy from the edge of the perforation if there is suggestion of a neoplasm or granuloma.

Treatment

The first objective is to cure the causative disease process before specific treatment of the perforation. Many perforations are asymptomatic and informed reassurance is all that is required. Treatment is usually indicated when there is troublesome crusting or bleeding. Medical treatment with 25% glucose in glycerol drops will loosen and help clear crusts. Barrier creams can help prevent drying and crusting. Silver nitrate cautery can be applied to bleeding granulations. Surgical closure of the perforation is difficult to achieve. A variety of operations including the use of split-skin grafts, buccal mucosa or sublabial myomucosal flaps, septal mucoperichondrial flaps, composite grafts from the pinna and moving septal cartilage to fill the hole have all been described. If the perforation continues to trouble the patient it is worth trying to plug the hole with a silastic septal button. Paradoxically, perforations that cause a whistle can be treated by enlarging them.

Follow-up and aftercare

This will depend on the cause of the perforation, the severity of the symptoms and the particular treatment the patient has been given. A patient with a silastic button should be seen at regular 4–6-monthly intervals to decrust and clean the prosthesis.

Further reading

Brain D. The nasal septum. In: Mackay IS, Bull TR (eds), *Scott-Brown's Otolaryngology*, Vol. 4, 6th edn. London: Butterworth, 1997.

Related topic of interest

Nasal trauma, p. 177.

SINONASAL TUMOURS

Tumours of the sinonasal region comprise a diverse group of benign and malignant neoplasms. The latter constitute a considerable challenge to the head and neck surgeon as they often present with advanced disease. Their low incidence and the lack of a consensus regarding staging has made comparison of treatment regimes between centres difficult.

Pathology

About 10% of head and neck cancer is sinonasal with an incidence in the UK and the USA of about 10 per million. It is about double this in Arabs, the Japanese and Africans. The male: female ratio in series varies between 1:2 and 1:5. Half of sinonasal cancer arises from the upper jaw, a quarter from the ethmoids and a quarter from the nasal cavity. Histologically 50% are squamous cell carcinoma, 15% anaplastic, 10% lymphomas and about 4% adenocarcinomas. Immunocytochemical analysis (in particular neurone specific enolase) of the small cell cancers (anaplastic and lymphomas) will reveal a proportion to be olfactory neuroblastomas. The association between the ethmoidal adenocarcinoma and hardwood workers is well documented. Workers handling chromate salts and those involved in nickel refining are at an increased risk of nasal malignancy. Chronic nasal pathology, including sepsis and Wegener's granulomatosis, and smoking cigarettes have recently been implicated as providing an increased risk of squamous cell carcinoma. Human papilloma virus genome has been identified and therefore implicated as an aetiological agent in non-dysplastic and dysplastic inverted papilloma and squamous cell carcinoma.

Classification

Both benign and malignant groups can be classified into epithelial, non epithelial, odontogenic, and fibro-osseous tumours.

1. *Benign.*
   Epithelial (papilloma, adenoma and inverted papilloma).
   Non-epithelial (fibroma, haemangioma, nasal glioma, Schwannoma, chondroma, haemangiopericytoma, chordoma, meningioma and osteoma).

2. *Malignant.*
   Epithelial (squamous cell carcinoma, adenocarcinoma, anaplastic carcinoma, transitional cell carcinoma, malignant melanoma, salivary gland malignancy in particular adenoid cystic carcinoma and olfactory neuroblastoma.
   Non-epithelial (fibrosarcoma, angiosarcoma, chondrosarcoma, rhabdomyosarcoma, and osteogenic sarcomas).

Important benign sinonasal tumours

Inverted papilloma, originally described by Ringertz, is the most important of this group forming about 5% of all nasal tumours. Macroscopically there is usually a papilliferous exophytic mass. Microscopically there are deep invaginations of epithelium into the stroma, with microcyst formation. The epithelium retains its basement membrane. Probably less than 2% undergo malignant change although there may be a synchronous sinonasal squamous cell carcinoma in up to a further 10%. This emphasizes the need for careful nasendoscopic follow up.

Osteomas most commonly arise from the frontal region where they may expand medially to block the frontal recess predisposing to a secondary mucocele or frontal sinusitis, inferiorly to displace the orbit, superiorly where they may erode the cribriform plate or posteriorly to erode the posterior wall of the frontal sinus and impinge on frontal lobe dura. They consist of hard cortical bone and require excision if symptomatic or enlarging.

Haemangiopericytomas may arise anywhere in the sinonasal region and have a spectrum of aggression, with a propensity to recur many years after apparent cure.

Malignant sinonasal tumours

Squamous cell carcinoma and adenocarcinoma both usually present at an advanced stage because their presenting symptoms of epistaxis, nasal obstruction and headaches occur only with a significant tumour mass. Further delays may arise because these symptoms are not usually associated with carcinoma by primary care physicians. Cheek swelling occurs only when the tumour has breached the anterior antral wall to impinge on periosteum. It is usually impossible to define a site of origin of the carcinoma due to its diffuse extent. This may include the cheek, orbit, nasal cavity and anterior cranial fossa. Five per cent of subjects will have a metastatic neck lymph node, usually upper deep cervical, on presentation. This indicates a poor prognosis but not necessarily incurability. A quarter of patients will die from distant metastases, most commonly the bronchus.

Adenoid cystic carcinoma is particularly difficult to eradicate because of its ability to spread via the branches of the trigeminal and olfactory nerves along perineurium.

Malignant melanomas comprise 1% of sinonasal carcinomas and usually arise from the septum or lateral nasal wall, where the prognosis is reasonable. Frontoethmoidal and antral malignant melanoma have a much worse prognosis. There is no relationship between Clark's classification (penetration of specific skin layers) and prognosis in this region although the latter is associated with Breslow's classification (thickness of the lesion in mm).

Olfactory neuroblastomas were undoubtedly under reported until recently when immunocytochemical stains for this tumour became available. It arises from neural crest stem cells, the precursors of olfactory cells, and microscopically resembles other small cell malignancies such as high grade lymphoma and anaplastic carcinoma. All ages are affected and urine vanillylmandelic acid (VMA), is not usually detectable. It always involves the cribriform plate so if resection is contemplated this must be via a craniofacial approach.

High grade T cell lymphoma (formerly lethal midline granuloma): see Related topic Non-healing nasal granulomata.

Staging

The UICC staging is as follows:

Tx   Primary tumour cannot be assessed.
T0   No evidence of primary disease.
Tis Carcinoma *in situ*.

Maxillary sinus.

T1   Tumour limited to the antral mucosa with no erosion or destruction of bone.

T2   Tumour causing bone erosion or destruction, except for the posterior wall, including extension into the hard palate and/or middle nasal meatus.

T3   Tumour invades any of the following: bone of posterior wall of maxillary sinus, subcutaneous tissues, skin of cheek, floor of medial wall of orbit.

T4   Tumour invades orbital contents beyond the floor or medial wall including apex and/or any of the following: cribriform plate, base of skull, nasopharynx, sphenoid sinus, frontal sinus.

Ethmoid sinus.

T1   Tumour confined to ethmoid with or without bone erosion.

T2   Tumour extends into nasal cavity.

T3   Tumour extends to anterior orbit and/or maxillary sinus.

T4   Tumour with intracranial extension, orbital extension including apex, involving sphenoid and/or frontal sinus and/or skin of nose.

Clinical features

1.   **Nasal cavity tumours.**   Epistaxis, nasal obstruction and a mass visible on nasendoscopy.

2.   **Frontal sinus.**   Features are similar to frontal osteomas except the history is shorter and more rapidly progressive.

3.   **Ethmoidal.**   Epistaxis, nasal obstruction and if the lamina papyracea is breached, proptosis, epiphora and diplopia. Nasendoscopy may reveal tumour extruding from the middle meatus.

4.   **Antral.**   Epistaxis, nasal obstruction, cheek swelling., headache if blocking the osteomeatal complex and atypical facial pain (suggesting involvement of the pterygo-palatine fossa or the infra orbital nerve). Oroantral fistula, ill-fitting dentures, trismus and ethmoidal symptoms occur with advanced disease.

Investigations

A high definition CT scan on both bone and soft tissue windows is the ideal to show soft tissue and bone involvement. A T2 weighted or STIR sequence MRI scan may distinguish tumour from inflammation, retained secretions and fat. Bone does not generate a signal.

Treatment

1.   **Inverted papilloma.**   The accurate identification of disease extent with CT and MRI imaging has allowed the advent of endoscopic resection for inverted papilloma. Recent studies have demonstrated recurrence rates no higher than with external approach surgery. There is significantly less morbidity by the endoscopic approach. The technique allows direct visualization of tumour and its extent can be accurately identified during surgery. It prevents an external scar, there is less blood loss and the hospital stay is shorter. Tumour limited to the anterior ethmoids or isolated middle turbinate or middle meatal lesion are ideal for endoscopic resection. Recent work

has also shown its application for tumours involving the posterior ethmoids and anterior wall of sphenoid. In essence provided the endoscope can visualize the distal extent of tumour during surgery then endoscopic resection is a reasonable and perhaps preferred alternative to external approach surgery. Post-operatively endoscopic inspection of the surgical cavity allows accurate monitoring of patient progress and early identification of recurrence. Wigand's figures for disease of similar extent are 17% recurrence rate for the endoscopic approach and 19% for external approach surgery at 2 years follow-up. Draf quotes a recurrence rate of 9% by the endoscopic approach. Limitations of the endoscopic approach include tumour extending into the frontal sinus and anterior wall of maxilla. Extensive experience and a high level of expertise in endoscopic sinus surgery is a prerequisite to undertaking the endoscopic approach.

2. **Carcinoma.** There are three main surgical options for carcinoma:
(a) *Lateral rhinotomy* for tumour limited to the lateral nasal wall, nasal cavity and ethmoid. An upper limb extension will allow tumour limited to the frontal ethmoidal region to be accessed.
(b) *Total maxillectomy.* For antral carcinoma. Reconstruction is by primary closure where possible. Split thickness skin grafts should line the exenteration cavity. Free flaps or a temporalis muscle swing flap will fill in the cavity and produce the optimum cosmetic result, but have the disadvantage that they may mask an early recurrence.
(c) *Craniofacial resection* is indicated when the cribriform plate is involved or breached. In general an orbital exenteration is indicated only if tumour breaches periostium to involve orbital fat. Adjuvant radiotherapy may be indicated depending on tissue margins.

Prognosis by stage is difficult for reasons already outlined. Overall a five-year survival of 40–50% would be reasonable.

Follow-up and aftercare

Ideally an orthodontist should take an impression of the maxillectomy cavity at operation in order to make a temporary obturator. Further review allows a fine tuning of the prosthesis to provide a light, comfortable, well fitting and easily removable obturator. Those who have a lateral rhinotomy or craniofacial cavity often have excessive crusting in the early post-operative phase. Glycerine and glucose nose drops and regular douching with saline will minimize this. Only the surgeon should extract crusts from the nares of the craniofacial patient as these may be attached to a fascia lata or temporalis fascia graft overlying the anterior cranial fossa. Follow-up which involves nasendoscopy to inspect the surgical cavity created or direct inspection of a maxillectomy cavity after obturator removal, laryngopharyngeal examination to exclude a second primary and neck examination to look for metastases should be monthly for the first post-operative year, bimonthly for the second, quarterly for the third and six-monthly until five years post surgery. Some surgeons thereafter review annually for a further five years.

Further reading

Lund VJ, Harrison DFN. Craniofacial resection for tumors of the nasal cavity and paranasal sinuses. *American Journal of Surgery*, 1988; **156**: 187–190.

Lund VJ, Howard DJ, Lloyd GAS, Cheesman AD. Magnetic resonance imaging of paranasal sinus tumors for craniofacial resection. *Head and Neck Surgery*, 1989; **11**: 279–283.

Donald PJ. Management of sinus malignancy. *Current Opinion in Otolaryngol and Head and Neck Surgery*, 1997; **5**: 73–78.

Brors D and Draf W. The treatment of inverted papilloma. *Current Opinion in Otolaryngology and Head and Neck Surgery*, 1999; **7**: 33–39.

Wilson J (ed). *Effective Head and Neck Cancer Management. Second Consensus.* British Association of Otolaryngologists, Head and Neck Surgeons, 2000.

Related topic of interest

Nasal granuloma, p. 170.

SINUSITIS

Predisposing factors

The commonest causes are nasal. Both the maxillary and frontal sinuses drain through narrow spaces and interstices into the middle meatus. The ethmoids also drain into this and the superior meatus. Any condition narrowing or blocking these may lead to secretion retention and poor ventilation, thus predisposing to consequent infection.

1. Local.
- Upper respiratory tract infection (acute infective rhinitis, i.e. common cold or influenza, tonsillitis or adenoiditis).
- Pre-existing rhinitis (allergic, vasomotor, rhinitis medicamentosa, etc.).
- Nasal polyps.
- Nasal foreign body.
- Nasal anatomical variations (septal deviation, abnormal uncinate process, middle turbinate or ethmoid bulla) narrow the infundibulum and predispose to its occlusion when there is intercurrent disease.
- Nasal tumour.
- Dental extraction or infection (diseases of the upper premolars and molars).
- Swimming and diving.
- Fractures involving the sinuses.

2. General.
- Debilitation.
- Immunocompromised host.
- Mucociliary disorders (e.g. Kartagener's syndrome, cystic fibrosis).
- Atmospheric irritants (dust, fumes, tobacco smoke).

Acute sinusitis

Acute inflammation of one or all the sinuses may occur (pansinusitis). The maxillary sinus is clinically the most commonly affected, followed by the ethmoid, frontal and sphenoid sinuses in that order.

Pathology

The majority of cases follow a viral upper respiratory tract infection which involves all of the respiratory epithelium including the paranasal sinuses. Such infections cause hyperaemia and oedema of the mucosa, which blocks the ostia. There will be cellular infiltration and an increase in mucus production.

The infection will also paralyse the cilia, leading to stasis of secretions predisposing to secondary bacterial infection. The usual causative organisms are *Streptococcus pneumoniae, Haemophilus influenzae* (pneumococcal and haemophilus infections accounting for 70% of cases in adults), *Streptococcus pyogenes, Moraxella catarrhalis,* and *Staphylococcus aureus*. *Klebsiella pneumoniae*, *Escherichia coli* and *Streptococcus faecalis* may spread from a dental source. Acute fungal infections (for example mucormycosis and aspergillosis) are rare, but may develop in immunocompromised or elderly diabetic patients.

Clinical features

The symptoms usually occur several days after developing an upper respiratory tract infection. The patient will have pain over the infected sinus, nasal congestion, fullness in the face, malaise and possibly a pyrexia. The fullness in the face and pain may be exacerbated by bending forward or stooping down.

Specific features may indicate the sinus that is infected. Pain developing in the cheek or upper teeth indicates maxillary sinus involvement. Frontal sinusitis produces pain in the forehead and tenderness below the eyebrows. Ethmoid sinusitis may cause pain between the eyes accompanied by frontal headache. Sphenoid infection may produce retro-orbital pain, or pain anywhere across the vault.

Anterior rhinoscopy may show red oedematous nasal mucosa and turbinates. Endoscopy with a 0° or 30° scope may reveal pus in the middle meatus or sphenoethmoidal recess. It may also be possible to elicit tenderness over the infected sinus. Percussion over the upper teeth may elicit tenderness, suggesting a dental origin of maxillary sinusitis.

Differential diagnosis

- Migraine.
- Dental pain.
- Trigeminal neuralgia.
- Temporal arteritis.
- Herpes zoster.
- Erysipelas.
- Sinonasal tumour.

Investigations

An elevated white cell count and erythrocyte sedimentation rate (ESR) will confirm an acute infection. Where possible pus from the nose should be cultured and blood cultures should be taken if there is systemic upset. Radiological investigation may show an opacity or fluid level, although plain X-rays are rarely if ever used (see Radiology). When there is doubt about the diagnosis, further confirmation can be obtained by a high-definition coronal CT scan, ideally using both soft-tissue and bone window settings.

Management

The aims of treatment are to resolve and limit the course of the acute infection, to prevent complications and to correct any precipitating factor.

1. *Medical treatment.* In the acute stages the patient should have:
- Bed rest and adequate simple analgesia (e.g. paracetamol).
- Broad-spectrum antibiotic (e.g. co-amoxyclav, clarithromycin). A second generation cephalosporin (e.g. cefuroxime) is recommended for penicillin-resistant pneumococci.
- A decongestant (e.g. pseudoephedrine or xylometa-zoline).

The patient should have a full 7-day course of the antibiotic. The decongestant may reduce nasal oedema, and hopefully open the natural ostia of the sinuses to allow free drainage. It can be given locally or systemically. The current practice of many rhino-logists is to shrink the mucosal lining, and aid infundibular drainage, by placing a pledget of cocainized cotton wool into the middle meatus for 20 minutes.

2. *Surgical treatment.* Functional endoscopic sinus surgery (see p. 108) is now considered to be the treatment of choice. If acute sinusitis fails to respond to medical treatment, then the patient may need antral puncture and washout. This will not only treat any infection in the maxillary sinus but will also promote drainage from the other sinuses. Any pus obtained should be cultured. If the patient has suffered recurrent infections it may be appropriate to perform an intranasal antrostomy for better and longer-lasting drainage. This is best performed with the aid of an endoscope. Frontal sinu-sitis which does not respond to these measures may requires trephine of the floor of the sinus via a small incision above the medial canthus. The ethmoid sinuses can be uncapped to promote drainage if they are specifically diseased and an anterior sphenoidotomy may be necessary for acute sphenoiditis.

The patient should be reviewed after resolution of the acute phase. Correction of any obvious precipitating factor (e.g. septoplasty for septal deviation) should be organized. It may be necessary to perform repeat antral washouts for some patients. Those surgeons who follow the philosophy of functional endoscopic sinus surgery claim that if definitive endoscopic sinus surgery is performed in the acute phase no further washout should be necessary.

Chronic sinusitis

Chronic inflammation of the sinuses usually follows recurrent acute sinusitis, but in some cases the onset is more insidious. There is no consensus view on what constitutes chronic sinusitis. It is usually considered to be *a condition in which sinusitis symptoms* (congestion, nasal discharge, postnasal drainage, facial pain) *and signs* (CT, endoscopy) *persist for weeks to months.* It has been stated that the incidence of this problem in the UK has been reduced by improvements in the general health of the population, diet, hygiene, and the introduction of antibiotics. Figures from the USA however, confirm that over the past decade, the incidence of sinusitis has increased. Chronic sinusitis accounts for over 85% of all clinic visits for sinusitis in adults.

Pathology

There is an increase in vascularity and vascular permeability. This leads to oedema and hypertrophy of the mucosa which may become polypoidal. Goblet cell hyperplasia and a chronic cellular infiltrate will occur. Ulceration of the epithelium will result in the formation of granulation tissue. Multiple small abscesses occur in the thickened mucosa and fibrosis of the submucosal stroma supervenes. The changes in the mucosa over this time may be irreversible, and when the original cause of infection has been treated the lining will not revert to normal.

The cardinal symptoms are nasal congestion, nasal or postnasal discharge and pain. A headache over the forehead, the bridge of the nose and the face is common. The patient may also suffer with anosmia, or even cacosmia (unpleasant smell), especially in infections of dental origin. Chronic irritation of the nasal airway and repeated rubbing may lead to a vestibulitis and epistaxis. Chronic pharyngitis and laryngitis with the patient complaining of a productive cough are often encountered. Clinical examination will usually show nasal inflammation or perhaps another obvious intranasal predisposing factor.

Differential diagnosis

It is not uncommon for general practitioners and those in other specialties to ascribe facial pain and headaches to sinus disease, often when it is not. The definition of chronic sinusitis becomes important in comparing studies on the disease, because different patient inclusion criteria may affect study results. It has been suggested that chronic paranasal sinus pain alone should not constitute chronic sinusitis.

The ENT surgeon is confronted as a rule with three different groups of headache patients:

(a) Those with headaches clearly connected to a sinus problem, such as inflammatory disease, neoplasm, barotrauma or another readily identifiable cause.
(b) Those with headaches clearly traceable to non-sinus causes such as migraine, neuralgias, cervical spine disorders, temporomandibular joint diseases, glaucoma, hypertension.
(c) Those whose problems are not clear and in whom there seems to be no overt indication of sinus disease. In this group of patients nasendoscopic examination with a high-definition coronal section CT scan may confirm that the symptoms are indeed sinus related.

Investigations

Only the combination of diagnostic endoscopy and high-definition coronal section CT scanning will provide the maximum information. One modality is said to enhance the accuracy of the other. Plain sinus radiographs are rarely indicated now because they may show varying degrees of opacification of the involved sinuses with mucosal thickening. Mucosal thickening occurs in 30% of individuals and its detection is often meaningless. Furthermore, some patients with sinogenic headaches may present with an atypical history and have negative findings on examination and plain sinus radiographs. This does not rule out a sinus cause for their problem.

The principal aims of treatment are to correct the predisposing cause, to ventilate the sinus and to restore normal mucosal lining in the sinus.

1. Medical. A course of broad-spectrum antibiotics in combination with a decongestant should be tried initially (though they should be avoided long-term). Any obvious predisposing factor, for example rhinitis or nasal polyps, should be treated with medical therapy (e.g. antihistamines, a steroid nasal spray, oral course of steroids).

2. Surgery

(a) *Functional endonasal sinus surgery.* Functional endoscopic sinus surgery is now the preferred alternative to the classical open surgical approaches to chronic sinusitis. Those who advocate this procedure claim that more accurate surgery can now be undertaken and that injury to the eye, optic nerve or dura is less likely. Stepwise removal of the ethmoidal cells extending to the posterior ethmoid and sphenoid sinus can be undertaken. The natural ostium of the maxillary sinus in the middle meatus can be cleared, opened and enlarged, as can any disease of the frontonasal duct.

(b) *Open sinus surgery procedures.* If irreversible changes have occurred to the sinus mucosa then some surgeons would consider it necessary to remove it. A wide range of procedures are available, so the choice of operation should be tailored to the requirements of the individual patient. Each procedure has its own limitations and specific complications. However, the more radical open procedures are still used and asked about in the examinations. They are listed below, but details of each procedure and its complications should be sought from an operative textbook.

- *Chronic maxillary sinusitis*: Caldwell–Luc procedure.
- *Chronic ethmoid sinusitis*: intranasal ethmoidectomy, external ethmoidectomy (Patterson's operation), transantral (Horgan's operation).
- *Chronic frontal sinusitis*: external frontoethmoidectomy (Howarth's operation), osteoplastic flap procedure (MacBeth's operation).
- *Chronic sphenoiditis*: via an intranasal ethmoidectomy, transantral to the posterior ethmoids then to the sphenoid sinus, via an external frontoethmoidectomy.

Fungal sinusitis

This is now being recognized more frequently, because of advances in diagnostic techniques (nasal endoscopy and CT scans) and increasing numbers of immunocompromised individuals. Fungal sinusitis can be divided into the following entities:

1. Mycetoma. These are masses of fungal debris that usually occur in the maxillary or ethmoid sinuses. Patients are typically immunocompetent and non-atopic. *Aspergillus fumigatus* is the most common organism isolated. Treatment is by endoscopic removal of debris and ventilation of the sinus. There is usually no requirement for antifungal or any other systemic therapy.

2. Allergic fungal sinusitis. Typically occurs in atopic immunocompetent young adults. Usually associated with nasal polyps and asthma. Associated fungi include *Aspergillus*, *Bipolaris* and *Curvularia*. Because of the potential for orbital and intracranial complications, appropriate treatment needs to be rapidly instituted. The mainstay of therapy is polypectomy and aeration of the sinuses. Systemic steroids and antifungal therapy (itraconazole), may also be useful.

3.   Chronic indolent sinusitis.   This should be suspected in a healthy patient presenting with chronic sinusitis resistant to conventional therapy. This is a slow progressive disease characterized by granulomatous infection. *Aspergillus fumigatus* is the most common organism isolated. Surgical debridement with removal of all debris from the sinuses is required. Amphotericin B is the drug of choice.

4.   Acute invasive (fulminant) sinusitis.   A rare entity that occurs in immuno-compromised individuals (diabetic ketoacidosis, chemotherapy patients, AIDS, leukaemia and lymphoma). *Aspergillus, Mucor* and *Rhizopus* are the associated organisms. Immediate treatment consists of intravenous antifungal therapy (amphotericin B) and radical surgical debridement, which can extend to a total maxillectomy and orbital exenteration. The earlier the treatment is started, the better the prognosis. The disease still carries a mortality rate of 50–80%.

Further reading

Durand M. The antibiotic treatment of sinusitis. *Current Opinion in Otolaryngology and Head and Neck Surgery,* 1997; **5**: 8–12.
Stammberger H and Wolf G. Headaches and sinus disease: the endoscopic approach. *Annals of Otology, Rhinology and Laryngology,* 1988; **97** (Suppl. 134).

Related topics of interest

SINUSITIS – COMPLICATIONS

In most cases sinusitis is uncomplicated and spread of infection beyond the walls of the sinus is uncommon. Complications may follow an acute infection, but are most frequent during an acute exacerbation of chronic sinusitis. They can be divided into:

- Orbital complications (orbital cellulitis and orbital abscess).
- Osteomyelitis (maxilla or frontal bone).
- Intracranial complications (meningitis, intracranial abscess, cavernous sinus thrombosis).
- Mucocele.
- Locoregional complications (pharyngitis, laryngitis, otitis media).

Orbital complications

These can occur at any age, but are more common in children. Peri-orbital cellulitis and orbital abscess usually result from direct spread of pus from the ethmoid sinuses. It can also spread from thrombophlebitis of mucosal vessels in any of the sinuses. The orbital septum forms a natural barrier which may localize the infection anteriorly as a preseptal cellulitis or posteriorly as orbital cellulitis.

Aching around the orbit is followed by oedema of the eyelids and later the conjunctiva. *Cellulitis* requires treatment with intravenous antibiotics and nasal decongestants to resolve the infection and limit further spread. The ethmoids are separated from the orbit by the thin lamina papyracea. A *subperiosteal abscess* results from direct spread from the ethmoids and collects between the lamina papyracea and the orbital periosteum. The swelling may displace the orbit lateral and down. With an *orbital collection* the eye will become proptosed and its movements progressively restricted to a complete ophthalmoplegia. The biggest anxiety is the risk of blindness as a result of tension and septic necrosis of the optic nerve. Early liason with an ophthalmologist is recommended. Visual acuity, red–green colour vision, visual fields, pupillary reflexes, and the optic disc should be examined. Colour blindness is an early sign. Absence of the ipsilateral and contralateral light reflex will occur with visual impairment. If the other eye is stimulated but there is no contralateral reflex, then the third cranial nerve (occulomotor) will have been affected. A CT scan will confirm the collection and extent of the disease. Urgent surgical drainage is indicated. An incision is made in the superomedial aspect of the orbit. Elevation of the orbital periosteum usually reveals the pus under pressure. An external ethmoidectomy is performed and a drain inserted. Synchronous infection of the maxillary sinus may require treatment with intravenous antibiotics and surgical drainage (usually an endoscopically fashioned middle meatal antrostomy and sinus washout).

Osteomyelitis

This only occurs in diploic bone and thus only in the maxilla of children and the frontal sinus of adolescents and adults. The common organism is *Staphylococcus aureus*. Osteomyelitis of the maxilla is rare and usually only seen in third world countries. It presents as a painful swelling of the cheek and lower eyelid. Treatment comprises intravenous antibiotics and debridement when necessary. Osteomyelitis of the frontal bone is more extensive and dangerous. There is a build-up of dull local pain with oedema of the forehead and the upper eyelids. A subperiosteal abscess of the forehead may form (Pott's puffy tumour). This is a life-threatening condition with a high risk of intracranial complications. High resolution CT scan and MRI will illustrate the extent of the problem. Prompt treatment with high doses of intravenous antibiotics, surgical drainage of the frontal sinus, and appropriate debridement is required.

Intracranial complications

The cavities of the frontal, ethmoidal and sphenoid sinuses are closely related to and separated by a thin wall of bone from the anterior cranial fossa. Infection may involve the brain and meninges from either direct spread or retrograde thrombophlebitis. Meningitis is the commonest complication, but encephalitis, intracranial abscess (extradural, subdural or cerebral) and cavernous sinus thrombosis may complicate sinus infections. The clinical features of meningitis are well known. A lumbar puncture may identify the causative organism, but it is essential to exclude raised intracranial pressure before this is done by looking for papilloedema.

Cavernous sinus thrombosis will cause a high fever, reduced conscious level and cerebral irritation. The eyes will proptose and an ophthalmoplegia of the cranial nerves which travel in the cavernous sinus will occur (III, IV, ophthalmic and maxillary branches of V and VI). An intracranial abscess may be more difficult to diagnose.

The important point is that the ENT surgeon should always maintain a high index of suspicion for all intracranial complications, particularly in sinusitis patients who become drowsy or show some neurological deficit. A CT scan with enhancement or MRI scan may assist in diagnosis. Intracranial complications should all be treated with high-dose intravenous antibiotics. An extradural or subdural abscess will require drainage by a neurosurgeon, together with drainage of the offending sinuses by an ENT surgeon. The mortality and morbidity after intracranial complications is considerable. Up to 25% of patients may die and nearly a third of surviving patients will suffer with epilepsy.

Mucocele

A mucocele may develop when the outlet from a sinus becomes permanently blocked. It occurs most commonly in the frontal sinus, but the ethmoid, maxillary and sphenoid sinuses can all be afflicted. There is an accumulation of sterile mucus which becomes increasingly viscous. The cyst gradually expands and exerts pressure on the sinus walls causing erosion. This leads to displacement of adjacent structures, especially the orbit. The main complaints are headache and swelling. These features can be dramatic if infection supervenes (pyocele). Diplopia and proptosis may result if the mucocele expands into the orbit. Radiographs will show enlargement of the sinus with thinning of the bone. CT scans will further delineate the extent of the disease if needed.

Treatment is surgical evacuation and drainage of the sinus. To approach the frontal sinus, the two options in common use are external fronto-ethmoidectomy

(Howarth's operation) and the osteoplastic flap procedure (Macbeth's operation). An endoscopic approach is an alternative in experienced hands.

Locoregional complications

Regional complications occur as a result of infection and inflammation spreading through the rest of the upper aerodigestive tract mucosa. Mucopus from sinusitis is carried back through the nasal airway into the pharynx and may cause a pharyngitis. Invasion of the subepithelial lymphoid tissue will produce a granular pharyngitis with visible nodules as the lymphatic tissue hypertrophies. Further downward spread may lead to irritation of the vocal cords causing a laryngitis. Sinusitis is also implicated as a cause and complication of tonsillitis and otitis media.

Further reading

Lund VJ. The complications of sinusitis. In: Mackay IS, Bull TR (eds), *Scott-Brown's Otolaryngology*, Vol. 4, 6th edn. London: Butterworths, 1997, 1–11.

Swift AC. The complications of sinusitis. In: *Diseases of the Head and Neck, Nose and Throat*. Jones AS (ed), London: Arnold, 1998: 868–883.

Related topics of interest

Sinusitis, p. 285; Functional endoscopic sinus surgery, p. 108.

SMELL AND TASTE DISORDERS

There are three chemosensory portions to smell and taste:
1. Olfaction.
2. Gustation.
3. Common chemical sensation.

Physiology

1. Olfaction (smell) is provided by a small area of olfactory epithelium in the vault of the nasal cavity. Odorant molecules (those molecule with the ability to bind and stimulate olfactory receptors) are carried into the nasal cavity with (inspiratory and expiratory) airflow. They may then dissolve in and diffuse through the overlying mucus or they may combine with specific odorant-binding proteins and be transported through the overlying mucus layer. The free molecules or odorant/protein complexes then attach to receptor proteins, resulting in the production of an intracellular secondary messenger (usually cyclic AMP), with subsequent cell depolarization and a neural action potential. Degradative enzyme systems appear to exist for stimulant breakdown after neural interaction. The olfactory neurones pass through the cribriform plate and sensory information passes to the olfactory bulb and then on to the thalamus, hypothalamus and cortex. Quite how this sensory information codes for smell is unknown. It is known, however, that different odorants have different rates and degrees of solubility in the overlying mucus. Not all olfactory receptors respond equally or at all to different odorants, neither are they equally distributed in the nasal cavity. It is likely that all these factors have a bearing on smell recognition. Recent research has postulated that there are certain 'groups' of smells that might be recognized by a relatively common mechanism.

2. Gustation (taste) is served by the taste buds, which are modified epithelial cells found throughout the oral cavity, although there are regional differences in their concentration and distribution. Bitter tastes are better perceived on the posterior tongue, sweet and salt on the anterior tongue and sour on the lateral border. Neural stimulation occurs after dissolving of the tastant in a similar fashion to olfaction although the neural pathways are more complex. Several different cranial nerves are involved, with their primary afferents synapsing in the tractus solitarius in the medulla, before sensation passes on to the thalamus and cortex.

3. Common chemical sensation (irritation and textural quality) is served by free nerve endings from branches of the trigeminal nerve in the oral cavity and nose with a contribution from the glossopharyngeal and vagus nerves in the oropharynx. These fibres are stimulated by (unpleasant) mechanical, thermal or chemical stimuli. Information is ultimately passed to the cortex via the thalamus.

Pathology

It is uncommon for common chemical sensation or taste to be lost; there is much redundancy in the neural supply and the sensory distribution is relatively wide. It is more likely that olfaction may be lost or impaired. Most losses of taste that patients complain of are in fact loss of olfaction. Olfactory disturbances tend to be more common with increasing age and fall into three main groups: impaired transport, sensory and neural.

The main causes of disorders of smell and taste are as follows:

1. Sinonasal disease (20–30%). (Transport). In most cases this is due to simple mechanical obstruction (polyps, mucosal swelling in rhinitis, etc.) preventing odorants from reaching the olfactory epithelium in the narrow nasal vault, although in some cases the local inflammatory response may alter the overlying mucus or the function of the receptor cells.

2. Following upper respiratory tract infection (15–20%). (Sensory). Probably due to damage of the peripheral olfactory receptors following infection with a neuropathic virus.

3. Head injury (20%). (Neural). Serious head injury can result in shearing of the olfactory filaments as they pass through the cribriform plate or direct contusion of the olfactory bulb or cortex.

4. Idiopathic (20%).

5. Others (15–20%). A multitude of other causes exist, including systemic disease, metabolic and connective tissue disorders, drug therapy, neurological conditions, toxin exposure, previous nasal surgery, radiotherapy and old age.

Clinical features

The patient may complain of loss (anosmia), diminution (hyposmia) or alteration, usually unpleasant (parosmia), in the sense of smell or taste. In this last case the patient is often confusing taste with flavour as taste is rarely lost. The majority of patients (60–75%) with sinonasal disease describe anosmia rather than hyposmia, as do those following head injury. Hyposmia is a more common symptom following URTI.

Investigations

A thorough history must be taken and any temporal relation to an upper respiratory infection or head injury noted. A full nasal examination including endoscopy will be required to establish any sinonasal disease. Radiological imaging (including CT scans) of the sinuses may be required. Further general investigations will be dictated by the clinical features. The sense of smell can be crudely tested using a variety of recognizable odours, e.g. peppermint, cloves, lemon or coffee. It is important that the test scents are not too pungent or irritant (e.g. bleach) as they may then be recognized by common chemical sensation. Some objective measure of olfaction is helpful. Commercial 'scratch and sniff' kits are available using a forced choice technique which greatly increase their sensitivity. For example, they can be useful for deciding if a patient is suffering from anosmia or is malingering.

Management

Sinonasal disease should be managed as appropriate to the condition. It has the best prognosis in terms of response to treatment. Reassurance regarding the absence of serious pathology should be stressed to the post-URTI and head injury groups. A small proportion in both groups (10–20%) will improve with the passage of time. Management of any systemic causes is as for that condition and drug-induced problems may require a change of medication. Little is known about the idiopathic group and certainly no treatments are available, but some surgeons will see if the patient has any response after a trial of using a steroid nasal spray. Some authorities claim that a trial of zinc supplements should be administered.

Follow-up and aftercare

This should be as appropriate for the underlying cause.

Further reading

Mott AE, Leopold DA. Disorders in taste and smell. *Medical Clinics of North America*, 1991; **75**: 1321–1348.
Getchell TV, Doty RL, Bartoshuk LM and Snow JB (eds). *Smell and Taste in Health and Disease.* New York: Raven Press, 1991.

Related topics of interest

Allergic rhinitis, p. 11; Halitosis, p. 115; Intrinsic rhinitis, p. 131; Nasal polyps, p. 174.

SNORING AND OBSTRUCTIVE SLEEP APNOEA

M. Pringle

Definitions

- Snoring: a noise generated as a result of partial upper airway obstruction during sleep.
- Apnoea: a period of no airflow at the nose or mouth for at least 10 s.
- Apnoea index (AI): the number of periods of apnoea per hour.
- Hypopnoea: 50% or greater reduction in normal tidal volume.

Sleep apnoea syndrome can be diagnosed if there are more than 30 apnoeic episodes in 7 h of sleep or if the apnoea index is more than 5. Sleep apnoea is classified as mild (AI = 5–20), moderate AI = 20–40) or severe (AI > 40). Sleep apnoea can be obstructive, central or mixed.

In obstructive sleep apnoea (OSA) there is complete upper airway obstruction yet the patient continues to make respiratory efforts to overcome this. In central apnoea, respiratory effort, and consequently airflow, ceases for a period of time. Central apnoea is due to a defect of autonomic control of respiration in the medulla or peripheral chemoreceptors resulting in a failure of respiratory drive. It is a symptom of serious neurological disease and is not considered further here.

Pathophysiology

The noise of snoring is produced by vibration of the soft palate and pharyngeal walls caused by turbulent airflow and the Bernouli effect from a partial obstruction. The obstruction occurs when the negative intraluminal pharyngeal pressure exceeds the ability of the dilators to hold the pharynx open. Any cause of airway narrowing from nares to glottis can contribute to increased airway resistance. Neuromuscular incoordination interfering with the reflex activity of the pharyngeal dilators associated with inspiration, increased compliance of pharyngeal tissues, the Venturi effect and the decreased muscle tone associated with sleep can all predispose to upper airway collapse. This obstruction has three effects:

1. hypoxia, which may cause cardiac dysrhythmias and if severe and prolonged may lead to pulmonary and systemic hypertension and cor pulmonale;
2. increased negative intrathoracic pressure and increased cardiovascular strain;
3. arousal, which is an attempt to overcome the obstruction and if frequent results in poor sleep quality.

As a consequence patients with severe OSA are at risk from increased mortality due to cardiovascular disease.

Clinical features

Snoring and OSA in adults is more common with increasing age, in men, in the obese and in those with a high alcohol intake. Snoring occurs in 10% of men under 30 years of age and 60% of men over 60 years of age, while OSA can be found in approximately 6% of men. In children it most commonly occurs around the age of 5 years when lymphoid hyperplasia is at its greatest. Snoring can be immensely socially disruptive and may lead to marital difficulties. OSA often leads to excessive daytime somnolence, morning headaches, personality change, intellectual deterioration, impotence and an increased risk of a road traffic accident.

It is important to establish whether the patient has simple snoring or OSA, to exclude any exacerbating factors (drugs, endocrine disorders, anatomical) and to identify the site and level of obstruction. A thorough history and examination is needed; while taking the history it is preferable to have the bed partner present.

Investigations

1. *Body mass index (BMI).* This measurement helps define degree of obesity. It is calculated by dividing the weight in kilograms by the height in metres squared (Kg/m^2). Normal BMI = 19–25, overweight = 26–30, obese = 30–40, very obese = > 40. Palatal surgery is far less effective in patients with a body mass index of > 30. This is probably because these patients are more likely to have OSA with multi-segmental or tongue base level collapse.

2. *General investigations.* These consider full blood count (FBC), thyroid function tests (TFT), chest radiograph, electrocardiogram (ECG).

3. *To identify sleep apnoea.* An overnight sleep study. Polysomnography is the gold standard and involves recording an electroencephalogram (EEG), electromyogram (EMG) (to detect periodic limb movements), ECG, airflow, abdominal and chest movements, oxygen saturation, body position monitor and microphone recording of the snoring. This is expensive in terms of time and equipment but is an ideal research tool. Effective screening sleep studies may be performed excluding EEG and EMG. One technique involves overnight video recording. Overnight pulse oximetry will detect all those with severe OSA but may miss some with moderate OSA. It does not detect arousal's (which are triggered by high negative intrathoracic pressure rather than hypoxia) and may miss 'high upper airways resistance syndrome' (HUARS).

4. *Site of obstruction.* To differentiate between palatal and tongue base or multi-segmental obstruction, a variety of tests have been developed including lateral cephalometry, sleep nasendoscopy, manometry, cine CT and somnofluroscopy. The latter two are research tools. Probably the most widely used test is the Muller manoeuvre. This involves positioning per nasally a flexible fibreoptic endoscope to the level of the tongue base with the patient in the sitting position and with the mouth closed. The patient inhales vigorously while the nares and mouth are occluded and the degree of hypopharyngeal collapse noted. The manoeuvre is then repeated with the endoscope positioned just above the soft palate (velopharyngeal level). In this way the level of obstruction can be identified in up to 85% or cases.

Treatment

Snoring and OSA are often multifactorial conditions with a variety of primary causative factors, hence there will never be one single universal cure for snoring. Accurate assessment is essential to guide treatment.

- *General.* Patients with simple snoring and mild OSA can be reassured that there is no evidence of long term health risk. For some patients this reassurance will be enough others will request further treatment. Weight loss is very important and advice with regard to alcohol and sedative medication are often helpful especially in patients with OSA.
- *Nasal obstruction.* Medical treatment of rhinitis, the use of the "Nozovent" nasal splint or Breathe Right nasal strips to open the nasal valve or surgical correction of a septal deviation, turbinate hypertrophy or nasal polyps may all help snoring by overcoming nasal obstruction, though this can not be guaranteed. If nasal CPAP or pharyngeal surgery are contemplated any nasal obstruction should be corrected first.
- *Oropharyngeal obstruction* causing simple snoring and OSA.

    i. Uvulopalatopharyngoplasty (UPPP) involves tonsillectomy and excision of the uvula. Laser palatoplasty involves excision of the uvula and scarring of the soft palate with the laser in a variety of ways to induce palatal stiffness.
    ii. LAUP (laser assisted uvulopalatoplasty) is a technique in which the uvula is vapourised by the laser and troughs created through the soft palate to each side of the uvula base to form a neouvula. LAUP is sometimes performed under a local anaesthetic. In appropriately selected patients all these procedures have a 70–80% success rate, though long term rates are around 50%. This may be related to later weight gain. This surgery can be very painful and complications include nasopharyngeal reflux and dry mouth.
    iii. Somnoplasty. A new technique in which low temperature radio-frequency energy is delivered via a needle placed into the soft palate. This results in an area of scarring and hence stiffening of the soft palate. It is recommended for certain individuals with simple snoring. Early results are encouraging but there are no long term studies.
    iv. Adenotonsillectomy. In children, OSA is in most cases adequately dealt with by adenotonsillectomy as this is the usual site of obstruction. With a history of OSA sedative pre-med should be avoided.

- In moderate to severe OSA due to tongue base and multisegmental airway collapse surgery is not particularly effective and anaesthetic risk is significant. Nasal Continuous Positive Airways Pressue (nasal CPAP) is the gold standard treatment. Air under pressure is delivered via a tight fitting nasal mask. The air acts as a pneumatic splint holding the upper airway open and preventing snoring and obstructive episodes. It can be extremely effective but compliance is often a problem.
- Maxillofacial.

    i. Mandibular Positioning Devices. This appliance is worn in the mouth overnight. It is like an upper and lower gum shield attached in such a way as to hold the lower jaw forward. This in turn draws the tongue base forward enlarging the pharyngeal airway. Long term effects on the temporo-mandibular joints are not known.

ii. Hyoid suspension techniques to advance the hyoid and hence move the tongue base forward have been tried with some success. In retrognathia mandibular osteotomies may be required. In patients with morbid obesity and life threatening obstructive sleep apnoea bi-maxillary and bi-mandibular advancement osteotomies have been performed together with significant success rates reported.

- Tracheostomy. In severe OSA, when all other forms of treatment have failed, a tracheostomy can be life-saving. Despite the procedure, it can significantly improve a patients quality of life.

Further reading

Croft C.B., Pringle M.B. Snoring and sleep apnoea. *Scott Browns Otolaryngology*, 6th edn. 1997; pp. 1–22.

Related topics of interest

Adenoids, p. 8; Tonsillectomy, p. 333; Tracheostomy, p. 336.

SPEECH AUDIOMETRY

In many animals the sense of hearing is adapted for a specific purpose. In the human, the ear is specifically tuned to the speech frequencies (500–4000 Hz). The main function of the human ear is therefore the perception of speech. Indeed, most of the handicap of hearing loss is due to loss of the ability to perceive the spoken word. Speech audiometry provides a measure of this ability and any corresponding deficit. Voice tests can be considered as a very basic form of speech audiometry. However, in general, speech audiometry implies the formal qualitative assessment of a subject's perception of speech. It measures the actual disability produced by the hearing impairment. It is useful in a variety of contexts including:

- Assessment and diagnosis of peripheral and central hearing disorders.
- Prediction of the usefulness of a hearing aid.
- Evaluation of the benefit which might be obtained by an operation (pre- and postoperative assessment).
- Medicolegal assessment.

Materials

1. **Instruments.** Testing is performed in a soundproof room using a cassette player or microphone with the volume controlled from the audiometer which presents speech material to the subject via loudspeakers or headphones. Speech material presented by the tester using a microphone is prone to variation in both intensity and accent. Standardized, prepared speech material presented by cassette and controlled by the audiometer is much more preferable. The use of headphones, as opposed to the free-field situation with loudspeakers, allows each ear to be tested individually and allows the non-test ear to be masked.

2. **Speech material.** Phonemes are the building blocks of speech and represent the smallest unit of recognizable speech sound (e.g. ay, aw, ah, etc.). There are 49 phonemes in the English language. Speech material is chosen to provide a representative balance of phonemes and can be presented as words, sentences or synthetic sentences which have no meaning. A great number of lists of appropriate speech material have been developed by various agencies e.g. Medical Research Council, Institute of Hearing Research, Fry, Boothroyd and Manchester junior word lists, and Bench, Koval and Bamford (BKB) sentences (University of Manchester).

Procedure

The subject is seated in a soundproof room and instructed in the test procedure. The recorded word lists are presented to the patient monaurally over headphones at various sound intensities. As speech audiometry is a suprathreshold test, masking of the non-test ear is required on all occasions. Masking sounds in speech audiometry are chosen to try and recreate an appropriate noise background such as speech, cocktail party and babble noise. Pink noise (equal energy for each octave over the hearing range) is often used when these are unavailable. The first presentation is usually at 20–30 dB greater than the pure-tone average for the frequencies 500, 1000 and 2000 Hz.

Subsequent presentations are usually made at +10, +20, –10 and –20 dB from this level, although more may be required. The patient is asked to repeat the words as accurately as possible and the percentage of words or phonemes which are correctly repeated at each sound intensity (dB) is calculated and plotted on a graph.

The graphical display is compared with the calibration graph for that particular machine, which will have been obtained by testing otologically normal individuals on that machine, using the same tapes and test environment. The recorded data can then be used to formulate certain scores and the shape of the graph used to give information regarding the type of deafness.

Scoring

(a) The optimum discrimination score (ODS) is the subject's maximum score, no matter how loud the volume is turned up. It is a measure of optimal performance and should be 100% when normal.

(b) The speech reception threshold (SRT) is the sound intensity (dB) at which the subject can correctly repeat 50% of the presented words.

(c) The half-peak level (HPL) refers to the sound level (dB) at which the discrimination percentage is half the ODS.

(d) The half-peak level elevation (HPLE) refers to the difference between the pathological and normal HPL. This is the dB level at which the patient achieves half the ODS in comparison with the level at which normal individuals achieve 50%. This is considered to be the most valuable diagnostic score.

Shape of the graph

If the hearing is normal all the words will be understood if they are played loudly enough. The result is a sigmoid-shaped curve with a steep, near-vertical portion in the middle. In patients with a conductive hearing loss all the words will be understood, but they must be played louder than for a normal subject. The curve is parallel to the normal but is shifted to the right (i.e. greater HPL) in proportion to the degree of hearing loss. The ODS is still 100% as discrimination is preserved.

In patients with a sensorineural hearing loss there is usually a loss of ability to discriminate speech, and consequently the ODS is often less than 100%. The gradient of the middle portion of the curve is often less and a plateau may be reached in which further increases in sound intensity do not improve discrimination. In severe cases 'roll over' may occur: beyond a certain point any further increase in sound intensity causes a reduction in the discrimination score. This type of curve is typical of a retrocochlear lesion.

Specific uses

1. **Non-organic hearing loss.** Speech audiometry can be used in the investigation of non-organic or feigned hearing loss. Two tests exist:

(a) *Delayed speech feedback* (DSF). The subject is asked to read text aloud. The speech is relayed to the test ear with a delay of 1–200 ms. If there is normal hearing in the test ear, stammering and a raised voice are almost inevitable.

(b) *Competition tests.* The patient is asked to repeat speech material delivered to the good ear while competing speech material is introduced to the test ear. If the hearing is normal, stuttering is likely when the competing material is 40 dB louder than the test material.

2. *Central function.* Speech audiometry can also be used as a test of central auditory function. This can be done using a variety of techniques, including speech messages in competing noise, competing messages and overlapping messages in each ear, accelerated, interrupted and filtered speech. For further details on this, the reader is referred to Keith and Pensak (1991).

Further reading

Ballantyne D. *Handbook of Audiological Techniques.* London: Butterworth-Heinemann, 1990.
Keith RW, Pensak ML. Central auditory function. *Otolaryngologic Clinics of North America*, 1991; **24**(2): 371–379.

Related topics of interest

Acoustic neuroma, p. 1; Non-organic hearing loss, p. 194; Clinical assessment of hearing, p. 45; Pure tone audiogram, p. 254.

SPEECH THERAPY IN HEAD AND NECK SURGERY

P. Young

The speech therapist is a member of the multidisciplinary rehabilitation team. The main aims of rehabilitation are to ensure that patients have optimal communication skills, oro-mandibular function and are able to swallow. The role of the speech therapist working with patients undergoing head and neck surgery is essentially threefold:

1. the rehabilitation of voice, following laryngectomy;
2. developing compensatory articulation strategies with patients who have had oral surgery;
3. assessment and therapy for patients who have dysphagia following head and neck surgery.

Voice rehabilitation following laryngectomy

Ideally laryngectomy patients (and their relatives) should be seen by the speech therapist for assessment, education and support pre-operatively. An oral examination and communication profile are carried out. Factors such as speech rate, volume, articulation, posture, tension levels, hearing, motivation and communication needs can have a significant bearing on the prognosis for rehabilitation of communication.

There are three options for alternative voice:

- electrolarynx;
- oesophageal voice;
- surgical voice restoration (SVR) with a voice prosthesis.

Electrolarynx

The electrolarynx is useful as a temporary measure before oesophageal voice is functionally adequate or before placement of a voice prosthesis. It can be a long-term option when the pharyngo-oesophageal (PE) segment is not viable, in cases of radical surgery where prosthesis placement is contraindicated, e.g. stomach pull-up, or when it is the patient's preference.

Efficient use of the electrolarynx is mainly dependent on neck status. Hard fibrotic post radiotherapy/surgery neck tissue will prevent transmission of sound into the oral cavity. Training is needed to develop accurate placement of the device, reduce speech rate, improve articulatory precision and to establish appropriate phrasing.

Oesophageal voice

Both oesophageal voice and SVR require a viable PE segment or neoglottis. The segment is composed of the inferior constrictor including cricopharyngeus and the upper oesophagus. There must be adequate apposition of the oesophageal mucosa to form a functional PE segment. The tonicity of the segment determines the quality of the voice achieved and the effort necessary to produce it.

The oesophageal speaker has to gain voluntary control of the PE segment in order to take air into the upper oesophagus. The air is then released, producing sound as it passes through the PE segment. It is then amplified by the resonating spaces and modified by the articulators in the normal way. There can be difficulties at any stage in this process. The patient has to learn to dissociate respiration from phonation. The acquisition of a functional oesophageal voice can take months of intensive speech therapy.

Surgical voice restoration

Oesophageal voice lacks the duration, fluency, consistency and volume which can be achieved with a voice prosthesis using pulmonary air. In SVR, when the stoma is occluded, expired pulmonary air passes through the one-way silicone valve in the tracheo-oesophageal wall, setting the PE segment into vibration. Voice prostheses are of two main types: the non indwelling type, e.g. Blom-Singer and Bivona, and much more commonly the in-dwelling type, e.g. Provox and Blom-Singer Groningen button. Indwelling valves, e.g. Provox II, can now be changed by a speech therapist/specialist nurse via the stoma, and certain adept patients can be trained to change their own valves.

Many centres now favour primary placement of the prosthesis during laryngectomy so that patients can leave the hospital with a voice. This means that much of the frustration, depression and strain on relationships caused by a lengthy period of postoperative aphonia can now be avoided.

When secondary placement is planned, the speech therapist or ENT surgeon carries out an air insufflation test (Taub and Bugner, 1973). A catheter is inserted via the nose to the level of the stoma and is connected to a housing, which is glued to the stoma, such that when the stoma is occluded pulmonary air is transmitted through the catheter to below the PE segment. The patient is asked to speak. The amount of air pressure needed to produce a voice and the fluency and durability of the voice achieved are noted. This test can also be carried out before commencing oesophageal voice training as it provides information about the tonicity of the PE segment.

After valve placement speech therapy involves: training in maintaining the valve, achieving accurate occlusion of the stoma, breath/voice co-ordination, and modifying the speech rate and phrasing to maximise intelligibility. Evaluation of the voice is carried out at regular intervals, including objective measurement of:

- duration, i.e. the number of syllables produced per breath on air charge;
- maximum phonation time: how long the patient can sustain a vowel on one breath;
- dynamic range (volume);
- availability of the voice, i.e. ease of initiation;
- pitch (where instrumentation is available).

Intelligibility and communication skills can be rated subjectively by naive listeners or by the speech therapist, who also rates tension levels, fluency, articulation, rate, voice quality, etc. Ultimately the success of voice rehabilitation is a measure of patients' satisfaction with their communication, i.e. to what extent are they able to use their voice with confidence in all situations.

There is no doubt that the best possible voice results are obtained with a voice prosthesis, but these are not without complications and the patient remains dependent on the hospital for maintenance of the voice. The available alternatives are not mutually exclusive, but individual ENT departments have to decide which is to be their method of choice and ensure that the other alternatives are available to patients if the first option is either contraindicated or unsuccessful.

Compensatory articulatory strategies following oral surgery

All patients should be seen pre-operatively so that the therapist can obtain a sample (preferably taped) of the patient's speech. Post-operatively, once healing is complete, patients are assessed using phonetically balanced word lists to establish an objective measure of their intelligibility across all the phonemes of English. The speech therapist then works on improving excursion and control of available articulators and systematic exploration of potential compensatory articulations which will improve the patient's ability to make phonemic contrasts and hence improve intelligibility, e.g. the use of a uvula sound as a substitute for /k,g/ phonemes in a glossectomy patient. These compensations are then practised for integration into spontaneous speech.

Surgical dysphagia

The speech therapist should see any patient pre-operatively when post-operative dysphagia is anticipated.

When healing is complete a bedside assessment of the swallow is carried out to identify the risk of aspiration. This includes:

- evaluation of the range, strength, speed and accuracy of movement of lips, tongue and palate;
- assessment of sensation in tongue, lips and palate;
- sample swallows observing oral manipulation, oral transit time, swallow initiation/delay, laryngeal elevation, clinical signs of penetration (substance entry into the airway above the vocal cords) and aspiration (before, during and after the swallow);
- the effect of modified textures, postures and manoeuvres on the efficiency and safety of the swallow.

Fees (fibreoptic endoscopic evaluation of swallowing) is useful to assess the anatomy, symmetry and clearance of the pharynx at rest and post swallow.

Access to videofluoroscopy or modified barium swallow is essential with this patient group. It permits full evaluation of oropharyngeal anatomy and impaired swallow physiology. It confirms whether aspiration is occurring, when, why and how much. The speech therapist can observe the impact of compensation techniques and therapeutic manoeuvres and make recommendations accordingly.

When alternative feeding methods are necessary to maintain nutrition, e.g. gastrostomy, the speech therapist continues to rehabilitate the swallow with the gradual re-introduction of oral intake when safe.

Follow-up and aftercare

Follow-up as an out-patient or on a domiciliary basis should be available for as long as is necessary for this patient group. Most speech therapy departments organise a club for their head and neck patients aimed at providing information, support and social activities on a long-term basis. Members of the club also carry out pre and post-operative visits to new patients.

Eating and talking are not only essential but pleasurable activities, and it is important not to underestimate the trauma suffered by patients who have problems with either of these functions. The aim of speech therapy is to achieve maximum rehabilitation and, where preoperative functional levels are not achievable, to assist patients to compensate and adjust to their new set of circumstances.

Further reading

Groher ME. Laryngectomy. In: Edels Y (ed). *Dysphagia – Diagnosis and Management*. London: Butterworths, 1984.

Logeman J. *The Evaluation and Treatment of Swallowing Disorders*. San Diego: College Hill Press, 1983.

Taub S, Bugner LH. Air bypass voice prosthesis for vocal rehabilitation of laryngectomees. *American Journal of Surgery*, 1973; **125:** 748–756.

Langmore SE, Schartz K, Olsen N. Fibreoptic endoscopic examination of swallowing safety. A new procedure. *Dysphagia*, 1988; **2:** 216–219.

Logeman J. *Manual for the Videofluoroscopic Study of Swallowing*. Austin TX: Pro-Ed, 1993.

Related topics of interest

Hypopharyngeal carcinoma, p. 124; Laryngeal carcinoma, p. 138; Laryngectomy, p. 143; Oral cavity carcinoma, p. 197; Oropharyngeal carcinoma, p. 203.

SPEECH THERAPY IN NON-MALIGNANT VOICE DISORDERS

P. Young

In recent years, significant progress has been made towards the understanding of the function and dysfunction of the human voice and applying this new knowledge and technology in the clinical evaluation and treatment of voice pathology.

Previously, ENT consultants would diagnose organic problems descriptively (e.g. vocal nodules) and other presentations where no structural changes could be observed would be classified as 'functional dysphonia'.

The latter group of voice disorders are characterised by habitual misuse of the voluntary muscles of the larynx and pharynx and have been classified by Morrison and Rammage (1994) as muscle tension dysphonias. They describe six typical glottic and supraglottic postures, visible on laryngoscopy which can be attributed to a particular pattern of underlying muscle misuse. If these patients are treated early, typical symptoms (e.g. pitch breaks, mild dysphonia and discomfort with prolonged talking) can be treated successfully. Untreated, these problems can progress to organic changes (e.g. nodules, chronic laryngitis, oedema, etc).

Referral to speech and language therapy

All patients with a voice disorder, with the exception of transexuals must be referred by an ENT surgeon. In the light of the above it is important that referral should include not only a description of the structure of the larynx and any organic changes, but also the glottic shape observed on phonation. Together with any relevant ENT findings and previous medical history, the patients occupation is important to note as most speech therapy departments will prioritise professional voice users for therapy.

Conditions that respond well to voice therapy

- Muscle tension dysphonias (e.g. posterior glottic chink, vocal cord bowing).
- False cord phonation (dysphonia plicae ventricularis).
- Psychogenic aphonia.
- Early/soft vocal nodules.
- Chronic laryngitis.
- Puberphonia.
- Reinke's oedema (mild).
- Globus sensation.

Conditions which do not respond well to voice therapy

- Occult cysts.
- Sulcus vocalis.
- Laryngeal papillomata.
- Reinke's oedema (severe).
- Hard, fibrous nodules.

Assessment

Joint ENT/speech and language therapy voice clinics are ideal for professional voice users. More time is allocated to each appointment, and using nasendoscopy, or rigid laryngoscopy with stroboscopy a detailed diagnosis can be made. Patients can view their larynx on a TV monitor, have a clear understanding of the diagnosis and try some therapy techniques on camera with clear visual feedback. This facility helps reduce anxiety, increases compliance and motivation in therapy.

Speech and language therapy assessment commences with an in-depth case history which highlights factors for therapy planning, e.g. the onset and course of the dysphonia, the patient's general health, any previous voice disorders and treatment, a profile of how the voice is used, and any predisposing factors, e.g. working conditions, relationship problems, traumatic life events.

Some specialist clinics now have access to instrumentation such as PCLX laryngograph, which allow the dysphonia to be repeatedly analysed in terms of physical and acoustic parameters. Traditional assessment is supplemented with objective analysis of pitch, i.e. the mode frequency, the frequency range used and a percentage irregularity measure (a measure of the periodicity of vibration, which correlates with perceived hoarseness). The laryngograph waveform gives quantitative and qualitative information about the closed phase of the vocal cord vibratory cycle.

These objective measures can be used:

- to provide a baseline before treatment (voice therapy or surgery) and to allow objective evaluation of improvement after treatment;
- as a therapy tool to provide instant visual feedback to the patient;
- for collection of data for comparative studies and for research and audit purposes.

Where sophisticated assessment facilities are not available, the therapist's assessment includes subjective evaluation of:

- breathing pattern;
- phonation: habitual pitch and range, quality, glottal attack, dynamic range (volume);
- resonance;
- articulation;
- palpatory assessment of laryngeal and pharyngeal tension;
- habitual misuse patterns;
- questionnaire for patient's own evaluation of problem.

Objectives for therapy together with an estimated number of sessions required are then set and agreed with the patient.

Therapy

The improved understanding of how phonation is affected by muscle tension imbalance has enabled the development of techniques to elicit specific muscle set responses. However therapy is tightly constrained in that techniques must be easy to teach and easy to learn and beneficial effects must be obvious in order to reinforce learning and maintain motivation (Casper, 1995).

The aim is to change behavioural patterns – to disrupt unhealthy motor engrams for voice and speech and establish and habituate healthy patterns. This is not a simple process as there is limited kinaesthetic and proprioceptive feedback from most of the larynx and vocal tract, and the patient has to bring previously automatic activity under conscious control in order to change it.

Although there are fundamental principles of therapy for a given disorder, therapy has to be tailored to the individual, taking into account the patient's age, sex, intelligence, culture occupation, general health, attitude to problem and communication requirements. Therapy may include the following approaches:

- manipulation of the affected musculature;
- deep relaxation techniques;
- use of facilitation techniques e.g. humming, yawn-sigh, nasalizing;
- programmes of therapy in which specific aspects of voice are worked on separately, e.g. pitch, resonance, or holistic programmes may be employed, e.g. the Accent method, in which separate features are not directly remedied but improve once a physiologically sound pattern of phonation is achieved;
- a psychotherapeutic approach aimed at releasing anxiety, fears, etc; which create tension leading to phonation problems.

Postoperative voice therapy is advisable in most conditions, even if it is not suspected that vocal misuse and abuse was the cause of the problem. Organic changes to the vocal cords often lead to maladaptive patterns of voice use which may persist postoperatively and lead to further problems.

Voice therapy with singers involves both speaking and singing voice and generally a programme of therapy helps to achieve an easy natural voice without strain. When the healthiest possible voice has been achieved the therapist may refer to a singing teacher, whose role is to develop technique and advise on singing style.

Occasionally group therapy may be appropriate, where patients with similar disorders and a background share common treatment needs.

Accurate diagnosis and management of voice problems takes account of laryngological, acoustic, perceptual, and palpatory case history findings. Voice therapy aims to release the natural voice and/or develop and refine control of specific aspects of voice production to achieve maximum vocal efficiency.

Further reading

Ramig LO, Verdolini K. Treatment efficacy: voice disorders. *Journal of Speech, Language & Hearing Research*, 1998; **41**: 101–116.

Carding PN, Horsley IA, Docherty GJ. A study of the effectiveness of voice therapy in the treatment of 45 patients with nonorganic dysphonia. *Journal of Voice*, 1999; **13**: 72–104.

Hillman RE. The efficacy of speech and language pathology intervention: voice disorders. *Seminars in Speech Language*, 1990; **11**: 297–309.

STRIDOR AND STERTOR

Definitions

- *Stertor* is noisy breathing caused by partial obstruction of the respiratory tract above the larynx.
- *Stridor* is noisy breathing caused by partial obstruction of the respiratory tract at or below the larynx.

Stertor

Aetiology

1. Congenital (present at birth).

- Nose — Choanal stenosis or atresia.
  External nasal deformity secondary to craniofacial abnormality.
  Dermoid, nasoalveolar, dentigerous and mucous cysts.
  Meningocele, encephalocele, meningoencephalocele.
- Nasopharynx — Craniofacial abnormality, especially Apert's syndrome and Crouzon's disease.
- Oropharynx — Micrognathia secondary to a craniofacial abnormality, especially Treacher Collins syndrome.
  Macroglossia, most frequently in those with Down's syndrome.
  Lingual thyroid and thyroglossal cyst.

2. Acquired.

- Trauma — Septal haematoma and secondary abscess.
  Nasal, septal and midfacial fracture.
- Inflammatory — Infective acute and chronic rhinitis.
  Acute and chronic adenoiditis.
  Acute tonsillitis, especially secondary to infectious mono-nucleosis.
  Parapharyngeal and retropharyngeal abscess.
  Ludwig's angina.
  Acute epiglottitis.
  Wegener's granulomatosis.
- Foreign body
- Allergy — Allergic rhinitis.
  Angioneurotic oedema of the floor of mouth.
- Neoplasia — Benign, e.g. simple nasal polyps, antrochoanal polyp, angiofibroma.
  Malignant, e.g. oropharyngeal and nasopharyngeal squamous cell carcinoma, nasal T-cell lymphoma.

Clinical features

Stertor is usually inspiratory but the accompanying features are diverse and depend on the cause. A full history should ascertain time of onset, symptom progression, aggravating and relieving factors, whether there is sleep apnoea, an intercurrent URTI or if trauma has occurred. Examination of the nose, throat (contraindicated in acute epiglottitis) and neck, pulse, temperature, respiratory rate and blood pressure may all be necessary.

Investigations

A lateral soft tissue neck radiograph or an MRI scan may be indicated to show the site of airway obstruction. In a child it is important to extend the neck to prevent the retropharyngeal soft tissue causing a pseudo-mass.

Treatment

Treatment depends on the cause, progression and severity of the stertor and on whether it is causing complications (see Related topics).

Complications

These are directly related to the airway obstruction and include right ventricular failure and pulmonary hypertension (sleep apnoea), central respiratory arrest (in the first 3 months of life neonates are obligatory nasal breathers), and acute total airway obstruction.

Stridor

Aetiology

1. **Congenital.**
- *Larynx*:

  Supraglottis Laryngomalacia, web, saccular cyst, cystic hygroma.
  Glottis Web, vocal cord paralysis.
  Subglottis Web, stenosis, haemangioma.
- *Trachea and bronchi*: Web, stenosis, tracheomalacia, tracheo and bronchogenic cyst, compression from vascular and other mediastinal tumours.

2. **Acquired.**
- Trauma Thermal and chemical, iatrogenic (intubation and surgical), blunt and sharp external.
- Inflammatory Acute laryngitis, acute laryngotracheobronchitis, diphtheria.
- Foreign body Laryngeal, tracheal, bronchial and external compression from an oesophageal foreign body.
- Allergy Angioneurotic oedema of the larynx or trachea.
  Extrinsic allergic alveolitis.
- Neoplasia Benign, e.g. laryngeal papillomatosis.
  Malignant, e.g. laryngeal or bronchial squamous cell carcinoma.

Clinical features

Typically, supraglottic stridor is inspiratory, the negative inspiratory intralaryngeal pressure indrawing the supraglottic soft tissues, passive opening occurring on expiration. Tracheal and main bronchial airway obstruction causes stridor because of turbulence of air flowing through a narrow but rigid airway that doesn't collapse. It may be inspiratory, expiratory or biphasic. In the smaller bronchi and bronchioles obstruction accentuates the physiological constriction occurring in expiration to cause an expiratory wheeze. A full history combined with examination of the nose, throat and neck is indicated if circumstances permit. This will usually allow a confident or a working diagnosis to be made. Immediate treatment or appropriate investigations can thus be instituted.

Investigations

A lateral soft tissue neck and chest radiograph, or a CT scan of the larynx and lungs may be appropriate. For certain conditions, including foreign body aspiration and innominate artery compression chest radiographs are very good at suggesting the correct diagnosis (86% in one study). It must be emphasized that in children with a bronchial foreign body, radiographs may be normal. Therefore if the history suggests there may be an aspirated foreign body then bronchoscopy is indicated even with a normal chest radiograph. A representative biopsy of a laryngeal or infralaryngeal mass may be indicated. Rigid endoscopy is still the gold standard of investigation as it allows the most complete examination of the aerodigestive tract. In one study of stridulous neonates, 87% had more than one abnormality including 33% with gastro-oesophageal reflux (see Related topics).

Treatment

This depends on the diagnosis and the severity of symptoms (see Related topics).

Further reading

Zerella JT, Dimler, McGill LC, Pippus KJ. Foreign body aspiration in children: value of radiography and complications of bronchoscopy. *Journal of Pediatric Surgery*, 1998; **33**(11): 1651–1654.
Walner DL, Donnelly LF, Quanounou S, Cotton RT. Utility of radiographs in the evaluation of pediatric upper airway obstruction. *Annals of Otolaryngology*, 1999; **108**: 378–383.

Related topics of interest

Paediatric airway problems, p. 232; Laryngeal carcinoma, p. 138; Laryngectomy, p. 143; Oropharyngeal carcinoma, p. 203; Nasopharyngeal neoplasm, p. 180; Adenoids, p. 8; Nasal malignancy, p. 174; Nasal granulomas, p. 170; Foreign bodies, p. 103.

SUDDEN HEARING LOSS

Sudden hearing loss is a significant subjective decline in the hearing acuity occurring either instantaneously or progressively over minutes or hours. Usually only one ear is affected and the aetiology often never identified. It can be classified into conductive and sensorineural causes.

Conductive causes

- External ear canal occlusion e.g. from wax or a foreign body.
- Infection e.g. otitis externa, acute otitis media or chronic otitis media.
- Ear trauma, from a direct blow, acoustic or barotrauma (see Related topics of interest).
- Iatrogenic.

Sensorineural

- Idiopathic.
- Iatrogenic.
- Serous and purulent labyrinthitis.
- Viral e.g. measles and mumps virus.
- Cerebellopontine angle tumours e.g. acoustic neuromas, cholesterol granulomas, congenital dermoids and meningiomas.
- Temporal bone fractures, in particular transverse fractures.
- Causes of perilymph fistula including round window rupture e.g from blast trauma or barotrauma.
- Menière's *disease* (primary endolymphatic hydrops) and secondary endolymphatic hydrops (which may cause Menière's *syndrome*).
- Ototoxic drugs, in particular aminoglycoside antibiotics, non-steroidal anti-inflammatory, beta-blocker, loop diuretic and chemotherapetic drugs.
- Central causes e.g. following a brain stem cerebrovascular accident.
- Autoimmune inner ear disease.

Clinical features

In subjects with an identifiable cause of a sudden hearing loss the diagnosis is usually made from a thorough otological and neurological history, examination and relevant special investigations. Nearly all those with a sudden conductive hearing loss will have a definitive diagnosis made but 60% of the sensorineural group will eventually be labelled as idiopathic of which 60% will recover spontaneously.

Management

All patients with a sudden bilateral sensorineural hearing loss should be admitted to hospital for several reasons:

(a) Close monitoring of the hearing by pure tone and speech audiometry is possible and desirable in order to determine whether the hearing is stable, improving or declining. This will provide a hearing prognosis and enable the patient's disability and handicap to be assessed.

(b) To allow rapid performance of relevant special investigations which may include electric response audiometry, MRI imaging, viral titres (two sets, six weeks apart) and syphilis serology in an effort to make a diagnosis.

(c) To provide rehabilitation in the form of (i) counselling from a hearing therapist, (ii) hearing aid and accessory aid provision (for example amplification of the TV, telephone bell, telephone receiver and door bell).

Treatment of the idiopathic group with vasodilators (e.g. betahistine), anticoagulants (e.g. heparin), blood viscosity lowering substances (e.g. dextran 40); steroids, antioxidants combined with steroids, and antibiotics is empirical. It is generally agreed by those who advocate such treatment that it should commence as early as possible after the onset of the hearing loss and certainly within the first few days of symptoms. Most treatments report a response rate of 60%, about the same as those who spontaneously recover with no treatment.

Those with a sudden unilateral hearing loss will have less of a disability and handicap, and do not require such urgent rehabilitation. As a general rule they do not require admission into hospital unless the aetiology (e.g. trauma, purulent labyrinthitis) dictates and they can be investigated as an out-patient.

Further reading

Byl F.M. Sudden hearing loss: eight years experience and suggested prognostic table. *The Laryngoscope*, 1984; **94**: 647–661.

Fisch U. Management of sudden deafness. *Otolaryngology and Head and Neck Surgery*, 1983; **91**: 3–8.

Kumar A, Maudelonde C, Maffee M. Unilateral sensorineural hearing loss: an analysis of 200 consecutive cases. *The Laryngoscope*, 1986; **96**: 14–18.

Fitzgerald DC & Marks AS. MRI in sudden sensorineural hearing loss. *Otolaryngology Head and Neck Surgery*, 1998; **118**: 737–738.

Related topics of interest

Otological aspects of head injury, p. 218; Labyrinthitis, p. 134; Acoustic neuroma, p. 1; Perilymph fistula, p. 244; Menière's Disease, p. 167; Ototoxicity, p. 228; Acute otitis media, p. 5; Chronic otitis media, p. 38.

THYROID DISEASE – BENIGN

J.C. Watkinson

Benign thyroid disease can be analysed from three different aspects which are often inter-related. These are thyroid goitre, hypothyroidism and hyperthyroidism. Patients with thyroid goitre are the most important from a surgical standpoint as it is this group that is often referred to ENT surgeons by general practitioners for primary management. In the United Kingdom, it is estimated that up to 15% of the population have a goitre. Within this group, approximately 8% have nodular thyroid disease of which 50% are solitary. Although thyroid nodules are common it is important to remember that thyroid cancer is extremely uncommon, with an incidence in the UK of between 1–2 per 100 000. The commonest way for cancer to present is as a solitary thyroid nodule. It is important to have as much information as possible on any patient prior to surgery. These cases are probably best dealt with by a multidisciplinary team including a head and neck surgeon, clinical oncologist and endocrinologist.

Classification of goitre

- *Simple (non toxic)* Diffuse, nodular, multinodular, and recurrent nodular.
- *Toxic* Diffuse, nodular, multinodular, and recurrent nodular.
- *Inflammatory* Hashimoto's, De Quervain's, Reidel's thyroiditis.
- *Neoplastic* Benign and malignant.
- *Rare goitres* TB, amyloid, syphilis, HIV and lithium.

1. Simple (non-toxic) goitre. These may be both physiological and pathological. Physiological goitres include puberty, pregnancy and with the contraceptive pill. The causes of pathological goitres include iodine deficiency. Nodular goitre may be solitary or multinodular. The differential diagnosis of the solitary thyroid nodule (apart from a colloid nodule) includes a follicular adenoma, thyroid cyst or carcinoma. Multinodular goitre can be associated with iodine deficiency which is endemic in patients living at high altitude such as the Alps or Himalayas. The majority of patients with multinodular goitre are euthyroid. An ultrasound scan will help confirm the diagnosis. This will also assist in delineation of the most prominent nodule, on which fine needle aspiration cytology can be performed. The benign nature of the disease may be confirmed in this way.

Patients with hypothyroidism may or may not have a simple goitre. Hypothyroidism may be congenital or acquired. The former is usually due to congenital absence or atrophy of the thyroid and untreated leads to cretinism. Rarely it is associated with inherited dyshormonogenesis such as Pendred's syndrome (which is the association of congenital hypothyroidism with high tone deafness). Acquired hypothyroidism is usually idiopathic or due to surgical ablation of the gland, post-treatment of thyrotoxicosis with radio-iodine, or Hashimoto's thyroiditis. Treatment is with thyroid hormone replacement. The starting dose is usually T4 100 µg/day. In the presence of subclinical hypothyroidism (high TSH > 10 mU/l, normal free T4), then treat with T4 (100 µg/day) if antibodies are positive, if there are convincing symptoms or a past history of radio-iodine treatment.

2. *Toxic goitre (hyperthyroidism).* Patients with thyrotoxicosis usually either have Graves disease or a solitary toxic nodule. Graves disease is caused by circulating thyroid stimulating immunoglobulins (IgG) which bind to thyroid stimulating hormone receptors (TSH receptor) to increase thyroid hormone production. These immunoglobulins are usually associated with thyroid eye disease which is caused by a specific antibody called exophthalmos producing substance (EPS) which targets retro-orbital tissue to cause oedema of fat and muscle. Graves disease may also be associated with signs of vitiligo, pretibial myxoedema and other autoimmune disorders such as pernicious anaemia.

Hyperthyroidism is usually treated either medically using tablets (carbimazole or Propylthiouracil) or with radioiodine. About 50% of patients will relapse following medical treatment. In these patients, together with those who have significant eye signs or who request surgery, an operation with a 'near total' or 'total' thyroidectomy is an alternative option. Radioiodine can also be used to treat large multinodular goitres in the elderly and infirm, when good shrinkage is achievable. Patients who have solitary toxic nodules are usually best dealt with surgically.

Some patients who have had a multinodular goitre for a long time can develop thyrotoxicosis (Plummer's disease). These patients are often elderly with co-existent morbidity such as ischaemic heart disease, and the rise in T4 is often associated with atrial fibrillation. Because of this, these patients usually have cardiac signs (and not eye signs) and are usually treated medically. Recurrent thyrotoxicosis is treated on its merits, but may require further treatment with either the same or another modality. Many patients (whatever their treatment) will be hypothyroid post-treatment and will be on long-term thyroxine replacement therapy.

3. *Inflammatory goitre.*
(a) Hashimoto's thyroiditis. This is most common in late middle-aged women. Antibodies are directed against thyroglobulin and/or microsomal peroxidase. They cause lymphocyte infiltration, atrophy and regeneration of the thyroid, and ultimately a goitre. The gland is usually firm, but rubbery. Initially patients are hyperthyroid, but may become hypothyroid as the disease progresses. Once the diagnosis is made, patients should be treated with thyroxine suppression and have thyroid function tests once a year. Rarely surgery may be required for an enlarged gland causing obstructive symptoms or when there is a fine needle aspiration cytology result that necessitates surgery. These patients are at a high risk of subsequently developing a thyroid lymphoma.
(b) De Quervain's thyroiditis is secondary to an acute viral infection. This is a flu-like illness, and associated with diffuse swelling and tenderness of the gland. There is usually both a transient hyperthyroidism and production of auto-antibodies.
(c) Riedel's thyroiditis is rare and associated with a woody hard, sometimes tender, irregular thyroid gland which histologically shows marked fibrosis. This is thought by some to signify a fibrotic reaction to an underlying carcinoma or lymphoma.

4. Neoplastic goitre.

This can be a benign adenoma or malignant tumour (see Related topic of interest).

5. Miscellaneous goitres.

For example sarcoidosis, tuberculosis, amyloid, HIV infection.

Clinical assessment

Depending on the cause and duration of the goitre, patients may be euthyroid, hyperthyroid or hypothyroid. A drug history is important because some are goitrogens, e.g. sulphonylureas. The goitre may produce discomfort on swallowing, dysphagia (implying oesophageal compression), or stridor (implying tracheal compression). It is important to confirm that the swelling moves with swallowing and to note its size, position and any retrosternal involvement. The latter is suspected from dullness to percussion over the manubrium. Examine the rest of the neck for nodes and perform indirect or fibreoptic laryngoscopy to check the mobility of the vocal cords.

Investigations

All patients with a goitre should have their thyroid function and thyroid antibody status checked. In addition, all euthyroid patients should have fine needle aspiration cytology performed and a vocal cord check is advised in those with any voice change, difficulty in swallowing and breathing and in those patients undergoing surgery. A chest X-ray may show tracheal deviation, mediastinal extension or lymphadenopathy, pulmonary metastasis or associated co-morbidity but the best way to assess upper airway obstruction is with a flow loop. Depending on the history, a serum calcium and calcitonin may be appropriate.

Ultrasound may be helpful in measuring tumour size, diagnosing multinodular goitres and excluding contralateral disease. It may also be used to evaluate complex cysts and can distinguish and identify purely cystic nodules. Only rarely is a cyst associated with a thyroid cancer. However, ultrasound cannot reliably distinguish between benign and malignant disease.

Radionuclide scintigraphy using I^{123} can be used to identify whether a nodule is 'hot' (takes up isotope) and therefore is functioning, or is 'cold' (and therefore not functioning). More than 90% of lesions identified with scintigraphy will not concentrate the radionuclide and therefore will appear 'cold'. These clinically solitary nonfunctional nodules may be an adenoma, carcinoma, a cyst or a dominant nodule in a non-palpable multinodular goitre and the likelihood of malignancy in a truly solitary 'cold' nodule is between 10% and 20%. If a cyst has been excluded on ultrasound, the likelihood of a solid cold nodule being malignant rises to about 50%. Truly functioning nodules (hot) are highly unlikely to be malignant.

Fine needle aspiration cytology is safe, cheap and reliable with a diagnostic accuracy of approximately 90% and is therefore the initial investigation of choice for a solitary thyroid nodule. The diagnostic strategy for evaluating the thyroid nodule is shown below.

A diagnostic strategy to evaluate the 'solitary' or 'dominant' thyroid nodule in a euthyroid patient

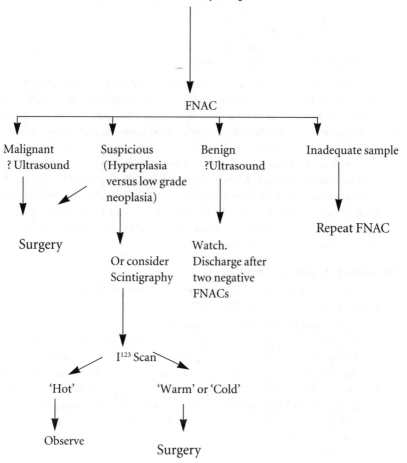

Anatomical imaging with CT or MRI is useful to assess both thyroid lobes, the neck for nodes, the visceral compartment of the neck, the mediastinum, the chest, the abdomen, and whole body staging for lymphoma.

Treatment

The indications for surgery are:

- Suspected malignancy.
- Cosmetic reasons.
- Tracheal or oesophageal compression.
- Thyrotoxicosis.

Types of surgery

The following operations can be performed on the thyroid gland:

- Lumpectomy.
- Hemithyroidectomy (total lobectomy).
- Subtotal thyroidectomy.
- Near-total or total thyroidectomy.

A lumpectomy is removal of the nodule alone with minimal surrounding thyroid tissue, while a total lobectomy completely removes one thyroid lobe with the isthmus. A subtotal thyroidectomy is bilateral removal of more than one half of the thyroid gland on each side plus the isthmus and is rarely performed nowadays. A 'near total' thyroidectomy is a total lobectomy and the isthmusectomy with removal of more than 90% of the contralateral lobe and is often done to preserve blood supply to parathyroids on one side. A 'total' thyroidectomy is removal of both thyroid lobes and the isthmus with preservation of the parathyroids and a completion thyroidectomy is a subsequent procedure to convert a lesser operation into a near total or total thyroidectomy. In general, the minimum operation that should be done on the thyroid gland is a total lobectomy.

Complications of thyroidectomy

As well as the hazards of any surgical operation there are specific potential local and general complications of thyroidectomy.

1. *Injury to related anatomical structures.*
   (a) Recurrent laryngeal nerve damage. The incidence of damage to the recurrent laryngeal nerve is approximately 2%. It is related to the experience of the surgeon and increased for operations involving malignancy and for revision surgery.
   (b) Damage to the external branch of the superior laryngeal nerve. The incidence is unknown but is increased in surgery for cancer, surgery for large goitres and can be reduced when operations are performed by an experienced surgeon and by use of a nerve stimulator.
   (c) Damage to the trachea.
   (d) Pneumothorax.

2. *Hormonal.*
   (a) Tetany (hypoparathyroidism which is secondary to parathyroid removal or bruising). This may recover and if so is covered with calcium replacements, but permanent damage is treated with replacement therapy using alphacalcidol.
   (b) Thyroid crisis (acute exacerbation of thyrotoxicosis).
   (c) Hypothyroidism (secondary to extensive removal of thyroid tissue).
   (d) Late recurrence of thyrotoxicosis (incomplete removal of the toxic gland to include the pyramidal lobe)

3. *Complications of the wound site.*
   (a) Haemorrhage which can be immediate or delayed. It can cause tracheal compression. Treatment is with evacuation.
   (b) Tracheomalacia (uncommon).
   (c) Wound infection.
   (d) Poor scar.

Follow-up and aftercare

In those patients who have had a hemithyroidectomy, thyroid function is checked at 6 weeks to check the contralateral lobe is functioning normally and if not a further blood test is done at 3 months. If there is still evidence of subclinical hypothyroidism, patients may well require long term thyroxine replacement therapy. This is particularly common in the elderly and in those who have positive thyroid antibodies. Patients who have had a 'near total' or 'total' thyroidectomy usually require immediate Thyroxine replacement therapy and all patients following thyroidectomy should have a vocal cord mobility checked so that the true incidence of cord paresis for one particular surgeon can be documented. Corrected serum calcium levels should be performed routinely 24 hours post-operatively to counteract iatrogenic hypoparathyroidism.

Further reading

Drury PL. The thyroid axis. In: Kumar PJ, Clarke ML (eds). *Clinical Medicine*, 2nd edn. London: Baillière Tindall, 1990; 798–809.

Related topic of interest

Thyroid disease – malignant, p. 322.

THYROID DISEASE – MALIGNANT

J.C. Watkinson

Aetiology

Carcinoma of the thyroid gland is not common. Several factors are now known to be important in its causation. These are:

- Natural diet deficient in iodine.
- Increased secretion of thyroid stimulating hormone.
- Male gender.
- A history of previous ionizing radiation.
- Genetic predisposition.
- History of previous thyroid cancer.
- Chronic lymphocytic thyroiditis.

Classification

There are various types of thyroid tumours and these are shown in Table 1 below.

Table 1. Classification of thyroid tumours

Benign	Malignant
	Primary
• Follicular cell adenoma	• Papillary carcinoma (80%)
• Hürthle cell adenoma	• Pure papillary
• Teratoma	• Mixed papillary-follicular
	• Follicular variant
	• Follicular carcinoma (10%)
	• Hürthle cell carcinoma
	• Medullary carcinoma (5%)
	• Anaplastic carcinoma
	• Lymphoma
	• Sarcoma
	• Squamous cell carcinoma
	Secondary
	• Kidney, lung, colon and breast

1. Papillary adenocarcinoma. Papillary adenocarcinoma (along with follicular adenocarcinoma) is a differentiated thyroid cancer and accounts for 80% of thyroid malignancy. It occurs in all ages and is the commonest type of thyroid cancer in children. It usually presents as a solitary thyroid nodule, but is often multicentric. Its various types are:

- Minimal (or microcarcinoma): less than 1 cm.
- Intrathyroidal: greater than 1 cm.
- Extrathyroidal: extending beyond gland capsule and/or lymph node metastases.

Papillary thyroid cancer either exists in a pure papillary form, as mixed papillary-follicular carcinoma or as the follicular variant papillary carcinoma. It is associated with a high incidence of cervical lymphadenopathy which may, on occasion, be the only initial presenting feature. Less than 10% will have distant metastases, which are usually to the lungs.

2. *Follicular adenocarcinoma.* Follicular adenocarcinoma occurs in older age groups between 40 and 60 years and is seldom seen under the age of 30. It is less common than papillary thyroid cancer (10% of all thyroid malignancy) and usually presents as a solitary thyroid nodule or occasionally with either distant bony metastases or cervical node involvement (about 10%). While papillary carcinoma can be identified on fine needle aspiration cytology, it is not possible to diagnose a follicular carcinoma using this technique since it cannot distinguish an adenoma from a carcinoma. Therefore, a diagnostic thyroid lobectomy is usually required.

3. *Medullary thyroid carcinoma.* This condition accounts for about 5% of all cases of thyroid malignancy. Medullary cancers arise from the parafollicular or C cells which secrete calcitonin and this can be a valuable tumour marker. It may occur as part of the multiple endocrine neoplasia (MEN) syndrome, as familial non MEN disease or in sporadic form. In patients with MEN, it is frequently bilateral (90%) and multifocal, and cervical node metastases are common. The autosomal dominant MEN IIa is associated with phaeochromocytomas (10%) and parathyroid hyperplasia (60%). MEN IIb is medullary carcinoma associated with mucosal neuromas, phaeochromocytomas and Marfan's syndrome. Genetic screening is now possible for familial disease using the ret proto-oncogene.

4. *Lymphoma.* Primary thyroid lymphomas are uncommon and account for fewer than 5% of all lymphoma cases. They usually present as a rapidly increased swelling of the neck in an elderly woman and there is often a history of Hashimoto's thyroiditis. The clinical presentation can be identical to anaplastic carcinoma and both these conditions should be excluded from each other by open biopsy. Once the diagnosis is made, patients require formal staging and treatment is with radiotherapy plus or minus chemotherapy.

5. *Anaplastic carcinoma.* These tumours are common in elderly women and many are superimposed on a long standing multinodular goitre. They present with rapid thyroid enlargement, are aggressively malignant and rapidly invade surrounding structures. They have a bad prognosis. Its histology comprises of swarms of small cells and can be difficult to distinguish from lymphoma, which has a good prognosis. Therefore, immunohistochemical staining for cytokeratin squamous cell marker, and CD4/CD8 lymphoid cell markers is required. Treatment of anaplastic carcinoma with radiotherapy is often ineffective, a tracheostomy may be required and most patients are dead within one year.

Investigations

All patients should have thyroid function tests and thyroid antibodies. Many will present with a solitary thyroid nodule so will have had FNAC. An ultrasound may be useful to measure the size of the primary tumour, to assess the contralateral lobe and to facilitate FNA in certain cases. Patients with advanced disease should be imaged with CT or MRI. Whole body staging for lymphoma is done with CT.

Staging

T1	Tumour < 1 cm.
T2	Tumour 1 cm–4 cm.
T3	Tumour > 4 cm.
T4	Tumour of any size extending beyond the thyroid capsule.

All categories may be subdivided into (a) solitary tumour, (b) multifocal tumour

N0	No regional lymph node metastases.
N1	Regional lymph node metastases.
N1a	Metastases in ipsilateral node.
N1b	Metastases in bilateral, midline, or contralateral cervical or mediastinal nodes.

Prognostic factors

There are a number of prognostic factors associated with differentiated thyroid cancer and these are listed below:

- Age.
- Sex.
- Tumour size.
- Tumour histology.
- The presence of nodal metastases, local invasion or distant spread.
- Extent of surgery.
- Thyroid hormone manipulation.
- Treatment with postoperative radio-iodine.

Patients over 45 do worse and women do better than men. Tumour size is important as is tumour histology with papillary tumours doing better than follicular and both of these do better than medullary. Nodal metastases carry a worse prognosis in the elderly and patients do worse in the presence of local or distant spread. The extent of surgery is important with survival rates being the best in a group of patients who have total thyroidectomy and radio-iodine ablation. The experience of the surgeon is also important.

Management

There are a number of treatment modalities for thyroid malignancy:

- Surgery.
- Radio-active iodine.
- External beam radiotherapy.
- Hormonal manipulation.
- Chemotherapy.

Papillary adenocarcinoma

The treatment of this cancer is with surgery and the outlook is excellent. Data from the Mayo clinic shows that patients who have tumours which measure less than 1 cm in size have an excellent prognosis and a 99% chance of living 20 years (the T1 lesion). In these cases it seems entirely reasonable to advocate a conservative approach with hemi-thyroidectomy, thyroid hormone suppression and serial thyroglobulin measurements. However, some may prefer to advocate total thyroidectomy and radio-iodine ablation. There is a risk that the tumour will be multicentric. As the tumour size increases, survival rates fall and certainly any patient with a tumour which measures greater than 3 cm or one with local or distant spread should be treated with total thyroidectomy and radio-iodine ablation. Treatment of the T2 lesion (1–4 cm) remains controversial but again following thyroid lobectomy for a suspicious FNA based on current data, it is reasonable after discussion with the patient to offer a conservative approach for tumours less than 3 cm in size when age and gender indicate a low risk patient.

Follicular adenocarcinoma

For follicular carcinoma, distant spread is more common so that tumours less than 1 cm which exhibit minimal invasion can be treated with conservative hemi-thyroidectomy but the rest (which will be the majority) require total thyroidectomy and radio-iodine ablation.

Treatment of differentiated thyroid tumours based on risk stratification

A risk stratification based on Gender, Age, Stage and Histology (GASH) is shown below:

- Gender.
- Age.
- Tumour size.
- Nodal and distant metastases.
- Tumour histology.

Patients can be divided into high risk or low risk (females under 45 are low risk) and there are low risk and high risk tumours (low risk tumours measure less than 1 cm in size). Those tumours greater than 1 cm and those associated with cervical or distant metastases are high risk.

This allows a surgical treatment strategy as shown in Table 2.

Table 2. Surgical treatment of differentiated thyroid cancer

Low risk patient with low risk tumour	Lobectomy
Low risk patient with high risk tumour	**? Lobectomy or total thyroidectomy**
High risk patient with low risk tumour	**? Lobectomy or total thyroidectomy**
High risk patient with high risk tumour	Total thyroidectomy

Those in bold text are an intermediate group.

All patients with differentiated thyroid cancer require a level VI dissection as part of the total thyroidectomy. At the time of surgery, the jugular vein is palpated and any suspicious nodes in levels II to V and VII are sent for frozen section and, if involved, a selective neck dissection of levels II to V or VII is carried out as appropriate. Clinically palpable disease requires at least a selective neck dissection involving these levels. Modified radical or radical neck dissections may be required.

Following total thyroidectomy, radio-iodine ablation of the residual normal thyroid tissue can be performed in the post-operative period after allowing TSH levels to rise. Protocols are available and patients are put on suppressive doses of T4 and an I^{131} whole body diagnostic scan carried out after ablation to confirm whether or not the treatment has been successful. Any uptake in the neck requires a therapy dose of I^{131}.

Medullary thyroid cancer

Treatment for this is surgical. A total thyroidectomy is done with a level VI dissection and any palpable nodal disease requires modified radical or radical neck dissection. It is usually possible to perform conservative surgery preserving at least the accessory nerve as well as sometimes both the sternomastoid muscle and the internal jugular vein. Usually level I does not need to be dissected in the untreated neck.

The treatment of anaplastic carcinoma and lymphoma has already been discussed.

Total thyroidectomy for cancer

The following points are important when performing the above operation:

- Adequate access is required via the appropriate incision. The strap muscles may need to be divided.
- Identify and attempt to preserve both recurrent laryngeal nerves.
- Any involved nerve should be resected.
- Parathyroid preservation is important.
- Access to the mediastinum may be required.
- Level VI dissection should always be done with a total thyroidectomy.
- Visceral extension into the larynx or pharynx may require extensive surgery.
- Major vessel involvement is uncommon but usually indicates inoperability.

Further reading

The management of the solitary thyroid nodule: a review by RM Walsh; JC Watkinson & J Franklyn. In: *Clinical Otolaryngology*, 1999. Vol. 24: 388–397.

Tumours of the thyroid and parathyroid glands. In: *Stell and Maran's Head and Neck Surgery*. 4th Edition. Butterworth-Heinemann, 2000.

Wilson J (ed). *Effective Head and Neck Cancer Management. Second Consensus.* British Association of Otolaryngologists, Head and Neck Surgeons, 2000.

TINNITUS

Definition

Tinnitus is the sensation of sound not brought about by simultaneously externally applied mechanoacoustic or electrical signals. This definition excludes vascular sounds and bruits.

Epidemiology

Tinnitus is a common experience with up to one third of the adult population experiencing it at some time in their life. Less than 1% of the adult population have tinnitus of sufficient severity to seriously affect their quality of life (although up to 8% may seek medical advice about it). The prevalence of tinnitus increases in association with a high frequency hearing loss although the association between severity of tinnitus and degree of hearing loss is very weak. Hyperacusis (as distinct from recruitment) is found as an associated symptom in about 40% of tinnitus sufferers. Hyperacusis can be defined as an undue sensitivity and distress to everyday sounds that would not normally trouble a 'normal-hearing' individual.

Pathophysiology

The cause of tinnitus is not known. In developing an understanding of tinnitus mechanisms two points should be borne in mind:

(a) There is a generated potential somewhere in the auditory system.
(b) This signal will undergo extensive auditory processing before it is perceived as tinnitus.

There are several hypotheses which attempt to explain these phenomena:

1. Altered auditory firing rate. There is some evidence that tinnitus is associated with an increase in the spontaneous firing rate of auditory nerve fibres. Hence the association with a high tone hearing loss.

2. Cross talk. It has been postulated that damage to the cochlea, by any mechanism, may cause damage to the myelin insulation between axons in the peripheral auditory system, leading to 'cross-talk' between them and thus to phase locking of spontaneous neural activity, experienced subjectively as tinnitus.

3. Central processing. Recent years have seen an increased appreciation of the role of central signal processing in tinnitus perception. A 'neurophysiological' model has been developed which suggests three phases in the aetiology of tinnitus:

- Emergence of the signal (perhaps due to local cochlea pathology).
- Detection and then (usually negative) perception, and finally.
- Persistence – due to autonomic arousal, anxiety and negative beliefs.

It has become clear in recent years that the 'problem' of tinnitus relates far more to the individual's psychological response to the abnormal tinnitus signal than to the signal itself. There is also evidence of increased central auditory gain in tinnitus sufferers and it may be this phenomena that explains the frequently associated hyperacusis.

Associated conditions

1. *Local causes.* Almost every ear disease and cause of deafness can be associated with tinnitus, and the great majority of tinnitus sufferers have some measurable hearing loss. Noise induced hearing loss seems to be particularly frequently associated with tinnitus as does Menières disease. Unilateral tinnitus may also be the only symptom of an acoustic neuroma.

2. *General causes.* These include cardiovascular disease (hypertension, cardiac failure), a hyperdynamic circulation as in anaemia and fever and drugs (particularly salicylates). Neurological conditions (multiple sclerosis, neuropathy) may also lead to tinnitus. Objective tinnitus may be found in palatal myoclonus, vascular malformations and exceptionally loud spontaneous otoacoustic emissions.

Clinical assessment

From the patient's history confirm that the patient is actually suffering with tinnitus and determine the character of the sound (intermittent or constant, pulsatile or non-pulsatile). It is also important to establish how much trouble the patient is having because this will dictate whether and how much treatment is necessary. Effects on sleep, mood and concentration are found most frequently.

A full ENT and cardio-vascular examination should be performed to ensure the patient is not hearing transmitted sounds or does not have a potentially remedial causes of tinnitus.

Investigations

1. Audiometric investigations.
- A pure tone audiogram is essential to document any hearing loss.
- Tinnitus pitch and loudness matching may be performed. Usually the pitch of the tinnitus is found to be at or around the frequency of the maximal hearing loss and the loudness is usually within 15 dB of the patient's pure tone threshold at that frequency. These tests make the assumption that the characteristics of an external sound can be meaningfully related to those of an internally generated sound. There is a consensus that psycho-acoustic tests of this kind give no useful information regarding tinnitus severity nor is there any relationship between perceived loudness of tinnitus and complaint behaviour.
- Loudness discomfort levels are useful if there is any co-existent hyperacusis. When measured sequentially they can indicate response to treatment.

2. It should be remembered that 10% of acoustic neuromas present with markedly asymmetrical tinnitus. MRI scanning will then be required.

3. In the absence of a clear diagnosis a full haematological screen to exclude anaemia, thyroid dysfunction, dyslipidaemias and hypoglycaemia can be helpful.

4. Objective pulsatile tinnitus may require angiography if a specific vascular lesion is suspected.

Management

Any underlying remedial cause should be treated first. Thereafter, if tinnitus persists, management is best undertaken by a dedicated team comprising otologist, hearing therapists, audiologists, and ideally, a clinical psychologist. Access to a local self-help group is useful to provide emotional support, lay counselling and relaxation therapy.

Modern treatment is described as habituation based therapy and consists of two main components: directive counselling and sound therapy. *Directive counselling* involves explaining the problem, countering negative beliefs and making efforts to ameliorate the tinnitus sufferer's reaction to the perception of their tinnitus signal. *Sound therapy* or sound enrichment involves the use of background sound, hearing aids and/or white noise generators (WNG) to raise the background 'sound floor' and thus reduce the prominence of the tinnitus signal.

- *Hearing aids.* These are useful for those patients who have a hearing loss. If an appropriate aid with maximal gain at around the frequency of the tinnitus is fitted, the increased awareness of the background sound tends to make the tinnitus less apparent.
- *White noise generators* (WNG). These produce a controllable and more palatable, broad-band sound. It is thought to act both by reducing the contrast between the tinnitus signal and background noise and improving the plasticity of the central auditory cortex and thereby facilitating a reduction in perception. These are particularly useful for individuals with a minimal or no hearing loss.
- *Combined hearing aid and WNG unit.* Useful for those with severe tinnitus and a hearing loss.
- A pillow radio or pillow speaker may help the patient get to sleep.
- Many other treatments have been tried (e.g. lignocaine, magnetic and ultrasonic stimulation, melatonin, ginko biloba amongst others) but success has been limited and adverse effects common.

Further reading

Coles RRA. Tinnitus. In: *Scott-Brown's Otolaryngology*, Butterworth-Heinemann, 6th edn, Vol. 2, Adult Audiology. D Stephens (ed). London: Chapter 18.

Jastreboff PJ and Hazell JWP. A neurophysiological approach to tinnitus: clinical implications. *British Journal of Audiology*, 1993; **27**: 7–17.

Related topics of interest

Evoked response audiometry, p. 78; Hearing aids, p. 117; Pure tone audiogram, p. 254.

TONSIL DISEASES

The tonsils are paired secondary lymphatic organs situated on the side of the oropharynx between the palatoglossal (anterior tonsil pillar) and palatopharyngeal folds (posterior tonsil pillar). They are part of Waldeyer's ring, a ring of lymphoid tissue consisting of the adenoids, the palatine tonsils and the lingual tonsils (which are embedded in the posterior third of the tongue). The ring as a whole is thought to have some protective function as a barrier against infection in the first few years of life. The tonsil is enclosed by a fibrous capsule, outside of which is a layer of areolar tissue. This separates the capsule from the pharyngobasilar fascia covering the superior constrictor muscle that forms the tonsil bed. The main blood supply of the tonsil is from the tonsillar branch of the facial artery.

Aetiology of acute tonsillitis

Although this is a common disease, its aetiology and pathogenesis are poorly understood. Acute tonsillitis is an infection which primarily affects the palatine tonsil. It is regarded as being distinctive from acute pharyngitis, which is most often a viral infection involving the lymphoid tissue on the posterior pharyngeal wall and may include the tonsil. Although the disease is seen in adults, it is most frequent in childhood, presumably because immunity to common childhood organisms has not been fully established. There is some doubt regarding the most common causative organisms in acute tonsillitis. It has been suggested that viruses (e.g. influenza, parainfluenza, adenoviruses, enteroviruses and rhinoviruses) may be responsible for tonsillitis in up to 50% of occasions. In many other cases it is felt that an initial viral tonsillitis may predispose to a superinfection by bacteria (β-*haemolytic streptococcus*, *Streptococcus pneumoniae*, *Haemophilus influenzae* and anaerobic organisms).

Clinical features

There may be a prodromal illness with pyrexia, malaise and headache for a day before the onset of the predominant symptom, which is a sore throat. Pain may radiate to the ears or may occur in the neck due to cervical lymphadenopathy. Swallowing may be painful (odynophagia) and the patient's voice may sound muffled. There may be trismus and dribbling. Some children may have abdominal pain and occasionally vomiting. The tonsils are found to be hyperaemic on examination with pus and debris in the crypts. There will be tender cervical lymphadenopathy, particularly the jugulodigastric nodes. Glandular fever, agranulocytosis, leukaemia and diphtheria must always be borne in mind. In general practice the clinical features usually make the diagnosis obvious without the need to resort to clinical investigations in the majority of cases. Cases that are referred to hospital are usually more severe, however, and it would be prudent to perform a Paul–Bunnell test, white cell count and a throat swab.

Management

Even though viruses are implicated as the pathogenic organisms in many cases, it is likely any patient who attends a medical practitioner with the clinical features of tonsillitis will be treated with antibiotics. Penicillin V is still the drug of choice, with erythromycin reserved for those patients allergic to penicillin. Ampicillin should never be used to treat acute tonsillitis in case the patient has infectious mononucleosis, when a generalized maculopapular rash may develop. The patient should have paracetamol for analgesia. Aspirin is contraindicated in children because of the risk of Reye's syndrome. Fluid replacement and bed rest are ancillary measures in the severe attack.

Complications of acute tonsillitis

1. *Local.*
- Severe swelling causing respiratory obstruction.
- Abscess formation:
  Peritonsillar (quinsy).
  Parapharyngeal.
  Retropharyngeal.
- Acute otitis media.
- Recurrent acute tonsillitis (chronic tonsillitis).

2. *General.*
- Septicaemia.
- Meningitis.
- Acute rheumatic fever.
- Acute glomerulonephritis.

Differential diagnosis of unilateral tonsil enlargement

- Asymmetry in a patient with recurrent bouts of acute tonsillitis.
- Neoplasia (squamous cell carcinoma or lymphoma).
- Apparent enlargement (peritonsillar abscess or parapharyngeal mass).

Differential diagnosis of ulceration of the tonsil

A working diagnosis can usually be determined from the history and clinical examination. Investigations include a full blood count, chest radiograph, serological tests and biopsy. Possible causes include:

1. *Infection.*
- Acute streptococcal tonsillitis.
- Diphtheria.
- Infectious mononucleosis.
- Vincent's angina.

2. *Neoplasm.*
- Squamous cell carcinoma.
- Lymphoma.
- Salivary gland tumours (adenoid cystic carcinoma or mucoepidermoid tumour).

3. *Blood diseases.*
- Agranulocytosis.
- Leukaemia.

4. **Other causes.**
- Aphthous ulceration.
- Behçet's syndrome.
- Acquired immunodeficiency syndrome (AIDS).

Further reading

Hibbert J. Acute infection of the pharynx and tonsils. In: Hibbert J (ed), *Scott-Brown's Otolaryngology*, Vol. 5, 6th edn. London: Butterworths, 1997; Chapter 4.

Hotaling AJ, Silva AB. Advances in adenotonsillar disease. *Current Opinion in Otolaryngology and Head and Neck Surgery*, 1993; **1**: 177–184.

Related topics of interest

TONSILLECTOMY

Indications for tonsillectomy

- Recurrent episodes of acute tonsillitis. (Surgeons differ in the definition of this. As a rule of thumb these episodes should last 5 days or more, five per year, for at least 2 years.)
- Previous episodes of peritonsillar abscess (quinsy).
- Suspected neoplasm (unilateral enlargement or ulceration).
- Part of another procedure (UVPP, access to glossopharyngeal nerve or styloid process).
- Gross enlargement causing airway obstruction (sleep apnoea syndrome).

Contraindications

These contraindications are not absolute, but surgery should be delayed until the particular problem is resolved. In some cases the decision to proceed with surgery should be reconsidered in the context of the potential problems.

- Recent episode of tonsillitis or upper respiratory tract infection (within 2 weeks).
- Bleeding disorder.
- Oral contraceptives.
- Cleft palate.
- During certain epidemics (e.g. polio).

Tonsillectomy and CJD

Concerns have been expressed about the potential for contamination of tonsillectomy instruments with 'prions' and subsequent development of Creutzfeldt Jakob disease (CJD). Although it is felt that the risk is extremely small, steps have been taken to minimize it. Current advice is that instruments which are in intimate contact with the tonsil (dissecting instruments, scissors, etc) should be disposable, but not the mouth gag or Draffins bipods.

Complications of tonsillectomy

1. **Peroperative.**
- Anaesthetic reaction.
- Haemorrhage.
- Damage to teeth.
- Trauma to the posterior pharyngeal wall (careless insertion of the tongue blade).
- Dislocation of the temperomandibular joint by over-opening the mouth gag.

2. **Immediate.**
- Reactionary haemorrhage.
- Anaesthetic complications.

3. Early.

- Secondary haemorrhage.
- Haematoma and oedema of the uvula.
- Infection (may lead to secondary haemorrhage).
- Earache (referred pain or acute otitis media).
- Pulmonary complications (pneumonia and lung abscess are rare).
- Subacute bacterial endocarditis (if the patient has a cardiac defect).

4. Late.

- Scarring of the soft palate (limiting mobility and possibly affecting voice).
- Tonsillar remnants (which may be the site of recurrent acute infection).

The most significant complication is haemorrhage, which occurs in approximately 2% of cases. Most of the deaths associated with tonsillectomy are directly or indirectly associated with this complication.

It is essential to ensure adequate haemostasis at the end of the tonsillectomy procedure as blood in the airway at this time may cause laryngeal spasm or can occlude the airway. The postnasal space should always be checked for a blood clot (the so-called 'coroner's clot'). Patients are nursed in the reverse Trendelenburg position (head down) so that blood trickles out of the mouth rather than being swallowed or aspirated.

Reactionary (primary) haemorrhage by definition occurs up to 24 hours postoperatively, but the vast majority occur within the first 8 hours. It is one of the reasons why some surgeons are opposed to day case tonsillectomy. Continuing haemorrhage will result in hypovolaemia, and if not corrected circulatory failure (shock) will be the consequence. The signs of reactionary haemorrhage are obvious: bleeding from the mouth, a gurgling sound in the throat on respiration, repeated swallowing, vomiting blood, a rising pulse rate and eventually a falling blood pressure and tachypnoea. Blood must be cross-matched and an intravenous infusion started. The tonsillar fossae should be inspected to identify a bleeding point. Any clot should be removed if possible and a gauze swab soaked in 1:1000 adrenaline applied to the fossa. If the bleeding continues, or there is any doubt, the patient should be prepared for a second anaesthetic and the bleeding point ligated under general anaesthesia. The second anaesthetic is hazardous and should only be administered by an experienced anaesthetist.

Secondary haemorrhage occurs some 5–10 days post tonsillectomy and is due to an infection of the fossae. If significant, the patient should be admitted to hospital for observation. A full blood count and cross-match should be performed. The infection and haemorrhage will usually settle after treatment with antibiotics (i.v. penicillin and metronidazole or erythromycin). It is unusual for such a patient to have to go back to theatre and when this is necessary the tonsillar fossae are found to be sloughy and friable and it is difficult to locate and ligate any specific bleeding point. It may be necessary to suture the faucial pillars together, or over Kaltostat or a gauze swab which is removed the next day.

Follow-up and aftercare

No specific follow-up is required after a routine, uncomplicated tonsillectomy. Patients who have suffered a significant haemorrhage should be reviewed within 2 weeks to check their haemoglobin. Patients who have a tonsillectomy for reasons other than recurrent acute tonsillitis should be followed up appropriately to their problem.

Further reading

Hibbert J. Acute infection of the pharynx and tonsils. In: Hibbert J (ed). *Scott-Brown's Otolaryngology*, Vol. 5, 6th edn. London: Butterworths, 1997, chapter 4.

Hotaling AJ, Silva AB. Advances in adenotonsillar disease. *Current Opinion in Otolaryngology and Head and Neck Surgery*, 1993; 1: 177–184.

Related topics of interest

TRACHEOSTOMY

A tracheotomy is an operation to make an opening in the trachea, while a tracheostomy means converting this opening to a stoma on the skin surface. Tracheostomy should, whenever possible, be carried out as an elective procedure. Many disorders are now managed by endotracheal intubation, and this should always be carefully considered first, but the decision for tracheostomy should not be left until it is too late. Children especially can deteriorate very suddenly. There is an old adage that states 'the time to do a tracheostomy is when you first think about it'. In many centres, percutaneous dilatational tracheostomy has emerged as the principle method for performing tracheostomy in the intensive care unit setting. This will also be discussed in this chapter.

Indications for tracheostomy

1. Airway obstruction. Advances in anaesthetics, including improved, less traumatizing types of endotracheal tubes, have reduced the number of potential tracheostomies. Upper airway obstruction is now the least common indication for tracheostomy.

- Congenital (subglottic stenosis, laryngeal web, laryngeal cysts).
- Trauma (foreign body, severe head and neck injury, swallowing corrosive, inhalation of irritants).
- Infection (acute epiglottitis, laryngotracheobronchitis, diphtheria, Ludwig's angina).
- Tumour (tongue, larynx, pharynx, trachea, thyroid).
- Vocal cord paralysis (thyroidectomy complication, bulbar palsy).

2. Protection of the tracheobronchial tree. This includes patients who need temporary protection of their airway (e.g. those patients undergoing head and neck surgery). Patients may benefit from a long-term tracheostomy if they suffer from any chronic condition (which are often neurological diseases) leading to inhalation of saliva, food, gastric contents or blood, or the stagnation of bronchial secretions. A cuffed tube will protect the airway from aspiration and allow easy access to the trachea for regular suction.

- Neurological diseases (polyneuritis, tetanus, myasthenia gravis, bulbar palsy, multiple sclerosis).
- Trauma (burns of the face and neck, multiple facial fractures).
- Coma (drug overdose, head injury, cerebrovascular accident).
- Head and neck surgery (oral or oropharyngeal resections, supraglottic laryngectomy).

3. Ventilatory insufficiency. Tracheostomy reduces upper respiratory dead space by about 70%, bypasses resistance to airflow in the nose, mouth and glottis, and allows the use of mechanically assisted respiration if necessary (intermittent positive-pressure ventilation).

- Pulmonary diseases (chronic bronchitis and emphysema, severe asthma, pneumonia).
- Neurological diseases (as above).
- Severe chest injury (flail chest).

Tracheostomy tubes

The selection of tracheostomy tube depends on the reason for the procedure and the postoperative requirements. A cuffed tube is preferred if the patient needs protection of the lower airway from aspiration or haemorrhage. Removable inner tubes facilitate cleaning and removal of crusted secretions while the outer tube maintains the airway. A fenestrated tube permits the passage of air upwards through the glottis, thereby allowing the patient to speak. Tube types can be divided into metal and synthetic.

1. Metal tubes. These usually consist of an obturator, an outer tube and an inner tube. They usually have an expiratory flap valve on the inner tube which allows phonation, but they do not have a cuff. Examples include the silver tubes of Chevalier Jackson and Negus. These are short and should only be used in patients with thin necks. The Durham tube has an adjustable flange so that it can be used in patients with either thin or very fat necks. The Koenig tube has a long flexible wire that can be used if there is a narrowing of the trachea. The Alder Hey tube is a typical example of a paediatric metal tube: both the inner and outer tubes are fenestrated and a valve is available to allow transglottic expiration and speech.

2. Synthetic tubes. Most of these are made from PVC, silicone or other synthetic plastics that are non-toxic. Examples include the Portex and Shiley tubes. These tubes can be connected to an anaesthetic connector or respirator. Nowadays they have low-pressure cuffs which can remain inflated for days, preventing aspiration and without causing pressure necrosis of the trachea. Paediatric synthetic tubes include the Franklin tube of Great Ormond Street, the Portex paediatric tube and the Shiley paediatric or neonatal tube. The Great Ormond Street tube and the Shiley are winged and sit comfortably in the infant's neck; the Portex is not winged but has square-ended flanges. None of the paediatric tubes have a cuff.

Postoperative management

1. Nursing care. Constant nursing attention is essential for at least the first 24 hours following the tracheostomy. The patient should be in a well-supported upright position; care must be taken in infants that the chin does not occlude the tracheostomy.

2. Suction. The patient will be unable to cough and clear secretions so suction should be applied regularly, by aseptic technique, to prevent a build-up of secretions in the trachea and bronchi. A sterile catheter is passed well down into each main bronchus in turn.

3. Humidification. Humidification of inspired air is essential to prevent drying of the airway, which encourages the formation of crusts and infection. Saline or sodium bicarbonate instillation into the trachea followed by immediate suction also helps to reduce the likelihood of such complications.

4. Apnoea. Some patients with chronic obstructive airways disease may develop apnoea following restoration of their airway. This is due to lowering of their Pco_2, with loss of stimulation of their respiratory centre. These patients need monitoring and the administration of carbon dioxide via a flowmeter through the tracheostomy if necessary.

5. Speech. A notebook or erasable pad should be provided for the patient to communicate. If the larynx is still functioning the patient can be shown how to speak by temporarily blocking the tube while exhaling. Patients with a permanent tracheostomy should if possible have a fenestrated tube with a speaking valve incorporated with the inner tube.

6. Swallowing. Some patients may experience problems, often because of the condition which necessitated the tracheostomy, but sometimes because of incoordination and the pressure of the tube's cuff. The tracheostomy tube may interfere with the normal mobility of the larynx during swallowing. Deflation of the cuff will sometimes help, but some patients may require a nasogastric tube.

7. Care of the tube. If there is an inner tube it should be taken out and cleaned whenever necessary; the outer tube must be held firmly while withdrawing the inner one. Replacement or cleaning of the outer tube is usually left for the first 5 days until a track has become established, then this should be done weekly or as required. If a cuffed tube has been used it should be inflated with the minimum amount of air that prevents an air leak, and it must have a low-pressure cuff to minimize the risk of tracheal stenosis. A spare tube of identical size and a tracheostomy dilator must always be available at the bedside in case a quick change is necessary. The first tube change is usually done about 48 hours after the tracheostomy and should always be performed by a doctor, preferably the surgeon who performed the procedure. Whenever the nursing staff perform subsequent tube changes it should be done when the whereabouts of a doctor is known in case of a problem.

8. Decannulation. The tracheostomy tube should be spigoted and removed as soon as is feasible. It should only be carried out when it is obvious that it is no longer required. The patient should be able to manage with the tube spigoted for a full 24-hour period, including a period of sleep. There may be difficulties in children who have had the tracheostomy for a long period of time, sometimes because of a psychological dependence on the tube. They also have a relatively smaller tracheal airway which may be partly blocked by granulation tissue, and surgical closure by excision of the scar tissue and the tracheocutaneous track may be required in some cases. After decannulation the patient should remain in hospital under observation for at least 2 days.

Complications

As with any operative procedure the complications of tracheostomy can be immediate (during the first 24 hours), intermediate (1–14 days) or late (>14 days). The following list can be a useful basis or plan for an examination answer.

1. **Immediate.**
- Anaesthetic complications.
- Damage to local structures (cricoid cartilage, recurrent laryngeal nerve, oesophagus, brachiocephalic vein).
- Cardiac arrest.
- Primary haemorrhage.

2. **Intermediate.**
- Dislodgement/displacement of the tube.
- Surgical emphysema.
- Pneumothorax.
- Obstruction of the tube or trachea (excessive crusting).
- Infection (perichondritis, wound infection, secondary haemorrhage).
- Tracheal necrosis (may lead to tracheal stenosis or tracheo-oesophageal fistula).

3. **Late.**
- Subglottic and tracheal stenosis.
- Decannulation difficulty.
- Tracheocutaneous fistula.
- Scar (hypertrophic or keloid).

Percutaneous tracheostomy

Percutaneous tracheostomy (PCT) has gained attention as an alternative to the standard tracheostomy technique. Despite its growing use, many otolaryngologists remain sceptical about its safety.

1. Technique. Several techniques are described but the Ciaglia modification of the Seldinger technique has the most support in the literature. Ciaglia's method involves a small vertical incision at the lower edge of the cricoid cartilage and blunt dissection is performed to the level of the trachea. Then there is a placement of multiple progressive dilators into the tracheal lumen over a wire that is introduced through this tract. Bronchoscopic guidance should be used when available, as it increases the safety of the procedure.

2. Indications/contraindications. The indications are the same as for conventional tracheostomy. The relative contraindications include: age less than 15 years, enlarged thyroid isthmus, previous tracheostomy, cervical spine fractures, evidence of coagulopathy, indistinct anatomic landmarks and previous laryngeal or neck surgery.

3. Complications. The main early problems are from bleeding and paratracheal insertion. This potentially lethal problem has been reported and associated with deaths. Bronchoscopic guidance is therefore advisable. The question of laryngo- tracheal stenosis as a long-term complication has not yet been adequately evaluated.

In reviewing the literature, some benefits appear to exist from the procedure, i.e. increased speed, smaller and more aesthetic wound, decreased operative bleeding and decreased rate of local wound infection. Costs also appear to be reduced – and this more than any other medical factor will guarantee its future use.

Further reading

Bradley PJ. The obstructed airway. *Scott-Brown's Otolaryngology*, Vol. 5, 6th edn. London: Butterworths, 1997, chapter 7.

Holtel MJ and Hall DJ. New techniques and advances in tracheostomy. *Current Opinion in Otolaryngology and Head and Neck Surgery*, 1999; **7**: 144–149.

Related topics of interest

Paediatric airway problems, p. 232; Paediatric endoscopy, p. 237; Stridor and stertor, p. 311.

TYMPANOPLASTY

Definition

Tympanoplasty is an operation to eradicate disease in the middle ear and to reconstruct the hearing mechanism with or without tympanic membrane grafting. Tympanoplasty may be combined with mastoid surgery when there is concomitant mastoid disease in patients with CSOM.

Myringoplasty is defined as an operation to repair or reconstruct the tympanic membrane. Strictly speaking it is not the same as a type 1 tympanoplasty because eradication of intercurrent middle ear disease is not included in the definition. They are, however, often used synonymously.

Classification

Wullstein in 1953 described five tympanoplasty reconstruction techniques after eradication of middle ear disease. A sixth was added by Garcia Ibanez in 1961.

1. ***Type 1.*** Reconstruction of the tympanic membrane with an intact and mobile ossicular chain.

2. ***Type 2.*** The malleus handle is absent. The tympanic membrane is reconstructed over the malleus remnant and the long process of the incus.

3. ***Type 3.*** The incus and malleus have been removed or eroded by disease. The tympanic membrane is reconstructed to lie on the stapes head to create a columella effect (myringostapediopexy). This is so called because in birds a single strut of bone, the columella, transmits sound from the tympanic membrane to the labyrinth.

4. ***Type 4.*** Only the stapes footplate remains. The footplate is exteriorized by leaving it exposed in the created mastoid cavity. The round window is acoustically separated from the oval window by reconstructing the tympanic membrane so that its superior margin lies on the promontory below the oval window, creating a round window baffle.

5. ***Type 5.*** The stapes footplate is fixed and a fenestration of the lateral semicircular canal is performed.

6. ***Type 6.*** Otherwise known as sono-inversion. There is an ossicular discontinuity. The round window niche is left uncovered and the tympanic membrane reconstructed so that its inferior edge lies on the promontory above the round window, thereby creating an oval window baffle.

In all of these procedures the aim was to aerate the middle ear by the Eustachian tube. This was difficult to achieve because the repaired tympanic membrane often became atelectatic and adherent to the medial wall of the middle ear. In addition, it became evident that an intact ossicular chain was important to achieve consistently good air-bone closure.

Ossicular chain reconstruction

Homograft tissue is now contraindicated because of the risk of CJD. Autograft reconstruction using cortical bone or remodelled incus is now usually preferred. An alternative is to use biodegradable porous hydroxyapatite tricalcium phosphate ceramics which have been shown to be replaced at least in part by osteogenic cells and host connective tissue. Porous polyethylene prostheses introduced by Shea in 1976 have produced results similar to hydroxyapatite, but there have been recent concerns regarding long term failure of the prostheses due to late fractures of the ceramic. There are several possible scenarios in reconstruction.

1.   A stapes footplate remnant is present with or without the malleus.   A myringostapediopexy or malleostapediopexy is performed using an autograft or ceramic total ossicular replacement prosthesis (TORP) to create the tympanic membrane or malleus-to-footplate assembly.

2.   The stapes superstructure is intact but there is an absent long process of incus.   The malleus handle may or may not be present. An autograft malleus-to-stapes assembly (incus transposition) or a ceramic partial ossicular replacement prosthesis (PORP) is used.

3.   There is an incudostapedial discontinuity secondary to an absent lenticular process and/or stapes head.   An incudostapediopexy using a cortical bone slither or a ceramic prosthesis as an incus-to-stapes assembly are the preferred methods of reconstruction.

To minimize extrusion of the ceramic implants some authorities recommend a slither of autograft tragal cartilage is interposed between the tympanic membrane and prosthesis. Closure of the air-bone gap to within 20 dB has been reported in up to 80% of patients using ceramic PORPs and 50% of patients using TORPS.

Follow-up and aftercare

The ear canal dressing is removed after 7–14 days. Nasal decongestants may improve Eustachian tube function in the short term and help ensure aeration of the middle ear cleft. Some authorities (e.g. Causse) advocate performing the Valsalva manoeuvre in the early postoperative period to achieve the same aim although there is a theoretical risk of displacing the prosthesis. Exertion and flying should be avoided until healing is achieved at 4–6 weeks, although some otologists allow both in the first post-operative week. Swimming is contraindicated until healing is complete. Diving may predispose to prosthesis displacement and should be avoided.

Further reading

Wullstein H. Theory and practice of tympanoplasty. *Laryngoscope*, 1956; **66**: 1076–1093.

Grote JJ. Biomaterials in otology. Proceedings of the First International Symposium 1983. Leiden, The Netherlands: Martinus Nijhoff Publishers, 1983.

Kerr AG and Riley DN. Disintegration of porous polyethylene prostheses. *Clinical Otolaryngology*, 1999; **24**: 168–171.

Related topics of interest

Mastoid surgery, p. 159; Chronic suppurative otitis media, p. 38; Cholesteatoma, p. 35.

TYMPANOSCLEROSIS

Tympanosclerosis is an abnormal condition of the middle ear, characterized by calcareous deposits in the tympanic membrane, tympanic cavity and occasionally in the mastoid.

Aetiology

The exact cause remains in doubt, but it appears likely that there is an abnormal healing process in response to multiple acute or chronic inflammatory episodes. Another important aetiological factor is tissue trauma, which is substantiated by the frequent occurrence of tympanosclerosis after myringotomy with or without insertion of ventilation tubes; this may be due to intraepithelial haemorrhage.

Pathogenesis

Three stages are recognized. In the initial stage, inflammatory processes cause an exudate, the formation of granulation tissue and damage to collagen fibres. This phase is generally considered reversible. The second stage is the reparative phase, characterized by fibroblast invasion. This results in excessive collagen synthesis and hyalinization, as a result of which fibres become indistinct, fusing into a homogeneous mass. Most authorities now consider the process to be irreversible, and in the third and final stage calcification and occasionally ossification may occur. It has been well established that the pathological changes of tympanosclerosis are situated in the lamina propria, which is the connective tissue component of tympanic membrane and mucosa.

Clinical features

It has been suggested that the term myringosclerosis be used when the process is confined to the tympanic membrane and the term tympanosclerosis be exclusively reserved to describe sequelae of chronic otitis affecting the ossicular chain. Morphologically, however, no differentiation can be made between the two conditions. Furthermore, the occurrence of plaques in the tympanic membrane may indicate the presence of more extensive disease in the middle ear in patients with a history of chronic otitis.

1. *Tympanic membrane.* Tympanosclerosis that is restricted to the tympanic membrane is most commonly seen, usually following myringotomy and ventilation tube insertion. It may occur in all age groups. Otoscopically, deposits present as sharply demarcated areas of white opaque, chalk-like material. Plaques usually occur only in the pars tensa, mostly situated in the anterior or posterior segments, varying in size. The clinical importance of this calcification is dependent on its size. In most cases there is little if any effect on the patient's hearing, even with quite extensive plaques. However, with very large plaques and those that impinge across the annulus, measurable hearing loss may result (20–40 dB). The condition occurs in approximately 5% of children with otitis media with effusion who have had no previous surgery. There is, however, a natural tendency for resolution in this group.

2. Middle-ear. Middle-ear involvement is much less common, but when it occurs is usually accompanied by a perforation of the tympanic membrane (85–100%). Interestingly, these ears are often dry. The patients are usually over 30 years of age and have had a long history of ear problems. The condition tends to be most prevalent in the oval window niche, epitympanum and promontory. These patients often have a significant hearing loss, which is invariably due to fixation of the ossicular chain.

Investigation

The clinical appearance of tympanosclerosis in either the middle-ear cavity or tympanic membrane rarely presents any diagnostic difficulties although it may occasionally look like a cholesteatoma. Examination under a microscope will nearly always resolve the issue. In cases of tympanosclerosis the involved ear is usually dry with a large central perforation, whereas in an ear with cholesteatoma the perforation or retraction pocket is usually marginal and often there is malodorous otorrhoea. An audiogram to assess any degree of (conductive) hearing loss is always useful.

Management

Tympanic membrane tympanosclerosis with an intact drum rarely requires treatment. Occasionally removal of a plaque may be required during myringoplasty, for a coexistent perforation, to aid healing.

Conductive hearing loss caused by tympanosclerosis can be treated with either a hearing aid or surgery. A hearing aid is safe and effective; surgery is controversial. The choice of procedure depends on the extent of middle-ear involvement but may include stapedectomy and/or attic mobilization or clearance. Studies that show initial improvement in hearing also demonstrate a deterioration in hearing levels with time. Furthermore, it has been shown that a number of patients suffer a postoperative sensorineural hearing loss.

Follow-up and aftercare

This should be appropriate to the patient's surgery and any active otological pathology.

Further reading

Wielinga EWJ, Kerr AG. Tympanosclerosis (review). *Clinical Otolaryngology*, 1993; **18**: 341–349.

Related topics of interest

Cholesteatoma, p. 35; Otitis media with effusion, p. 213; Tympanoplasty, p. 341.

VERTIGO

T.H.J. Lesser

Definition

Vertigo is the hallucination of movement. It is the cardinal symptom of disease of the vestibular system including its central connections.

The 'sense' of balance is very basic and phylogenically predates sight and hearing. When this basic system goes wrong, the patient is left disabled. Sir Terence Cawthorne said that 'labyrinthine disturbance may make one feel like the end of the world has arrived and I am told by sufferers from sea sickness that in the acutest phase of their distress they wish that it had'. Remembering this enables us to understand the distress of these patients. It also, in combination with the very basic nature of the sense of balance, explains the many symptoms such as muzzy head, loss of memory and anxiety that are associated with vestibular disorders. These are secondary effects from the vertigo and often remain after the vertigo has gone.

Anatomy and physiology

The vestibular sense organ consists of the three semicircular canals, the saccule and the utricle. These are membranous tubes within the dense temporal bone. The membranes are fluid filled and have cells with cilia which bend as the fluid moves relative to them. This excites or depresses the nerve cells and alters the tonic input into the brain. The semicircular canals are at right angles to each other and detect changes in angular acceleration. The utricle and saccule have otoconia embedded in a gel overlying the cilia and are positioned to detect linear acceleration.

The nerve impulses from the labyrinth go to the vestibular nuclei in the brain stem. Here they are integrated with two other inputs that enable us to balance. The two other inputs are vision and proprioception, from the joints, skin and muscle receptors. The neck and ankles are the most important proprioceptive inputs. Approximately 70% of balance is due to visual input, 15% from proprioception and 15% from the vestibular system. The brain stem computerizes these three inputs and with the help of the cerebellum maintains the balance and co-ordination of the head and body.

Pathology and clinical syndromes

Non-vestibular disorders such as cardiovascular, metabolic, musculoskeletal or ocular disease may cause dizziness or a sense of light-headedness, though not usually vertigo. Vestibular disorders are either central or peripheral. Central disease includes cerebrovascular disease, migraine, multiple sclerosis, brain tumours and very rarely vertebrobasilar insufficiency. The last hardly ever causes vertigo as a presenting symptom. Indeed, if the vertebral or basilar artery is constricted, dysarthria, visual phenomena, diplopia and weakness of one side of the body are usually the presenting signs. Cervical vertigo frequently occurs and is more likely to be due to disordered proprioceptive input from the neck. Iatrogenic vertigo caused by drugs (aminoglycosides, diuretics, co-trimoxazole, metronidazole) is common due to either ototoxicity or a central effect. Non-organic dizziness and vertigo also exist and may be associated with hyperventilation. These causes aside, we are left with the peripheral causes of vertigo, of which there are three main symptom complexes.

1. **Benign positional vertigo** commonly occurs after a head injury or ear infection and is a rotatory vertigo with a particular head movement. There are no other otological manifestations. It is diagnosed by the Hallpike manoeuvre.

2. **Menière's syndrome** comprises paroxysmal fluctuating hearing loss, vertigo and tinnitus, each attack lasting many minutes or hours.

3. **Acute vestibular failure** consists of marked vertigo for many hours or days often preceded by an upper respiratory tract infection.

Acoustic neuroma usually presents with a unilateral sensory hearing loss, but this is often accompanied by tinnitus and occasionally there is a non-specific dizziness. Middle-ear disease such as cholesteatoma can also cause vertigo, as can inner ear infections such as syphilis.

Clinical features

It is often difficult for patients to describe their sensations, and in taking a full and accurate history the symptom of vertigo must be differentiated from other types of dizziness such as fainting, light-headedness, claustrophobia, or some peripheral (musculoskeletal) dysequilibrium. A full description of the sensation should be obtained with reference to precipitating factors (e.g. neck movements), associated symptoms (e.g. deafness, tinnitus) and frequency and duration of the attacks. A previous history of trauma should be noted. Previous medical history, medication, and alcohol ingestion should also be considered in the context of possible causes or aggravation of the symptoms.

An otological and neurological examination is mandatory in all cases of vertigo. In particular middle-ear disease is looked for and nystagmus on finger following or after the Hallpike test. Gait assessment including Romberg's and Unterburger testing is important (see Vestibular function tests). A general medical examination may be required if the symptoms dictate.

The Hallpike manouvre

Positional nystagmus is best elicited by this positional test. The patient is positioned sitting on a bed and the procedure is explained. This explanation should include a reassurance to the patient that they will not be allowed to fall whatever happens. The patient is told to keep their eyes open and look straight ahead. The head is held firmly between the examiner's hands and turned 45° to the right or left. The patient is then rapidly laid backwards, with their head over the edge of the bed, 30° below the horizontal. The patient is asked if this provokes symptoms similar to those they have been describing and the eyes are observed for nystagmus. If neither occurs after 30 seconds then the patient is returned to the upright position and again asked if there is any vertigo and the eyes examined for nystagmus. If no symptoms or nystagmus are elicited the process is repeated but with the head to the other side.

Benign paroxysmal positional nystagmus elicited by the Hallpike manoeuvre usually has a latent period of 5 seconds before the onset of rotatory nystagmus, a fast component to the nystagmus directed towards the undermost ear, an associated vertigo which distresses the patient; and the nystagmus fatigues rapidly. This contrasts with nystagmus of central origin, which appears immediately, causes little or no vertigo and persists indefinitely if the head position is maintained. If there are no symptoms or nystagmus after the Hallpike manoeuvre, it is very unlikely that head positioning or neck extension has any role in the cause of the patient's vertigo.

Investigations

Vestibular testing consists of pure tone audiometry, evoked response audiometry, electronystagmography with caloric stimulation, optokinetic and positioning stimulation, and posturography (see Related topics). MRI with gadolinium enhancement is the radiological investigation of choice.

Management

1. **Vestibular rehabilitation.** This is now considered to be the mainstay of treatment in many vestibular disorders. The first step is to counsel the patient regarding their symptoms, to provide reassurance and to explain the importance of persisting with treatment. This is followed by a series of habituating exercises performed regularly to enable tolerance mechanisms to occur in the brain stem. It is known that structural changes occur to allow vestibular compensation such as a modification of the distribution and sensitivity of cholinergic synapses. These allow a new equilibrium situation to occur. With adequate counselling as many as 80% of patients with vestibular disorders will benefit from vestibular rehabilitation to encourage vestibular compensation. Specific manouvres and exercises are used for BPPV. The Epley (liberatory) manouvre works as a single treatment in up to 80% of patients. Brandt–Daroff exercises encourage habituation and succeed in 95% of cases when used with determination. In addition to vestibular rehabilitation, patients may also benefit from spectacles to improve their visual acuity or a walking stick to aid peripheral balance function and to give them more confidence.

2. **Medical treatment.** This consists of lifestyle changes (e.g. less alcohol) and drugs. The latter are usually vestibular sedatives such as prochlorperazine or cinnarizine, histamine analogues such as betahistine, or antidepressants.

3. **Surgery.** This is usually used for episodic peripheral vertigo diagnosed as Menière's syndrome and consists of endolymphatic sac shunting, vestibular neurectomy or labyrinthectomy. A middle-ear infusion of an aminoglycoside via a cannula in the round window is used by some. Occasionally surgery is used for benign positional vertigo when posterior semicircular canal obliteration or singular neurectomy is done.

Further reading

Luxon LM. Rehabilitation and management of balance and vestibular disorders. In: *Diseases of the Ear*. 6th edn. Ludman and Wright (eds). London: Arnold, 1998; 233–241.

Related topics of interest

VESTIBULAR FUNCTION TESTS

An individual maintains balance by coordinating sensory information provided by (1) the vestibular system, (2) the eyes and (3) the proprioceptors in the muscles of the limbs, trunk and neck. These sensory organs connect directly with the brain stem and the cerebellum and then with the cerebrum. The clinical correlate of this is that the assessment of any disorder of disequilibrium must be based on a multidisciplinary approach. A comprehensive history is essential, together with a complete general medical examination, with particular attention to the eyes, the ears, the central nervous system and the locomotor system.

Having established the need for a general medical approach to the problem of unsteadiness, it is necessary to identify the presence or absence of a vestibular component. Clinically, tests based on (a) the vestibulo-ocular reflex and (b) vestibulospinal reflexes can be performed.

Tests of the vestibulo-ocular reflex

Eye movements are generated in response to visual signals and vestibular activity. The central vestibulo-ocular and visuo-ocular pathways are intimately related, and both pathways share the common final pathway of the oculomotor nerve. If visually controlled eye movements are normal (e.g. saccades and the smooth pursuit system), derangement of the vestibulo-ocular reflex may correctly be ascribed to vestibular dysfunction. However, if visually controlled eye movements are abnormal, care must be taken in the interpretation of vestibulo-ocular responses.

Saccades

Saccades are rapid eye movements, which correct errors in the direction of gaze, and bring the desired object of fixation to the fovea in the shortest possible time. Central nervous system disease may cause abnormalities of latency, accuracy or velocity of saccades. Saccadic eye movements may be assessed by asking the patient to look back and forth between the examiner's index fingers, separated either horizontally or vertically.

Smooth pursuit

This system is responsible for maintaining gaze on a moving target, by comparing the eye velocity with that of the target velocity and producing a continuous match of eye and target position. It may be examined clinically by asking the patient to follow a pendulum swinging from side to side. Bilaterally impaired smooth pursuit is usually a non-specific abnormality observed in a fatigued patient or one who is on certain medication (alcohol, antidepressants, anticonvulsants or benzodiazepines). Unilateral impairment is a more reliable marker of central nervous system pathology.

Nystagmus

Nystagmus is an involuntary, rhythmical oscillation of the eyes away from the direction of gaze, followed by a return of the eyes to their original position. It can be either physiological or pathological.

- Physiological nystagmus refers to nystagmus observed in normal subjects. It will be present in the majority of normal individuals if the irises of the eyes are deviated horizontally further than the punctum of the lacrimal sac: an important point to remember when testing for spontaneous nystagmus. Physiological nystagmus can also be induced by thermal (caloric) or rotational stimulation.

- Pathological nystagmus may be congenital or acquired. Congenital nystagmus is present from birth. It is nearly always dependent on optic fixation and so disappears when this is removed by asking the patient to wear Frenzel's glasses. Acquired nystagmus is described as ocular, vestibular or central in origin.

1. Ocular nystagmus. This tends to be pendular. It is common in congenital blindness, but may occur without any defect of vision. Miner's nystagmus is a form of the ocular variety.

2. Vestibular nystagmus. This consists of a slow movement of the eyes in one direction followed by a quick return in the opposite direction. The slow component is produced by impulses from the vestibule. The fast component, or recovery movement, is a central correcting reflex. The direction of the nystagmus is named according to the direction of the fast component, e.g. a nystagmus whose quick component is to the right is called a nystagmus to the right. Nystagmus is most marked when the patient looks in the direction of the fast component and is lessened or abolished when looking in the direction of the slow component. Vestibular nystagmus can be spontaneous or positional.

(a) Spontaneous nystagmus can be elicited by asking the patient to follow a finger held 60 cm away to the left and then the right, and then up and down. Increasing degrees of severity of spontaneous nystagmus are recognized. First-degree nystagmus is present only when the eyes are deviated in the direction of the fast component. Second-degree nystagmus is present when the patient looks straight ahead. Third-degree nystagmus is still present when the patient looks in the direction of the slow component.

(b) Positional nystagmus is usually rotatory and accompanied by rotatory vertigo. Positional testing is described in detail elsewhere. Basically, tests for positional nystagmus are done in the upright and supine positions with the head turned to either side. A nystagmus which is fatiguable and short-lasting is usually associated with a peripheral pathology (e.g. benign paroxysmal positional vertigo). A nystagmus which is not associated with vertigo and does not fatigue is more likely to be associated with a central lesion.

Specific tests based on the vestibulo-ocular reflex

1. Rotation tests. The nystagmus induced by acceleration and deceleration in a rotating chair is recorded. The test has the disadvantage of stimulating both labyrinths simultaneously. The test is also criticized because the stimulus is considered excessively violent, and it has found limited clinical application.

2. Caloric tests. In spite of improved imaging of the temporal bone and the advent of evoked response audiometry, this remains a popular investigation. It is also a popular topic in the Fellowship examination (see Caloric tests).

3. *Electronystagmography (ENG).* This technique is based upon the positive potential which exists between the cornea and retina. Electrodes are attached to the skin at each outer canthus close to the eyes. Changes in the corneoretinal potentials are recorded at the electrode sites as the eyes move from straight-ahead gaze. The changes in electric potential are used to follow nystagmus, and after amplification are recorded permanently on a moving paper strip. Full ENG testing includes a series of tests including different head positions, eyes open and closed, and caloric tests.

Test of the vestibulospinal reflex

Tests based on the vestibulo-ocular reflex are regarded as the most essential part of the investigation of the vestibular system. In contrast, tests of vestibulospinal function are commonly neglected in the evaluation of patients with balance dysfunction. Clinically vestibulospinal function is tested by examining stance and gait.

Romberg test

The Romberg test is used to assess a patient's ability to stand, feet together, arms by the side, with eyes open and then closed. The patient may fall towards the side of a recent peripheral vestibular lesion.

Unterburger test

This is performed by asking the patient to walk up and down on the spot for 30 seconds, with eyes closed and arms outstretched in front, with hands clasped together. Body rotation of more than 30°, or forward or backward displacement of more than 1 metre, is regarded as abnormal.

Gait testing

Gait is assessed by watching the patient walk normally with eyes open and then closed. A hemiplegic gait, cerebellar ataxic gait, Parkinsonian shuffle, or high stepping gait with loss of proprioception may become apparent. With eye closure some patients with uncompensated vestibular lesions will veer towards the affected side.

Specific tests based on the vestibulo-spinal reflex

Objective balance assessment has potential clinical use in the investigation of dizzy patients as a complement to existing tests. Posturography is the recording of postural sway. Several techniques have been used to evaluate such postural stability, but the most commonly used are force platforms. The data have enabled the effects of various sensory modalities upon balance to be identified, and some claim they allow various pathological conditions to be differentiated. A few of the more recent platforms have been used to rehabilitate patients with balance dysfunction by way of visual feedback. The high cost of many balance platforms has prohibited their use in both research and clinical practice.

Further reading

Omahoney CF, Davies R. Vestibular investigations. In: *Diseases of the Ear*, 6th edn. Ludman H and Wright T (eds.) London: Arnold, 1998; 87–104.

Schwaber MK. Vestibular function analysis. *Current Opinion in Otolaryngology and Head and Neck Surgery*, 1993; **1**: 35–39.

Related topics of interest

Caloric tests, p. 27; Vertigo, p. 346.

VOCAL CORD PALSY

Anatomy

The roots of the vagus emerge from the pons and medulla to gain a trunk and exit the skull through the jugular foramen. The vagus gives two important branches for voice production: the superior and the recurrent laryngeal nerves. The superior laryngeal nerve branches into the external laryngeal nerve, supplying the cricothyroid muscle, a cord adductor, and the internal laryngeal nerve, which is sensory to the laryngeal mucosa above the vocal cords. The recurrent laryngeal nerve arises high in the chest on the right, looping around the subclavian artery to reach the tracheo-oesophageal groove, but on the left arises at the level of and looping around the aortic arch to reach the same groove. The nerve enters the larynx below the cricoid cartilage and the lateral origin of cricopharyngeus and so cannot be injured above this level. It supplies the remaining intrinsic laryngeal muscles and is sensory to mucosa below the cords.

Pathology

A vocal cord palsy may be unilateral or bilateral, and the movement the cords cannot initiate is described as an adductor or an abductor palsy. There are two theories describing the position of the vocal cord, neither of which is entirely satisfactory.

1. Semon's law   states that, for any lesion affecting the recurrent laryngeal nerve, the fibres supplying the adductors are more susceptible to injury. The cord should lie in a median position if this were true.

2. The Wagner–Grossman theory   proposes that, because the superior laryngeal nerve supplies the cord adductor cricothyroid, a low lesion of the recurrent laryngeal nerve will allow the vagus to exert an overall abductor effect on the vocal cord. However with a lesion affecting the origin or above of the superior laryngeal nerve, the cord will lie in the cadaveric position. The fact that a cord palsy caused by a left apical bronchial carcinoma produces a median positioned cord somewhat discredits this theory.

A vocal cord palsy may arise from pathology of:

(1)   The recurrent laryngeal nerve, e.g. iatrogenic, pressure damage or a neuropathy.
(2)   The cricoarytenoid joint, e.g. rheumatoid arthritis.
(3)   The intrinsic muscles which move the vocal cord, e.g. a myopathy or infiltration by a malignancy.

In practice, recurrent laryngeal nerve palsy accounts for the majority of cases.

Aetiology

1. Malignant disease (30%)   especially of the bronchus, oesophagus, thyroid and nasopharynx.

2. *Iatrogenic (25%)*   especially thyroid and parathyroid, oesophageal, pharyngeal pouch and left lung surgery.

3. *External trauma (15%)*   e.g. from road traffic or sporting accidents and stab or gunshot injury.

4. *Idiopathic (15%)*   in which no cause is identified but which may be related to infection with a neuropathic virus.

5. *Others (15%)*   e.g. neurological disorders, myopathies, Orton's syndrome and inflammatory disease.

Clinical features

A breathy voice with a poor cough suggests an uncompensated adductor palsy. A voice which becomes weak or hoarse with use suggests an abductor palsy or a compensated adductor palsy. Stridor suggests a bilateral abductor palsy. Aspiration can occur with any palsy if the sensory supply to the larynx is compromised. Symptoms related to the cause may be present, such as haemoptysis or dysphagia.

Investigations

A CT scan from the skull base to the aortic arch is the first and most useful investigation. Further investigations are then chosen as appropriate to the underlying cause. Evaluation of the paralysis itself is assessed during phonation and respiration, ideally using videostroboscopic endoscopy.

Management

1. *Unilateral abductor palsy.*   In most cases no treatment is necessary because the normal cord compensates to produce a near-normal voice which tires with use. Speech therapy may be helpful.

2. *Bilateral abductor palsy.*   Many patients surprisingly are not stridulous unless they develop an upper respiratory tract infection. Others are stridulous and the treatment options are: an endoscopic laser cordectomy or arytenoidectomy or both, or a permanent tracheostomy. A neuromuscular pedicle procedure using the ansa cervicalis and a strap muscle has been described (by Tucker) but has not been widely adopted.

3. *Unilateral adductor palsy.*   When the cause is idiopathic or there is a chance of spontaneous resolution, a wait of at least a year is necessary. Speech therapy can be helpful to achieve compensation. For surgical treatment, any improvement in voice will be at the expense of the airway, so judgement is required to achieve the optimum compromise. Treatment consists of a cord medialization procedure which includes:

- Injection of Teflon (available on a named-patient basis as it may cause granulation tissue formation) or a collagenase-resistant collagen (e.g. GAX collagen), which is injected just lateral to the vocalis muscle at two sites: just anterior to the vocal process and midway between this and the anterior commissure.
- An anterior, external thyroplasty (e.g. Isshiki), posterior thyroplasty (e.g. Woodman's operation) or a suture technique (e.g. Downie's arytenoidoplasty).

4. *Bilateral adductor palsy.* Most patients will aspirate and often the cause is a neurological or myopathic disorder so that medialization procedures do not usually help the cause. A permanent tracheostomy or even a laryngectomy as a last resort may be required.

Follow-up and aftercare

This is required:

(a) To exclude an occult carcinoma.
(b) To observe spontaneous resolution.
(c) To enable a stable situation to be reached with regard to the voice and airway.

Aftercare will be necessary for those patients requiring a tracheostomy.

Further reading

Tucker HM. Human laryngeal reinnervation. *Laryngoscope*, 1976; **86**: 769–779.
Woodson GE, Miller RH. The timing of surgical intervention in vocal cord paralysis. *Otolaryngology and Head and Neck Surgery*, 1981; **89**: 264–267.

Related topics of interest

Lasers in ENT, p. 147; Stridor and stertor, p. 311; Tracheostomy, p. 336.

INDEX